The MRCGP Clinical Skills Assessment (CSA) Workbook

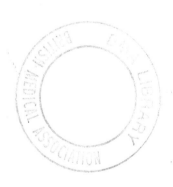
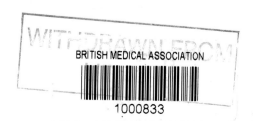

The MRCGP Clinical Skills Assessment (CSA) Workbook

MONAL WADHERA
BSc MBBS MRCP DRCOG MRCGP DFRSH AHEA
General Practitioner, London
GP Tutor, London Deanery
NIHR In Practice Fellow

and

RAJEEV GULATI
BSc MBBS MRCP MRCGP DRCOG AHEA
General Practitioner, London
FY2 Supervisor, London and Eastern Deaneries

Edited by
KALPANA SHARMA
BSc MBBS DCH DRCOG FRCGP
General Practitioner, London
Programme Director, West Middlesex VTS
MRCGP CSA Examiner

Foreword by
JOHN SPICER
Head, School of General Practice
London Deanery

Radcliffe Publishing
London • New York

Radcliffe Publishing Ltd
2nd Floor
5 Thomas More Square
London E1W 1YW
United Kingdom

www.radcliffehealth.com

Electronic catalogue and worldwide online ordering facility.

British Library Cataloguing in Publication Data
A catalogue record for this book is available from the British Library.

ISBN-13: 978 184619 269 2

The paper used for the text pages of this book is FSC® certified. FSC (The Forest Stewardship Council®) is an international network to promote responsible management of the world's forests.

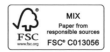

Typeset by Pindar NZ, Auckland, New Zealand
Printed and bound by TJ International Ltd. Padstow, Cornwall, UK

Contents

Foreword

A sea change occurred in the world of general practice training in mid-2007. For the first time a formal 'curriculum' was issued as a guide to teachers and learners, defining what was deemed necessary in knowledge, skills and attitudes to be a general practitioner (GP) in the United Kingdom. Its source was the Royal College of General Practitioners.

With this curriculum (more precisely a 'syllabus', but let us not be too precise) came a set of assessment modules that GP trainees have to pass to gain their status as lawfully practising GPs. Core knowledge is now assessed by a machine-marked paper, and skills and attitudes are assessed in the workplace. Key clinical skills are examined by Clinical Skills Assessment (CSA): a series of simulated patient interactions, run as close to a standard consulting session as is possible. It is a derived form of objective structured clinical examination (OSCE) used extensively in the undergraduate medical sphere.

Whilst the CSA is perceived and functions as an entry level credentialing module, it is actually a test of how any doctor can show appropriate skills in context. It may have uses for other groups of doctors, perhaps those who are struggling with their standards, or even those who want to use its structure for continuing professional development.

What the authors have developed in this text is a guide to excellence in this assessment method: how it runs, how it is structured, how it is marked. Anyone anxious about performance and success in the CSA (and all of us are) will find it a practical way to prepare and pass.

Because the CSA is a practical exam, it takes practise to prepare and the best preparation is the everyday business of general practice, augmented by reflection and discussion thereafter. In that fact lies the key to all examinations for general practice in the UK; there is no better preparation than dealing with patients and their problems, and using those interactions as a springboard to knowledge and skill acquisition.

At the time of writing, UK general practice faces a period of unprecedented change in its structure and function. GPs may be adopting the ways of the commissioner of secondary care services, a role not hitherto undertaken in such depth. But what has been called the 'stuff of general practice' – the consultation between a patient and a GP, in the presence of the suffering (in one way or another) of the former – will never go away. And it is this that the CSA seeks to assess.

The cases described in this book are the stuff of general practice, all rooted in day-to-day experience. They proceed from the simulated patient to the evidential basis of care, taking in key clinical aspects, decision-making, and social and psychological issues. Lubricating all of these things are the interpersonal skills that candidates need to demonstrate. And it is the latter that forms a strong determinant of patient satisfaction.

The authors have constructed a text that is, among other things, an examination preparation support. But it is also a book to assist in maintaining quality in primary care and for that reason any GP will find merit in considering its pages.

John Spicer
Head, School of General Practice, London Deanery
General Practitioner, Croydon
January 2011

About the authors

Dr Monal Wadhera qualified from Imperial College at St Mary's with MBBS in 2002, having completed a BSc in Cardiovascular Medicine in 1999. She completed the MRCP in 2005 and decided on a career in general practice. She trained on the West Middlesex VTS and qualified in 2007, achieving the Member of the Royal College of General Practitioners (MRCGP) with distinction. She was awarded the 'Great Expectations' Bursary by the Royal College of General Practitioners (RCGP) in 2007.

Monal is a sessional GP in London and has a keen interest in medical education. She is a GP Tutor with the London Deanery, the Clinical Lead in Professional Development at Hammersmith & Fulham PCT and has recently been awarded the NIHR In-Practice Fellowship. She achieved a distinction in the Certificate in Learning and Teaching at Queen Mary University of London, and a merit in the RCGP Leadership Programme. She is currently enrolled in the MA in Clinical Education at the Institute of Education, University of London.

Monal is an Examiner for medical students at Queen Mary University of London, and has written two previous revision guides for the MRCP examination. She is an Associate Member of the Higher Education Academy and has been involved in postgraduate and undergraduate teaching. She has recently become a GP Appraiser, which she enjoys greatly. Outside of medicine, her interests include reading, travelling, writing and yoga.

Dr Rajeev Gulati qualified from University College London with MBBS in 2000, and a BSc in Psychology in 1997. He achieved a Merit for Outstanding Performance in MBBS Written Finals and a Certificate of Merit in Clinical Pharmacology. He completed his MRCP in 2003 and then worked as a registrar in general and emergency medicine. He subsequently pursued a career in general practice and trained on the Northwick Park VTS. He completed the MRCGP during his registrar year in 2006.

Rajeev is a full-time GP Principal in a busy training practice in North London and is an Associate Member of the Higher Education Academy. He is an FY2 Trainer, and is actively involved in teaching medical students and GP registrars at the practice. He is an Examiner for final year medical students at King's College School of Medicine. He was also a teaching fellow whilst working as a medical registrar at Chelsea & Westminster Hospital.

Rajeev completed the Certificate in Learning and Teaching at Queen Mary University of London and is enrolled to do the TTT course at the London Deanery. He has also taught at revision courses for medical students and junior doctors for The Royal Society of Medicine. His other teaching commitments include organising a monthly clinical training programme at his surgery. He has also written two revision guides for the MRCP exam. His general interests include golf, travelling and he has recently taken up playing the guitar.

Dr Kalpana Sharma qualified from King's College Hospital Medical School with MBBS in 1982, having completed a BSc in Biochemistry in 1979. She became a GP in 1987 and has been a GP Principal in Southall, Middlesex, for 20 years. She was awarded FRCGP in 2004 for her commitment to general practice.

Kalpana has a keen interest in medical education, and has been the Programme Director for West Middlesex Hospital VTS for 15 years. She has also substantial experience of being a GP trainer within her practice. She was awarded the Paul Freeling Award by the RCGP in 2007 for her commitment to postgraduate GP vocational training.

Kalpana has been an examiner for the MRCGP CSA examination for three years, and was recently appointed as a National Clinical Assessment Service (NCAS) Assessor. In addition, she is involved in undergraduate teaching, GP mentorship and has undertaken GP appraisal since 2002. Her passions include reading, travel and supporting Arsenal.

Dedications

We would like to dedicate this book to Anya Kamla Gulati. Although her time in this world was too short, she will live in our hearts forever.

We would also like to dedicate this book to our grandparents, parents and families, whose continued love and support has nurtured where we are today and where we will be tomorrow.

Monal would particularly like to thank her late grand-mother, Jyotsna Wadhera, who gave her the gift of chasing her dreams. Her memory lives on strongly. Monal is extremely grateful for the care and unconditional love of her parents, Pramila and Naresh Wadhera. Mum and dad, you're the best, and I love you lots! A special thanks to Rudresh and Gurjit Wadhera, who are always inspirational with their words and actions. Your countless cups of tea proved vital! Baby Devan offered hours of entertainment and life perspective when writing the book. And a final mention to Raj, who wrote this book with me – you have been fantastic to work with, and I look forward to a hot samosa with you and Abha very soon!

Raj would particularly like to thank his wife, Abha Gulati, whose support, input and patience (lots of it!) have been invaluable. Her enthusiasm and encouragement throughout the process of writing this book were a tremendous source of inspiration. Abha, I will always love you and could not have done this without you! Raj is also grateful to his mum, Santosh Gulati and his sisters and brother, Neena Sohal, Ashwini Kumar Gulati and Kiran Harding. All of you have provided me with unconditional love and care through all of the highs and lows over the years. My father, the late Jai Kishan Gulati, continues to provide great strength and perspective on life's challenges. All of you mean so much to me. Monal, it has been a total pleasure to write this book with you too. Abha and I look forward to that hot samosa with you, perhaps accompanied by a glass of wine or two!

Acknowledgements

Working together on this book has been a great learning experience. We shared many moments of laughter despite our hard work, and hope we have created a high-quality book for the CSA exam.

We would like to thank Dr Kalpana Sharma, whom we know as Nan, for her unprecedented guidance and support as editor. Nan has mentored us throughout this project and been approachable at all times (even at midnight!). We have found her authenticity and high standards in general practice and medical education invaluable and greatly appreciated her encouragement, given whilst maintaining a sense of humour.

We are also grateful to Dr John Spicer, Head of the General Practice School at the London Deanery, for contributing the Foreword to this book, and are greatly encouraged by his words.

We are also appreciative of Jonathan Bevan, David Mendel, Kati Hajibagheri Chintal Patel, Nina Vadgama, Wai Weng Yoon, Arif Zafar, and who contributed towards the book and helped us format the cases and new ideas. Dr Robert Zabisco and Anthony Gonsalves also offered some fantastic suggestions.

We would like to acknowledge Iain Moir at the National Institute for Health and Clinical Excellence (NICE), Karen Joseph at the Driver and Vehicle Licensing Agency (DVLA), Graeme Paterson at the National Archives, Geoff Hacket at the British Society of Sexual Medicine and Edwair Weir at the National Clinical Guideline centre for their time spent on providing us with copyright permissions.

Finally, we would like to thank Camille Lowe and the team at Pindar for completing the typesetting, as well as Michael Hawkes, Gillian Nineham and the team at Radcliffe Publishing.

List of abbreviations

5-HT$_1$	Serotonin
A+E	Accident and emergency
ACE	Angiotensin converting enzyme
ACL	Anterior cruciate ligament
ACR	Albumin:creatinine ratio
AF	Atrial fibrillation
AFP	Alpha-fetoprotein
AIDS	Acquired immune deficiency syndrome
ALP	Alkaline phosphatase
ALT	Alanine aminotransferase
ARB	Angiotensin receptor blocker
AST	Aspartate aminotransferase
BCG	Bacillus Calmette–Guérin
bd	Twice a day
BHS	British Hypertension Society
BMA	British Medical Association
BMI	Body mass index
BNF	British National Formulary
BP	Blood pressure
CABG	Coronary artery bypass graft surgery
CAD	Coronary artery disease
CBT	Cognitive behavioural therapy
CHF	Congestive heart failure
CIN	Cervical intraepithelial neoplasia
CK	Creatinine kinase
CKD	Chronic kidney disease
CNS	Central nervous system
COC	Combined oral contraceptive
COPD	Chronic obstructive pulmonary disease
CPR	Cardiopulmonary resuscitation
CRP	C-reactive protein
CSA	Clinical skills assessment
CSM	Committee on Safety of Medicines
CT	Computed tomography
CVA	Cerebrovascular accident
CVD	Cardiovascular disease
CXR	Chest X-ray
dBP	Diastolic blood pressure
DC	Direct current
DENs	Doctor's educational needs
DIC	Disseminated intravascular coagulation
DMARD	Disease-modifying antirheumatic drug
DOT	Directly observed therapy

DPP4	Dipeptidyl-peptidase 4
DVLA	Driver and Vehicle Licensing Agency
ECG	Electrocardiogram
ED	Erectile dysfunction
EDD	Expected date of delivery
EF	Ejection fraction
eGFR	Estimated glomerular filtration rate
ENT	Ear, nose and throat
ERCP	Endoscopic retrograde cholangiopancreatography
ESR	Erythrocyte sedimentation rate
FBC	Full blood count
FEV$_1$	Forced expiratory volume in 1 second
FSH	Follicle stimulating hormone
FVC	Forced vital capacity
G6PD	Glucose-6-phosphate dehydrogenase
GFR	Glomerular filtration rate
GGT	Gamma-glutamyltransferase
GI	Gastrointestinal
GLP-1	Glucagon-like peptide-1
GMC	General Medical Council
GP	General practitioner
GUM	Genitourinary medicine
HAART	Highly active antiretroviral therapy
HD	Huntington's disease
HGV	Heavy goods vehicle
HIV	Human immunodeficiency virus
HL	Hodgkin's lymphoma
HPV	Human papillomavirus
HRT	Hormone replacement therapy
IBD	Inflammatory bowel disease
IBS	Irritable bowel syndrome
ICP	Intracranial pressure
ICS	Inhaled corticosteroid
Ig	Immunoglobulin
IM	Intramuscular
INR	International normalised ratio
IOP	Intraocular pressure
ITU	Intensive treatment unit
IUCD	Intrauterine contraceptive device
IUS	Intrauterine system
IV	Intravenous
IVDU	Intravenous drug user
IVF	In-vitro fertilisation
JVP	Jugular venous pressure
kg	Kilogram(s)
L	Litre(s)
LA	Left atrium
LABA	Long-acting β_2 agonist
LAMA	Long-acting muscarinic antagonist
LARC	Long-acting reversible contraception
LDL	Low-density lipoprotein
LFTs	Liver function tests
LH	Luteinising hormone
LMN	Lower motor neurone

LMP	Last menstrual period
LTOT	Long-term oxygen therapy
LV	Left ventricle
LVF	Left ventricular failure
MCPJ	Metacarpophalangeal joint
MDT	Multidisciplinary team
MI	Myocardial infarction
MMR	Measles, mumps and rubella
MND	Motor neurone disease
MRCGP	Member of the Royal College of General Practitioners
MRI	Magnetic resonance imaging
MS	Multiple sclerosis
MTPJ	Metatarsophalangeal joint
NHS	National Health Service
NICE/NIHCE	National Institute for Health and Clinical Excellence
NIHR	National Institute for Health Research
NIPPV	Non-invasive positive pressure ventilation
NIV	Non-invasive ventilator
NNRTI	Non-nucleoside reverse transcriptase inhibitor
NRT	Nicotine replacement therapy
NRTI	Nucleoside reverse transcriptase inhibitor
NSAID	Non-steroidal anti-inflammatory drug
O_2	Oxygen
OCD	Obsessive-compulsive disorder
od	Once a day
$PaCO_2$	Partial pressure of carbon dioxide
PBC	Primary biliary cirrhosis
PCL	Posterior cruciate ligament
PCOS	Polycystic ovary syndrome
PCR	Polymerase chain reaction
PCT	Primary care trust
PD	Parkinson's disease
PEG	Percutaneous endoscopic gastrostomy
PEP	Post-exposure prophylaxis
PHQ9	Patient health questionnaire
PI	Protease inhibitor
PIPJ	Proximal interphalangeal joint
PMR	Polymyalgia rheumatica
PMS	Premenstrual syndrome
PPAR	Peroxisome proliferator-activated receptor
prn	Pro re nata or as needed
PSC	Primary sclerosing cholangitis
PUNs	Patient's unmet needs
PUVA	Psoralen combined with ultraviolet A (UVA) treatment
PV	Per vaginam
qds	Four times a day
RA	Rheumatoid arthritis
RBCs	Red blood cells
RCGP	Royal College of General Practitioners
RR	Respiratory rate
SABA	Short-acting β_2 agonist
SAH	Subarachnoid haemorrhage
SAMA	Short-acting muscarinic antagonist
sBP	Systolic blood pressure

SC	Subcutaneous
SFH	Symphisis-fundal height
SLE	Systemic lupus erythematosus
SSRI	Selective serotonin reuptake inhibitor
STD	Sexually transmitted disease
STI	Sexually transmitted infection
TB	Tuberculosis
TCA	Tricyclic antidepressant
tds	Three times a day
TFT	Thyroid function test
TIA	Transient ischaemic attack
T_LCO	Carbon monoxide lung transfer factor
TNF	Tumour necrosis factor
TOP	Termination of pregnancy
TRH	Thyrotropin releasing hormone
TSH	Thyroid stimulating hormone
TURP	Transurethral resection of prostate
UK	United Kingdom
UMN	Upper motor neurone
UPSI	Unprotected sexual intercourse
URTI	Upper respiratory tract infection
USA	United States of America
USS	Ultrasound scan
UTI	Urinary tract infection
VTS	Vocational training scheme

List of permissions

The publications listed below are reproduced in part within this book with the permission of their copyright holders.

Station 1.2
National Institute for Health and Clinical Excellence. Chronic Kidney Disease: early identification and management of chronic kidney disease in adults in primary and secondary care: NICE guideline 73. London: NIHCE; 2008. www.nice.org.uk/CG73 (accessed 20 November 2010).

Station 1.3
DVLA. *DVLA Guidelines: 'For Medical Practitioners: at a glance guide to the current medical standards of fitness to drive'*. Swansea: DVLA; 2010.

Station 1.10
National Institute for Health and Clinical Excellence. Irritable Bowel Syndrome in Adults: diagnosis and management of irritable bowel syndrome in primary care: NICE guideline 61. London: NIHCE; 2008. http://guidance.nice.org.uk/CG61 (accessed 19 November 2010).

Station 1.13
National Institute for Health and Clinical Excellence. Chronic Obstructive Pulmonary Disease (Update): NICE guideline 101. London: NIHCE; 2010. http://guidance.nice.org.uk/CG101 (accessed 21 November 2010).

Station 2.1
National Institute for Health and Clinical Excellence. Atrial Fibrillation: NICE guideline 36. London: NIHCE; 2006. http://guidance.nice.org.uk/CG36 (accessed 19 November 2010).

Station 2.3
Food Standards Agency. *Food Handlers: fitness to work*. London: Food Standards Agency; 2009.

Station 2.9
National Institute for Health and Clinical Excellence. Heavy Menstrual Bleeding: NICE guideline 44. London: NIHCE; 2007. www.nice.org.uk/CG44 (accessed 19 November 2010).

Station 2.11
British Society for Sexual Medicine. *British Society for Sexual Medicine Guidelines on the Management of Erectile Dysfunction*. Fisherwick: British Society for Sexual Medicine; 2007. Available at: www.bssm.org.uk/downloads/BSSM_ED_Management_Guidelines_2007.pdf (accessed 12 December 2010).

Station 3.3
National Institute for Health and Clinical Excellence. Type II Diabetes: NICE guideline 66. London: NIHCE; 2008. www.nice.org.uk/CG66 (accessed 19 November 2010).

Station 3.4
National Institute for Health and Clinical Excellence. Glaucoma: NICE guideline 85. London: NIHCE; 2009. www.nice.org.uk/nicemedia/pdf/CG85 (accessed 19 November 2010).

Station 3.8
National Institute for Health and Clinical Excellence. Obsessive-compulsive Disorder and Body Dysmorphic Disorder: NICE guideline 31. London: NIHCE; 2005. www.nice.org.uk/CG031 (accessed 25 November 2010).

Introduction

About the exam
The CSA in context of the MRCGP
There are three components to the MRCGP exam:
- Applied Knowledge Test (AKT).
- Clinical Skills Assessment (CSA).
- Workplace-Based Assessment (WPBA).

This book concentrates on the CSA exam. As its name suggests, the CSA is a clinical exam that provides simulated clinical scenarios, designed to recreate a typical surgery that you may encounter in your everyday practice.

The format of the MRCGP exam was changed in 2007. Prior to then, it was not necessary to obtain the MRCGP to become a GP. Instead, trainees had to successfully complete a multiple-choice exam, a written paper and video tape a series of consultations from everyday practice (occasionally, instead of the videos, trainees sat a 'simulated surgery'). With the advent of the new MRCGP exam in 2007, the multiple-choice paper was modified into a new format now known as the AKT. The video and essays were replaced by the WPBA and the CSA. Passing the MRCGP exam is now compulsory to become a GP.

Aims of the CSA
The CSA aims to examine trainees' clinical skills. It also specifically examines the communication skills of candidates. The WPBA also tests these skills during the trainees' registrar year. The CSA exam helps to ensure that a formalised, more standardised measure can be used to assess candidates.

Objectives of the CSA
The RCGP have outlined a curriculum for GP trainees, called *The RCGP: GP curriculum statements*, first produced in January 2007 (available at: www.rcgp-curriculum.org.uk/rcgp_-_gp_curriculum_documents/gp_curriculum_statements.aspx [accessed 6 January 2011]). The CSA is intended to emphasise certain areas of the curriculum, namely:
- primary care management
- problem-solving skills
- comprehensive approach
- person-centred care
- attitudinal aspects
- clinical practical skills (an additional area not in the curriculum).

These areas were adopted into a 'blueprint', that forms a framework from which the RCGP can select areas to test in the CSA.

A range of these skills are tested in the CSA exam, and alongside these skills a range of clinical conditions are also incorporated into the exam. Examples of the clinical conditions being tested include:
- musculoskeletal conditions
- neurological conditions

- gastrointestinal (GI) conditions
- psychiatric conditions
- infectious diseases
- sexual health conditions.

Spread of cases
As mentioned, there is a wide range of clinical conditions involving patients of different ages and ethnicities (children are generally represented by their fictional parents), some of which are acute and others chronic. When writing the cases, the RCGP tests specific parts of its blueprint – bear this in mind when revising and planning your approach to each case.

Marking of cases
The examiner marks each case in terms of three domains or areas. This creates an overall numerical mark for the case. Each domain carries the same number of marks.
    The domains are:
- **Information gathering:** adopting a targeted history and examination (if required) to elicit a diagnosis and management plan.
- **Clinical management:** showing the ability to manage primary care conditions in a logical, integrated manner. This should take account of the patients' individual circumstances and incorporate evidence-based methods.
- **Interpersonal skills:** adopting recognised consultation methods to follow a patient-centred consultation. Consideration of the patients' ideas, concerns and expectations, as well as any ethical considerations.

The marks are awarded as: **clear pass**, **marginal pass**, **marginal fail** or **fail** for each domain. As well as marking the domain scores, the examiners will also separately rate the candidate as a pass, a fail or a borderline, overall.

Structure of the exam
The CSA exam consists of 13 simulated scenarios. Each consultation lasts 10 minutes, with a 2-minute break between each case. A bell will sound at the end of 10 minutes. The candidate remains in the same room while the actor and examiner rotate around the different rooms. During a consultation the examiner remains silent and out of the candidate's view. Exceptions to this might be if the examiner needs to hand the candidate an examination card or to tell them that a particular part of the examination can be assumed as normal.
    In the 2-minute break, the candidate has the chance to read the notes for the next consultation, which are prepared in a folder on the desk.
    The RCGP has recently announced that all 13 stations will count towards the overall mark, instead of the previous 12 out of 13 cases. The borderline group method will be used to set the pass mark on the day. This is an established and robust standard-setting method, which allows for day-to-day variability in the difficulty of case mixes. For each case, the overall numerical case marks of the candidates in the borderline group are averaged. These averaged scores are then aggregated across all the 13 cases to create the 'cut score', i.e. the approximation between a passing and a failing score. The final, actual, pass mark has an adjustment to the cut score to take account of the standard error of measurement (SEM).

Examiners and actors
The examiners are GPs who have received special training to become examiners. They attend regular training workshops to calibrate their marking values to ensure there is adequate standardisation and objectivity across the exam. The examiners have detailed notes of what is expected of the candidates in any given case. Marking sheets include details of the blueprint domains being tested, and room for general feedback. The actors are fully briefed and trained to participate in this role. They are not there to trip you up, although not all the information will be handed to you on a plate, so ensure you listen to what they say and pay attention to any cues they give you!

Where and when to take the CSA

The CSA exam is currently carried out in Croydon, in a purpose-built accommodation over three floors. The college has plans to move its headquarters to a central London site and to run the CSA from these new premises within the next few years. There are currently four sittings per year. The exam is available to ST3 doctors. The RCGP recommends at least six months of working in the National Health Service (NHS) system as a GP registrar before sitting the CSA.

How to prepare

The best way to prepare for this exam is through the cases you see everyday: see as many patients as you can; list your patient's unmet needs (PUNS) and doctor's educational needs (DENS); get involved with daily activities, such as dealing with hospital correspondences and blood results, as well as home visits. Specific methods to help with revision are outlined below.

- Arrange joint surgeries with your trainer to have your consultations constructively critiqued.
- Respond to any feedback from video consultations or from your e-portfolio. See these as a learning exercise – we all find it daunting to watch ourselves on screen!
- Read the *British Journal of General Practice* and the *British Medical Journal*. The GP journals have articles geared towards GP registrars, but also discuss clinical guidelines and common ethical dilemmas.
- NICE guidelines are easily available online, and it is important to become familiar with the common ones, e.g. those concerning hypertension, chronic obstructive pulmonary disease (COPD), diabetes.
- Several courses are available. Trainees often find courses help them to gain confidence, and also provide an opportunity to carry out mock exams.
- It also goes without saying that a useful revision aid, such as this one, is an extremely good way of keeping ahead of the game.

Top tips for exam day

- Carry a doctor's bag with you. Carry equipment as if you were doing a home visit. There will only be basic equipment in the room so come prepared and it is better to use equipment you are familiar with. Carry an up-to-date *British National Formulary* (BNF) as well.
- Dress smartly but comfortably for the exam.
- Use the two-minute break between consultations to read the available patient notes; write down what you think the examiners are looking for and what the main points to ask are.
- When it comes to the physical examination, state to the patient in simple terms what you intend to do. The examiner might hand you a card with the salient findings, or you might be expected to perform an examination or use a piece of equipment, e.g. a peak flow metre.
- Ensure you watch the time. Conduct a focussed history and examination. Do not waste time getting bogged down in systems reviews or areas that are not relevant.
- Treat the actor as you would a real patient. Be kind and respectful.
- Get a good night's sleep the night before, arrive at the venue in good time and, most importantly, remain calm and relaxed.

About the book

This book has been written with the very close involvement of a MRCGP examiner. Dr Kalpana Sharma has been involved at each stage of writing, including in the choice and design of each case, its content and the revision notes at the end of each case. Her involvement has been integral to ensuring the material presented is at the standard required for the real exam.

How to use this book

We have written a variety of representative CSA cases, each of which is formatted and written as it would be presented in the exam. These cases can be approached alone or with a partner (i.e. by taking turns at being the actor and doctor).

Structure of the book

This book includes 3 circuits of 13 cases each, giving a total of 39 cases. This has allowed us to give examples of many different kinds of cases. Each circuit includes the variety and spread of cases you would expect in the actual exam to comply with the CSA blueprint.

Structure of the cases

Candidate's and actor's notes

The opening section to each case includes the most relevant points from the patients' notes and any relevant hospital correspondences for the candidate to use. If you are playing the doctor, it is best to take 2 minutes to write notes and consider what the case might be about. Often there is very little to go on from these notes, but it is important to absorb what is written, perhaps highlighting any potentially important points. The actor's notes provide a detailed brief for the actor, and guide them through potential issues, such as details of the history, the patient's expectations and also how the actor should react if certain situations arise during the consultation. It is useful to read the examples of these in this book to get a feel for what they include in the exam. The next step is to role play the scenario in 10 minutes. Following this, refer to the remaining sections to reflect on how the case went.

The three domains

Following the candidate's and actor's notes, the rest of the case is written according to the three domains, namely **information gathering**, **clinical management** and **interpersonal skills**. We have included the ideal points that you would be expected to cover in the exam setting. With regards to interpersonal skills, we have written this section by drawing on the key components of the case, emphasising the best communication methods to employ and example quotes you might use. Do not feel restricted by this. It is only a guide.

Tutorial

The cases end with a tutorial relating to the case, followed by further reading that we feel might be useful and relevant. The tutorial may cover factual information, relevant clinical guidelines or theories relevant to the case.

Once you have practised a range of cases from the book, we would encourage you to apply the case structure, or 'skeleton', used here to interesting cases you come across in your own daily practice. You may wish to practise such cases with colleagues, and decide together on the best way to approach the three domains.

O⊷ Key summary

- The CSA exam takes account of three domains – information gathering, clinical management and interpersonal skills.
- Remember to listen to the patient, as they will often provide the relevant cues that need to be elicited in order for you to pass the case comfortably.
- The best way to prepare is in your everyday practice.
- Approach the cases in this book as you would the exam.
- Enjoy!

Further reading

- Simon C, Everett H, van Dorp F. *Oxford Handbook of General Practice*. 3rd ed. Oxford: Oxford University Press; 2010.
- Royal College of General Practitioners (RCGP). *GP Training*. London: RCGP; n.d. Available at: www.rcgp.org.uk/gp_training.aspx (accessed 21 July 2010).
- Royal College of General Practitioners (RCGP). *Marking the Clinical Skills Assessment: changes for September 2010*. London: RCGP; n.d. Available at: www.rcgp-curriculum.org.uk/mrcgp/csa/changes_to_the_csa_-_faqs.aspx (accessed 13 December 2010).

- McKelvey I. The consultation hill: a new model to aid teaching consultation skills. *Br J Gen Pract.* 2010; **60**(576): 538–40.
- Neighbour R. *The Inner Consultation: how to develop an effective and intuitive consulting style.* 2nd revised ed. Oxford: Radcliffe Publishing; 2004.
- Pendleton D, Schofield T, Tate P, *et al. The Consultation: an approach to learning and teaching.* Oxford: Oxford University Press; 1984.
- Stott NCH, Davis RH. The exceptional potential in each primary care consultation. *J R Coll Gen Pract.* 1979; **29**(201): 201–5.
- Silverman JD, Kurtz SM, Draper J. *Skills for Communicating with Patients.* Oxford: Radcliffe Publishing; 1998.

Circuit 1

Station 1.1

Actor's notes

Background
- You are Andrew Woodhouse, a 57-year-old journalist.

Opening statement
- 'Doctor, I want to talk to you about how I want to die.'

History
- You were diagnosed with motor neurone disease (MND) one year ago after investigation for muscle weakness in your hands and legs. The specialist explained that your overall condition will deteriorate and eventually you will lose complete independence.
- You want to die with dignity and want to know what your options are.

Ideas, concerns and expectations
- You are struggling to type because your hands are weakening. This is extremely frustrating, because your mind is still active. You are concerned that your condition is deteriorating and you will end up 'like a vegetable', dependent on others for the smallest of things.
- You have some negative ideas and are scared about the last few days of your life because you recall how undignified your father's death was. You do not want to spend your last days in hospital, reliant on strangers who do not remember your name.
- You are especially concerned that you will become so weak in the last few days of your life that you may end up 'fighting for breath' or 'choking to death'.
- You have heard about certain medical centres that 'end your life' so you can die peacefully, and have come to discuss this with the GP, so you can die with dignity at a time of your choosing.

Further history candidate may elicit
- You were diagnosed with MND after seeing a specialist because you were finding it difficult to type and write. Your legs felt weak, and you often tripped over. Now, you are struggling with everyday tasks like buttoning your shirt and opening doors.
- You are passionate about writing but now only work part time because you are struggling to type and write – you know you will have to give up your job soon.
- Your legs are getting weaker. Last week, you were incontinent because you could not walk quickly enough to the toilet. Your wife had to help clean and wash you. You felt humiliated.
- Your father died of lung cancer 10 years ago and spent his last days in hospital, in pain. He was left incontinent for hours because the nurses were too busy to help, and the doctors would repeatedly 'stab him' with needles, 'like a pin cushion'. You remember holding your father's hand in the last few days of his life, as he said 'Please just let me die'.
- Last week, you went to the hospital for a follow-up appointment with the neurologist.

- Whilst waiting to be seen, you spoke to another patient with MND who sat next to you in a wheelchair. He told you patients with MND can 'die fighting for breath' or 'choke to death', and also mentioned that there were 'medical centres', which helped to 'end your life'. You asked the neurologist about this but he seemed reluctant to talk about it.
- You want to know more about these 'medical centres'. You did ask your family to get you some information about these centres, but they refused, saying this was an 'awful idea'.
- Your family are extremely supportive, and you have a loving wife who organises days out and special treats for you. You spend most weekends with your family, laughing together.
- You are not depressed – you just want others to respect your decision to die with dignity.

Medical history
- MND.

Drug history
- Riluzole 50 mg bd.

Social history
- You have been a journalist for a national newspaper for 34 years and now work part time.
- You have never smoked but do have the odd glass of wine on the weekends.
- You live with your wife in a house with stairs that you manage, very slowly. She helps you with washing, dressing and shopping, although you try to remain as independent as you can.
- You have two children who live nearby. They are planning to move back into the family house to offer more support to you and your wife.

Family history
- There is no family history of MND.
- Your mother died of a stroke last year and your father died of lung cancer 10 years ago.

Approach to scenario
- Your primary concern is about dying with dignity. You want the doctor to understand that it is 'my life, my death and my choice'.
- You ask the GP about the 'medical centres' that help you end your life because you feel 'this is the only reasonable option I can think of, Doctor'.
- You are disturbed by the loss of independence you face, and want to function normally for as long as possible. In particular, you want to continue writing for the newspaper – this gives you 'a reason to live'.
- You are struggling with wearing your clothes, and felt humiliated by the recent episode of incontinence when you could not get to the toilet quickly enough.
- You welcome any thoughts or suggestions the doctor has to offer to help maintain your independence, e.g. with writing and wearing clothes.
- You are particularly scared at the thought of 'fighting for breath' or 'choking to death'.
- If the doctor appears compassionate, empathic and explains that there are various ways to maintain your independence, keep you comfortable and prevent you from suffering in the last days of your life, you are willing to consider other alternatives, such as an advance directive.
- If the doctor does not come across well and does not show any understanding of your predicament, you become angry and ask 'How would you feel if you were in my situation?'

Information gathering

Presenting complaint

a History of motor neurone disease

- What symptoms did he present with?
- When was it diagnosed?
- What treatment is he having?
- Has he developed any complications? For example:
  — muscle spasms
  — difficulty swallowing
  — speech problems
  — choking sensation
  — breathing difficulties.
- Which symptoms bother him most?

b Assisted suicide

- What has he heard about assisted-suicide centres?
- Why is he considering assisted suicide?
- Does he know it is illegal in this country?
- Is he under pressure from his family?
- How does he think his family will react?
- Has he considered having an advance directive?
- What does he know about end-of-life and palliative care?

c Assess for depression

- Any thoughts of suicide or self-harm.

Medical history

- Other comorbidities.
- Previous episodes of depression.

Family history

- MND or other chronic diseases.

Drug history

- Current medications.
- Check if he has access to large quantities of drugs that could be taken as an overdose.

Social history

- Occupation.
- Marital status.
- Dependents.
- Support mechanisms.
- Home circumstances (house/flat/bungalow).
- Current activities of daily living (shopping, dressing, washing).

Patient's agenda

- Explore his understanding of MND.
- Explore the impact of MND on his personal and professional life.
- Explore his concerns regarding end-of-life care.
- Explore his understanding of assisted suicide and the implications this would have on his family.
- Explore his understanding of palliative care and advance directives.

Clinical management

1 Overview

- Explain that physician-assisted suicide is illegal in the UK, even though there are specialised centres in some countries in Europe (e.g. Dignitas in Switzerland) that people can attend to get assistance to end their life.
- Emphasise that there are many ways to manage the complications of MND to help preserve his independence as long as possible, and that it would be possible to exert his autonomy and remain in control during the last stage of life without resorting to euthanasia or physician-assisted suicide.

2 Management of motor neurone disease complications

- Explain there are a range of treatments to help manage the complications of MND, and focus on areas that concern him most of all, such as voice-activated software or use of a Dictaphone to help him continue writing, and incontinence pads, which could be useful as mobility deteriorates.
- Stress the role of multidisciplinary teams (MDTs) such as occupational therapy who could provide him with a wide range of home adaptations to facilitate independence.

3 End-of-life care

- Reassure him that terminal care has significantly changed since his father's death.
- Underline the role of the palliative care team as specialists who deal with end-of-life care.

a Place of death

- Explain that he has the option of dying at home or in a hospice (which offers personal care) with his loved ones around him – hospital is not the only option.

b Discuss fears about end of life

- Reassure and try to alleviate the patient's fear about 'fighting for breath' or 'choking to death', explaining this is rare and most people with MND die peacefully.
- **Sensitively** explain that patients with MND usually die because of a chest infection or because the respiratory muscles become 'too weak to work', leading to reduced consciousness and coma. The moment of death comes peacefully as breathing slows and finally ceases.
- Explain that there are a number of medications that can prevent him from suffering (*see* page 9).
- Reassure him that all appropriate medications can be kept in the house to prevent delay in administration, and will be available when needed.
- Inform him of the Breathing Space Kit produced by the MND Association, which provides information to guide the carer to administer the medication in an emergency.

c Advance directives

- Explain that an advance directive is a 'living will'. This is a legal document he can write in advance of the terminal phase of his illness to protect his autonomy.
- This allows him to consent to, or refuse, medical treatment when he is too ill to communicate his decisions himself. Through the advance directive, he can:
  - (i) name a proxy to express his wishes in the event of a life-threatening illness
  - (ii) request that life-sustaining treatment, such as resuscitation, is withheld when he deteriorates
  - (iii) make specific requests regarding his future treatment, e.g. he wants to be treated at home or in a hospice, and does not want to be admitted to hospital
  - (iv) express the type of treatments he would prefer in certain circumstances, e.g. if he develops pneumonia, he can request **not** to have antibiotics.
- Advise him to seek legal advice about the advance directive and to discuss it with his family.

4 Follow-up

- Offer him a follow-up appointment to discuss this further once he has had time to reflect on the choices discussed. Suggest he can bring his wife with him for you to speak to.
- Offer leaflets or information printed out from the Internet on advance directives and end-of-life care.
- Offer to give him the telephone number of the Motor Neurone Disease Association, as it can also offer help.

Interpersonal skills

- Assisted suicide and euthanasia are emotive topics. The challenge in this case is to explore the patient's reasons for considering assisted death. It is important to exclude depression and coercion from family members.
  - 'How are you and your family coping?'
  - 'Have they suggested assisted suicide to you? Is this something they want or you want?'
- In many cases of chronic or terminal illness, early referral to palliative care can help manage complications. Involvement of the MDT can provide the patient and carers with invaluable aid, providing methods for the patient to stay as independent as possible.
  - 'I can appreciate that you want to maintain your independence. There are specialised teams, such as the occupational therapists, who can help modify your home to make it more suitable for you. They have all sorts of devices to help you, such as shoe aids to help you put your shoes on easily, and special cutlery to help you eat by yourself.'
  - 'Clothes and shoes with Velcro can be easier to manage than buttons or shoes with laces.'
  - 'Would these options be useful to you?'
  - 'Could you use a Dictaphone to record your thoughts and ask someone to type up your notes? How about voice-activated software?'
- Many terminally ill patients are fearful of fighting for breath or choking to death, and it is important to provide them with adequate reassurance.
  - 'Most people with MND usually die peacefully – the "breathing" muscles become weaker, and consciousness decreases, leading to a coma or "deep sleep". Breathing reduces and finally stops. With the help of medication, this process is usually very peaceful.'
  - 'The palliative care team will work with us to take appropriate steps to make sure you have a dignified, peaceful death.'
- Advance directives are a means of a patient maintaining control over their medical care in situations where they may lose capacity.
  - 'Another alternative to these medical centres is making a "living will", or advance directive. This is a legal document that helps you keep control of your medical care if you reach a stage when you cannot communicate what you want.'
  - 'For example, one of the common complications for MND sufferers is to develop pneumonia. You can choose whether or not you would like antibiotics to treat the infection. Choosing antibiotics may lengthen your lifespan, but you may opt for withholding antibiotics, and letting nature take its course.'
- During this station, it is important to show empathy to the patient, understand his concerns, explore his ideas on assisted suicide, discuss alternatives with him and respect his autonomy.

O—┅ Key summary
- Recognise that assisted suicide is illegal in this country but is legal in other countries.
- Outline methods to help a patient retain independence for as long as possible.
- Be familiar with end-of-life care and the role of the palliative and MDTs.
- Explain the purpose of an advance directive and how it may be useful.
- Involve the patient throughout the consultation and in the proposed management plan, remaining empathic and sensitive to their situation at all times.

Motor neurone disease

- MND is a progressive neurological disease that is usually fatal within 2–3 years. Death often occurs due to bronchopneumonia.
- Patients present with upper and lower motor neurone dysfunction due to the degeneration of anterior horn cells and cranial nerve nuclei.
- There are no signs of sensory loss, ocular movements are not affected and there are no cerebellar or extrapyramidal features.

Clinical features

- Muscle wasting, weakness and fasciculation causing difficulty in manipulating objects, gait disorder and a tendency to trip.
- Bulbar involvement causing dysarthria and dysphagia.
- Respiratory muscle involvement leading to dyspnoea and orthopnoea.

Clinical patterns of motor neurone disease

TABLE 1.1 Clinical patterns of MND

TYPE	DESCRIPTION
Amyotrophic lateral sclerosis	50–65% of cases • LMN signs in the arms • UMN signs in the legs • Most cases are sporadic • 5–10% of cases are familial
Progressive muscular atrophy	10–25% of cases • Affects distal muscles • Asymmetrical limb wasting and weakness • LMN signs predominate
Bulbar palsy	25% of cases
Progressive bulbar palsy	• LMN signs • Weak and fasciculating tongue • Nasal speech
Pseudobulbar palsy	• Spastic tongue • Spastic dysarthria • Labile emotions
Primary lateral sclerosis	<2% of cases • Signs progress from UMN to LMN

Investigations

- Electromyography shows a pattern of severe, chronic denervation.
- Other investigations normally include blood tests, magnetic resonance imaging (MRI) of the brain and sometimes muscle biopsy to exclude the possibility of other neurological conditions.

Management options

TABLE 1.2 Management options for patients with MND

COMPLICATION	MANAGEMENT
Writing	Voice-activated software or Dictaphone
Muscle weakness	Physiotherapy Walking aids and splints Occupational therapy to provide home aids, e.g. • Hands-free telephones • Modification of door handles, locks and switches • Can openers, modified cutlery, cups and plates
Incontinence	Incontinence pads Catheter may be useful in due course
Dysarthria and dysphonia	Speech therapy Communication aids such as speech synthesisers
Drooling	Drugs, e.g. hyoscine, glycopyrronium and anticholinergics
Dysphagia	PEG tube Dietician to consider food consistency and supplements
Muscle cramps	Quinine
Muscle spasticity	Drugs, e.g. baclofen and diazepam Physiotherapy to prevent contractures and improve joint mobility
Dyspnoea	Drugs, e.g. morphine orally or diamorphine SC/IM/suppositories to help ease fear, anxiety and breathlessness Physiotherapy to aid mobility Chest physiotherapy for breathing exercises Referral to respiratory physician to consider NIPPV
Choking	Drugs, e.g. diamorphine, midazolam, haloperidol, lorazepam and glycopyrronium bromide
Depression	Antidepressants Counselling services Input and support from the Motor Neurone Disease Association
Respite care	Referral to local hospice-based team

Treatment
- NICE (2001) suggests the use of riluzole, a glutamate antagonist, to treat amyotrophic lateral sclerosis. Treatment of complications with multidisciplinary involvement is crucial.

Further reading
- Motor Neurone Disease Association website. www.mndassociation.org/ (accessed 20 November 2010).
- Directgov. *Your Right to Refuse Future Medical Treatment.* Directgov; n.d. Available at: www.direct.gov.uk/en/governmentcitizensandrights/death/preparation/dg_10029683 (accessed 20 November 2010).
- Fallon M, Hanks G, editors. *ABC of Palliative Care.* 2nd ed. Oxford: Blackwell Publishing; 2006.
- National Institute for Health and Clinical Excellence. *Guidance on the use of riluzole (Rilutek) for the treatment of motor neurone disease* London: NICE; 2001. Available at: ww.nice.org.uk/nicemedia/live/11415/32139/32139.pdf (accessed 20 November 2010).

Station 1.2

Candidate's notes

Name	Amy Lody-Pine
Age	75
Medical history	Hypertension
	Osteoarthritis
Medication	Bendroflumethiazide 2.5 mg od
	Ibuprofen 400 mg tds
	Paracetamol 1–2 tablets qds prn
Allergies	Nil
Last consultation	Saw GP six months ago for painful knees
	Knee radiographs revealed osteoarthritis
	Advised paracetamol and ibuprofen
	Annual BP check one month ago: 145/95 mmHg
	Advised to have annual blood test and check home BP
	Blood test revealed impaired renal function
	Sent letter from practice to have repeat blood test in two weeks and then to come for review appointment

Blood results

1st Set		2nd Set	
Sodium	139 mmol/L	Sodium	142 mmol/L
Potassium	4.5 mmol/L	Potassium	4.7 mmol/L
Urea	6.8 mmol/L	Urea	4.5 mmol/L
Creatinine	145 µmol/L	Creatinine	148 µmol/L
eGFR	57 mL/min/1.73 m^2	eGFR	55 mL/min/1.73 m^2
FBC	Normal		
LFTs	Normal		
Fasting glucose	Normal		
Fasting cholesterol	Normal		

Actor's notes

Background
- You are Amy Lody-Pine, a 75-year-old Caucasian, who is retired.

Opening statement
- 'Hello doctor. I've come for my blood tests.'

History
- You saw your GP one month ago to have your blood pressure (BP) checked. He asked you to have your annual blood test.
- You had your blood test and called the practice for the results the following week.
- The receptionist advised you that the doctor wanted you to repeat the blood test in two weeks but did not explain why.
- You had the repeat blood test and telephoned for the results again. This time the receptionist advised you that the doctor wanted to see you to discuss the blood results.
- You have come today to speak with the doctor about your blood results.

Ideas, concerns and expectations
- You are worried that the blood tests are abnormal and concerned that this suggests a serious problem.
- You are alarmed to hear that your kidneys are not functioning normally. You want to know how to stop your kidneys from deteriorating and how to keep them 'healthy'.
- You have had a friend who requires dialysis three times a week because 'his kidneys are failing' and are concerned that you will need dialysis in the future.
- You are worried that if you stop taking ibuprofen, the pain in your knees will stop you from playing tennis, and you will lose mobility.

Further history candidate may elicit
- Your knees have been painful for some months. You saw the GP who advised you to have X-rays of both your knees; these showed arthritis.
- You also mentioned that you have occasional right-sided hip pain. The doctor explained this was due to arthritis too. He advised you take paracetamol or ibuprofen for the pain.
- You tried paracetamol initially, but found ibuprofen controls the pain better. You take one or two tablets of ibuprofen daily. If you play tennis or walk long distances, you take it three times a day.
- You were diagnosed with hypertension two years ago – it was picked up incidentally by your GP when you visited to have your cholesterol checked.
- Since then, you have been taking a 'water tablet' daily. You are concordant with your medication.
- You saw the GP one month ago for your annual BP check and to have a blood test.
- You were told that your BP was higher than normal and asked to check your BP at home twice a day with a monitor provided by the surgery. You have brought the home readings with you today.
- You had a blood test but were asked to repeat it – you are unsure why.
- Your friend's husband has started dialysis for 'kidney failure'. Your friend is finding it difficult to cope with repeated journeys to the hospital and cannot go on holiday because her husband needs his dialysis.

Medical history
- Hypertension.
- Osteoarthritis.

Drug history
- Bendroflumethiazide 2.5 mg od.
- Ibuprofen 400 mg tds.
- Paracetamol 1–2 tablets qds prn.

Social history
- You do not smoke or drink alcohol. You are retired, having worked as an architect in the past.
- You are enjoying retirement and keep busy by travelling with your husband, playing tennis, taking long walks in the country and reading.

Family history
- Your father died nine years ago after a heart attack. Your mother died seven years ago, following a stroke.
- You have three children who are all married and have children themselves. They live locally.

Approach to scenario
- You are worried when the doctor tells you that your kidney function is not normal.
- You want to know how severely your kidneys are affected and why.

- You want to know if you will need dialysis, and how this can be avoided.
- You would like to know what can be done to prevent any further deterioration.
- If the doctor mentions that the tablets you are taking may cause kidney impairment, you ask why you were not informed of this prior to taking the tablets.
- You are worried about stopping the ibuprofen because your knees can be very painful. You are concerned that if you stop the ibuprofen, the pain will not be controlled and you will have to stop playing tennis and going for long walks.
- If the doctor is considerate and explains other painkillers are available, you will agree to change to another painkiller.
- You are concerned your BP is high despite the tablets you are taking. You are happy to change to an alternative.
- You wonder if any further investigations are needed, such as a 'scan' to look at the kidneys.
- You ask if you need to see a kidney specialist.
- If the doctor is able to reassure you and explain why this is not needed at this stage, you are prepared to hold off further investigations and referral.
- If the doctor does not come across well and does not reassure you adequately, you become upset and demand to see a 'kidney specialist'.

Information gathering
Presenting complaint
a Blood test
- Confirm that the reason for the initial blood test was for annual review.
- Ask if she knows why she had to repeat the blood test.

b Renal failure
- Ask about:
  — loin pain
  — haematuria
  — dysuria
  — nocturia
  — urinary frequency.

c Blood pressure
- Ask how long she has had high BP.
- Ask whether she has had headaches.
- Ask about home BP recordings (high or normal).
- Ask about concordance with current antihypertensive treatment.

d Osteoarthritis
- Which joints are affected?
- What is the impact of joint pain on her lifestyle?
- Which analgesics are effective and how often are they needed?

Medical history
- Hypertension.
- Diabetes.
- Recurrent urinary tract infections.

Family history
- Adult polycystic kidney disease.
- History of hypertension, diabetes and renal failure.

Drug history
- Use of antihypertensive drugs.
- Use of nephrotoxic drugs, e.g. non-steroidal anti-inflammatory drugs (NSAIDs), gentamicin.

Social history
- Occupation and family circumstances.
- Hobbies and recreational activities.

Patient's agenda
- Explore her understanding of osteoarthritis.
- Explore her concerns about the joint pains and painkillers.
- Explore her fears about renal failure and dialysis.

Examination
- Offer to recheck her BP, dipstick the urine, perform fundoscopy.
- Offer to examine her hips and knees.
- 'If it's okay with you, I will recheck you, check your hips and knees, look at the back of your eyes and test your urine.'

Examination card	
Blood pressure	BP today is 152/97 mmHg
	Home BP readings are between 145/90 and 155/95 mmHg
Fundoscopy	Normal
Urine dipstick	Normal
Hip and knees	Normal with full range of movement and no joint swelling

Clinical management
1 Explain the results of the blood tests
- Explain that the first blood test showed mild renal impairment (chronic kidney disease [CKD] stage 3), which was confirmed in the second blood test.
- Check her understanding of renal impairment and discuss any concerns she raises.
- Suggest the likely cause of her renal impairment is the combination of hypertensive disease with the use of nephrotoxic drugs – bendroflumethiazide and ibuprofen.
- Apologise that she was not made aware of the potential side effects of the drugs on the kidneys.
- Reassure the patient that CKD is common >75 years, with nearly 50% having CKD 3 to 5.
- Explain that, in view of only mild impairment with causes such as diuretic and NSAID usage, and a history of hypertension, the best course of action would be to use alternative analgesics and antihypertensives.
- Reassure her that an ultrasound scan (USS) and referral to a specialist are not required in this instance.
- Check how she feels about switching medications and holding off further investigations and referral at this stage.

2 Discuss management of chronic kidney disease stage 3
a Blood pressure
- Explain that her BP needs to be better controlled to prevent any further potential renal damage or complications (such as myocardial infarction [MI] or stroke).
- Advise her to:
  — keep systolic blood pressure (sBP) <140 mmHg (target range 120–139 mmHg)
  — keep diastolic blood pressure (dBP) <90 mmHg.

13

- Suggest stopping bendroflumethiazide as this can cause renal dysfunction.
- Start an angiotensin converting enzyme (ACE) inhibitor.
- Explain that this antihypertensive has reno-protective properties.
- Explain that the dose will need to be titrated to the maximum tolerable.
- Advise the patient that renal function will need to be monitored, and a blood test should be performed in one to two weeks to ensure there is no further deterioration of renal function.
- Advise the patient that cough is a common side effect with ACE inhibitors.

Note:
- According to NICE guidelines, in patients with CKD stage 3 and hypertension:
  — Patients with angiotensin receptor blockers (ACR) <30 mg/mmol should be offered a choice of antihypertensive.
  — Patients with an ACR >30 mg/mmol should be offered ACE inhibitors or an albulmin:creatinine ratio (ARBs).
- However, in this case, the ACR level is not known, so **ideally** an ACE inhibitor would be initiated.

b Urine sample
- Reassure her that her urine dipstick was normal.
- Ask her to provide a urine sample to send to the laboratory to help assess renal function by measuring the protein in the urine (ACR).

c Stop nephrotoxic drugs and offer alternative analgesia
- Discuss the benefits (pain relief) and risks (renal and gastric complications) of ibuprofen.
- Suggest stopping ibuprofen.
- Offer a topical NSAID.
- Offer alternative oral analgesics such as Co-dydramol.

3 Follow-up
- Advise a repeat blood test in one to two weeks to assess renal function on the ACE inhibitor.
- Offer a follow-up appointment to discuss the blood and urinary ACR results, and to recheck her BP, amending the antihypertensive as needed.
- Provide her with information leaflets on CKD.

Interpersonal skills
- This station assesses the candidate's knowledge of managing CKD in primary care.
- In addition, the candidate is expected to reassure the patient that she is unlikely to develop severe renal failure or need dialysis treatment.
  — 'Your kidney function is only slightly lower than it should be. This is very common for people who are 75 years or older – nearly half of all men and women over the age of 75 years have mild kidney impairment like you.'
  — 'It is extremely unlikely that your kidneys will deteriorate more seriously, or that you will need dialysis.'
  — 'However, it is important that we ensure you are not on medications that affect the kidney. It is also important to control your BP because this will help prevent any further kidney damage.'
- CKD stage 3 is common. Renal ultrasound or referral to a renal specialist is unnecessary. Therefore, the candidate would be expected to negotiate with the patient to hold off ultrasound and referral, as part of the gatekeeper role of being a GP.
  — 'I can understand that hearing your kidneys are not working 100% is alarming. However, I want to reassure you that this is both common and usually not a cause for concern.'
  — 'I would suggest that we aim to change your medications, control your BP and recheck

your blood tests in three weeks. Sending off a urine sample would be useful because we can test for protein, which helps to assess kidney function.'
— 'If your kidney function continues to decline, then of course we would need a kidney specialist to see you. However, at this stage, they are unlikely to suggest anything else than what I have recommended. How does this sound to you?'

○⚷ **Key summary**
- Know how to manage CKD stages 1–5.
- Reassure the patient that this is common and unlikely to lead to severe kidney failure.
- Explain the need for optimising BP control and avoiding nephrotoxic drugs.
- Understand the patient's concerns about pain control for osteoarthritis, explaining the risks and benefits of NSAID use.
- Negotiate with the patient to hold off ultrasound and referral to a specialist at this stage.

Chronic kidney disease (NICE, 2008)
- CKD is common and frequently unrecognised since it is asymptomatic until its late stages.
- Advanced CKD carries a higher risk of mortality.
- Thirty per cent of people with advanced kidney disease are referred late to nephrology services, resulting in increased morbidity and mortality.
- Treatment can prevent or delay the progression of CKD, and reduce the development of complications such as cardiovascular disease.

Stages

TABLE 1.3 Stages of chronic kidney disease

CKD STAGE	eGFR (mL/min/1.73 m²)	DESCRIPTION	TESTING FREQUENCY
1	>90	Normal or increased GFR, with other evidence of kidney damage	12 monthly
2 (Mild)	60–89	Slight decrease in GFR, with other evidence of kidney damage	12 monthly
3A 3B (Moderate)	45–59 30–44	Moderate decrease in GFR, with or without other evidence of kidney damage	6 monthly
4 (Severe)	15–29	Severe decrease in GFR, with or without other evidence of kidney damage	3 monthly
5	<15	Established renal failure	6 weekly

Evidence of chronic kidney damage
- Other evidence of chronic kidney damage includes:
  — persistent microalbuminuria
  — persistent proteinuria
  — persistent haematuria (after exclusion of other causes, e.g. urological disease)
  — structural abnormalities of the kidneys demonstrated on ultrasound scanning or other radiological tests, e.g. polycystic kidney disease, reflux nephropathy
  — biopsy-proven chronic glomerulonephritis.

Renal ultrasound
- Offer a renal ultrasound to all people with CKD who have:
  — stage 4 or 5 CKD
  — progressive CKD

— visible or persistent invisible haematuria
— symptoms of urinary tract obstruction
— family history of polycystic kidney disease and are >20 years old
— been considered by a nephrologist to require a renal biopsy.

Referral to specialist

- Take into account the individual's wishes and comorbidities when considering referral.
- People with CKD in the following groups should normally be referred for specialist assessment:
  — stage 4 and 5 CKD +/− diabetes
  — ACR ≥70 mg/mmol, unless known to be due to diabetes and already appropriately treated
  — ACR ≥30 mg/mmol and haematuria
  — rapidly declining estimated glomerular filtration rate (eGFR) (>5 in 1 year or >10 within 5 years)
  — poorly controlled hypertension despite the use of ≥4 antihypertensive drugs
  — people with, or suspected of having, rare or genetic causes of CKD
  — suspected renal artery stenosis.

Cardiovascular disease risk reduction

- Statins should be used for primary prevention of CVD in all patients.
- Offer statins for the secondary prevention of CVD disease irrespective of baseline lipid values.
- Offer antiplatelet drugs for the secondary prevention of cardiovascular disease.

Blood pressure control

TABLE 1.4 Blood pressure control in chronic kidney disease

	RECOMMENDED BLOOD PRESSURE
No diabetes	sBP <140 mmHg (target range 120–139 mmHg) dBP <90 mmHg
Diabetes or ACR ≥70	sBP <130 mmHg (target range 120–129 mmHg) dBP <80 mmHg

Antihypertensive use

TABLE 1.5 Choice of antihypertensives in chronic kidney disease

	INDICATIONS	ACTIONS
Diabetes	ACR >2.5 in men **or** >3.5 in women +/− hypertension	Offer ACE inhibitors/ARBs
No diabetes	Hypertension and ACR <30	Offer choice of antihypertensive as per NICE
	Hypertension and ACR ≥30	Offer ACE inhibitors/ARBs
	ACR >70 +/− hypertension or cardiovascular disease	Offer ACE inhibitors/ARBs

- Treat with ACE inhibitors first. Move to ARBs if ACE inhibitors are not tolerated.
- Titrate ACE inhibitors/ARBs to the maximum tolerated therapeutic dose before adding second-line agent.
- Test eGFR and serum potassium before treatment starts.
- Repeat one to two weeks after treatment starts and after each dose increase.

Chronic kidney disease in people without diabetes

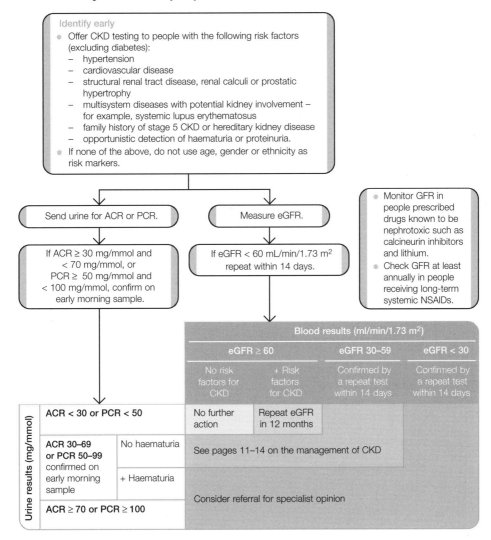

FIGURE 1.1 Algorithm for treatment of CKD in people without diabetes

(Reproduced with permission of National Institute of Health and Clinical Excellence)

National Institute for Health and Clinical Excellence. Chronic Kidney Disease: early identification and management of chronic kidney disease in adults in primary and secondary care. London: NIHCE; 2008. www.nice.org.uk/nicemedia/live/12069/42119/42119.pdf (accessed 20 November 2010).

Chronic kidney disease in people with diabetes

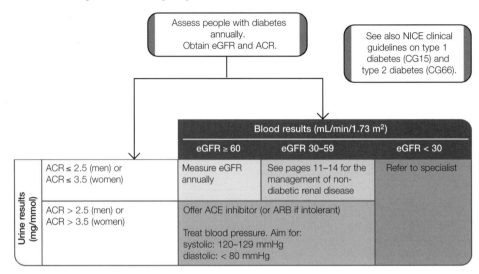

FIGURE 1.2 Algorithm for treatment of CKD in people with diabetes

(Reproduced with permission of National Institute of Health and Clinical Excellence)

National Institute for Health and Clinical Excellence. Chronic Kidney Disease: early identification and management of chronic kidney disease in adults in primary and secondary care. London: NIHCE; 2008. www.nice.org.uk/nicemedia/live/12069/42119/42119.pdf (accessed 20 November 2010).

Further reading

- The Renal Association. *The UK eCKD Guide*. Petersfield: The Renal Association; n.d. Available at: www.renal.org/whatwedo/InformationResources/CKDeGUIDE.aspx (accessed 20 November 2010).
- National Institute for Health and Clinical Excellence. Chronic Kidney Disease: early identification and management of chronic kidney disease in adults in primary and secondary care. London: NIHCE; 2008. www.nice.org.uk/nicemedia/live/12069/42119/42119.pdf (accessed 20 November 2010).
- Steddon S, Ashman N, Chesser A, *et al. Oxford Handbook of Nephrology and Hypertension*. Oxford: Oxford University Press; 2006.

Station 1.3

Candidate's notes	
Name	Harjeet Kaur
Age	24
Medical history	Miscarriage three months ago
Medication	Nil
Allergies	Nil
Last consultation	Three months ago following miscarriage

Actor's notes

Background
- You are Harjeet Kaur, a 24-year-old Sikh lady who is a housewife.

Opening statement
- 'Hello Doctor. I can't hear very well.'

History
- For the last two days, you have not been able to hear properly from your left ear.
- You can hear 'whooshing' noises in the left ear.
- The ear is not painful, and you do not have any fever.
- There was some bleeding from the ear initially but not now.

Ideas, concerns and expectations
- You are worried because you cannot hear properly.
- You are concerned that if you do not hear your husband speak to you, he may become upset, which could lead to an argument. A few days ago, he threatened to kill you. You are terrified and unsure of what to do next, or who to speak to.
- You are scared of leaving your husband – you cannot support yourself financially and are concerned how your community will react if you did. You believe you will not be allowed to stay in the UK if you leave your husband, and will cause shame to your family if you return to India.
- You have seen the doctor several times before but felt that the consultations were hurried, even after your miscarriage.
- You are unsure of what to expect from the doctor today, but want to know if your hearing will return.
- You would value any support the doctor can give you.

Further history candidate may elicit
- Your hearing reduced significantly after your husband, Jugdeep, hit you two days ago. He came home from work and became angry when he found you on the telephone to your mother in India.
- He abused you, shouting that you should not call your relatives now you were married because he was your family now, and calling India was too expensive.
- You tried to explain that you called your mother because you received a letter today from your brother telling you that she had been in hospital for hip surgery following a fall.
- At this point, Jugdeep became even angrier, saying you should not answer back. He then hit you on the head several times, and on the left ear, which started to bleed. He kicked and

punched you multiple times on the arms and legs. He told you he would kill you if you 'misbehaved' again.
- Jugdeep was verbally abusive to you soon after you got married. After a few months, he started to hit you. The violence is occurring more frequently – every few days. The abuse always happens at home.
- There are no witnesses and you have not spoken to anyone because you feel you are to blame – if you did what you were told, maybe he would not hit you.
- Three months ago you became pregnant. Jugdeep got angry – he did not want children so soon. He hit you very hard in your abdomen. You subsequently miscarried. You were devastated.
- You did try to speak to the GP before, when you came about the miscarriage. The GP rushed through the consultation then, and did not seem interested in you.
- You are not currently pregnant. You have not thought of ending your life but feel confused and scared as to what to do next.
- Jugdeep has never hit you with an object, or tried to strangle you.
- You have never called the police and are unaware of any services available to help you.

Medical history
- You had a miscarriage three months ago. This was your first pregnancy.

Drug history
- Nil.

Family history
- Your parents and two brothers live in India. You have no family in the UK.

Social history
- You had an arranged marriage to Jugdeep six months ago. You were living in India before and moved to the UK after the marriage. You were happy to marry Jugdeep – he seemed like a 'nice boy'.
- You do not drink alcohol or smoke.
- You have a degree in economics from Punjab University but your husband refuses to let you work.
- You spend your days cooking and cleaning the house. You have no friends in the UK.
- Your in-laws have introduced you to their community. They always seem to be complaining the house is not clean enough and there is not enough food. They live locally with their younger son.
- Your husband works as a pharmacist. He has lots of friends and sees them regularly without you.
- He drinks heavily two to four times a week when he goes out with his friends. When drunk, he has forced you to have sex. He does not have a criminal record as far as you know.

Approach to scenario
- You are worried about your hearing loss, but are very scared of your husband.
- You have poor self-esteem and come across as fearful.
- During the consultation, you appear timid, have poor eye contact and speak softly.
- If the doctor asks you how the injury occurred, you tell him/her that you 'fell over' when you were cleaning and hit your head on the floor.
- If the doctor is sensitive, caring and approaches the topic of domestic violence, you will open up slowly and explain how the injury really happened.
- You provide small amounts of information at first, but if the doctor shows empathy, you answer the questions with more detail, admitting that you feel ashamed.
- You will not introduce the topic of domestic violence yourself, and if the doctor does not approach the subject, you do not bring it up.

- You feel alone and isolated. You welcome any offer of advice or support since you do not have family or friends in this country.

Information gathering
Presenting complaint
a Ear symptoms
- Ask if she can hear at all from the left ear.
- Ask about earache, fever and discharge.

b Domestic violence risk assessment
i Background
- History of abuse (past and present).
- Is there emotional +/– physical +/– sexual abuse?
- Is the abuse becoming more frequent, intense or severe?
- Are there any children being harmed?
- Is she pregnant?
- Extent of the injuries.
- Is she about to leave her partner?
- How much at risk does she feel?
- Does she have a physical disability or mental health problem?

ii Facts about the abuser
- Does the abuser:
  — misuse alcohol or drugs?
  — have a criminal record?
  — use or threaten to use weapons?
  — have a mental health problem?
- Has the abuser threatened to kill or attempted strangulation?

iii Assess for depression
- Any thoughts of suicide or self-harm.

iv Other information
- Place of, and witnesses to, assault.
- Explore if she has an alternative place to stay.
- Sources of emotional support (family and friends).
- Attempts to contact police, refuges or consideration of separation.

Medical history
- Including history of serious injuries following domestic violence.
- History of physical disability or previous mental health problems.

Family history
- History of domestic violence in her own family.

Drug history
- Current or past use of contraception.

Social history
- Occupation.
- Financial situation.
- Enquire about alcohol and smoking.
- Friends, relatives and support mechanisms.

Patient's agenda
- Explore her concerns about her hearing.
- Explore her fears about her marital situation.
- Explore her cultural and religious beliefs about marriage.

Examination
- Offer to examine her ears.
- 'Is it okay if I look in your ears to see if there is any damage or infection?'

Examination card
Ear examination   Bruising behind the left ear
Ruptured left tympanic membrane with dried blood in the ear canal
Right ear canal and tympanic membrane are normal

Clinical management
1 Provide information
- Offer information sensitively, checking the patient's understanding as you go along.
- Reassure her that confidentiality will be maintained. (This is especially important if the partner is also a registered patient at your practice.)*
- Make it clear that the abuse is **not** her fault, and that 'violence in the home is illegal, just as is violence on the street'.
- Emphasise she is a victim of crime, has legal rights and a right to safety.
- Let her know she is not alone – 25% of women experience abuse.
- Encourage her to see there is life after abuse – other women have created safer lives for themselves and so can she.
- Discuss the physical and emotional consequences of chronic abuse.
- Ask what **she** would like you to do, explaining agencies may be able to help where you cannot.
- Provide written information about legal options and help offered by:
    — police domestic violence units
    — Women's Aid National Helpline
    — local women's refuges and shelters
    — social service and local authority housing departments.
If children are involved, a referral to social services is needed.

2 Decide on a plan of action
- Respect her autonomy, self-determination and self-esteem.
- Explore the potential cultural reasons that prevent her from leaving her husband.
- Discuss if she wants to leave her partner or stay with him.
- If she wants to leave her partner, provide her with details of local services available, and offer help in contacting them.
- If she chooses to return to her partner:
    — Give her the phone number of a local Women's Refuge or Women's Aid.
    — Advise her to keep some money and important financial and legal documents hidden in a safe place in case of an emergency.
    — Advise her to avoid places such as the kitchen when the abuse starts, where there are potential weapons.
    — Help her to plan an escape route in case of emergency.
    — Educate her about calling 999 if needed. Advise her to confide in a neighbour who can call 999 if they hear the abuse.

3 Attend to her physical health needs
- Explain that her left eardrum is perforated.
- Advise her to keep the ear dry.
- Reassure her that in most cases the eardrum will heal and hearing will return to normal.
- Explain there is a risk of infection and she should return for antibiotics if earache or discharge occur.
- Offer to start her on contraception – include options such as depot preparations so her partner is not aware, if she prefers.

4 Follow-up
- Offer her a follow-up appointment to review the eardrum and her situation at home.
- Explain a small number of patients with perforated eardrum need to be referred for surgery.

Interpersonal skills
- In this case, the patient has presented with an injury suggestive of domestic violence.
- The candidate would be expected to suspect domestic violence in view of the bruising around the ear, traumatic injury and overall demeanour of the patient.
- Having suspected domestic violence, the candidate would need to discuss this delicately and sensitively with the patient, using communication skills including open questions, active listening and demonstrating empathy.
- After examination, the candidate could ask the patient:
  — 'Mrs Kaur, unfortunately your left eardrum is torn, which is causing the problem with your hearing. One of the reasons people develop a hole in the eardrum is because someone has hurt them. Has this happened to you?'
  — 'What do you think your options are?'
- Domestic violence is a challenging subject. It is important to:
  — Ask questions in a gentle, non-threatening way.
  — Allow for silence, giving her time to speak.
  — Encourage her that she has options available.
  — Explore reasons for staying with her partner, including cultural or religious beliefs.
  — Respect the patient's autonomy regarding future action, and not to pressurise her into following a particular course of action.
- Do not be afraid to ask direct questions.
  — 'Are you scared at home?'
  — 'Has your partner ever hit you?'
  — 'Have you been forced to do anything sexually that you did not want to do?'

O⚊ Key summary
- Be familiar with how domestic violence may present – bruises, perforated tympanic membranes, depression or repeated attendances to a doctor for minor illness.
- Ensure you inform the child-protection team or social services if children are involved.
- Treat patients for both the **physical** and **emotional** consequences of domestic violence.
- Emphasise that domestic violence is illegal, and inform them of their legal rights and the support services available to them.
- Offer to contact services on their behalf if required and encourage a follow-up appointment.

Domestic violence
- Domestic violence occurs in all parts of society, accounting for a quarter of all violent crime.
- Partner abuse is as common among same-sex couples as heterosexual couples.
- Particularly vulnerable groups are women with low socio-economic status or mental illness.
- Domestic violence is more likely to begin or escalate during pregnancy.
- If language is a barrier, always use a professional interpreter, not a relative or friend.

Statistics

- Two women are killed every week by a current or former partner.
- Twenty per cent of women in England and Wales say they have been physically assaulted by their partner at some stage.
- Thirty per cent of domestic violence cases start during pregnancy.
- Fifty-two per cent of child-protection cases involve domestic violence.
- Ninety per cent of domestic violence happens with the child or children in the same or next room.

Note:
- These are reported cases, and therefore probably underestimate true incidence.

Examples of domestic abuse

a Physical
- Such as shaking, smacking, punching, kicking, starving, tying up, stabbing, suffocating, throwing things, using objects as weapons and female genital mutilation.

b Sexual
- Such as forced sex, forced prostitution, refusal to practise safe sex and sexual insults.

c Psychological
- Such as intimidating, insulting, isolating the victim from friends and family, criticising and treating the victim as an inferior.

d Financial
- Such as not letting the victim work, undermining efforts to find work or study, refusing to give money, asking for an explanation of how every penny is spent and making them beg for money.

e Emotional
- Such as swearing, undermining confidence, making racist remarks, making the victim feel unattractive, calling them stupid or useless and eroding their independence.

Effects of domestic abuse

TABLE 1.6 The physical and psychological effects of domestic violence

PHYSICAL EFFECTS	PSYCHOLOGICAL EFFECTS
Death	Suicide
Bruising	Self-harming behaviour
Tiredness	Fear
Poor nutrition	Guilt
Broken bones	Depression
Chronic pain	Post-traumatic stress disorder
Miscarriage	Increased misuse of drugs and alcohol
Maternal death	Loss of self-confidence
Premature birth	Loss of hope
Babies with low birth weight or stillborn	Low self-worth
General poor health	Panic or anxiety
Burns or stab wounds	Eating disorders

Reasons why women stay with an abuser

A woman may:

- still love the abuser
- be afraid of the abuser
- be financially dependent on the abuser
- think there is a chance their partner will change
- want their children's father to be around as they grow up
- be anxious about living alone, not being able to cope or the unknown
- suffer chronic post-traumatic stress and be unable to make critical decisions
- be convinced by the abuser that they are worthless and no one else will care for them.

Barriers to disclosing domestic violence

Women often do not disclose domestic violence because:

- Nobody may have ever asked.
- They might be worried about stigma surrounding domestic abuse.
- They might be afraid of the consequences of telling someone.
- Some women do not recognise their situation as domestic abuse.
- The consequences of talking might seem worse than staying silent.
- The perpetrator may have threatened worse abuse if she talks to someone.
- They might be worried about losing their children if social services are involved.
- There might be cultural or religious barriers.

Freephone, 24-hour National Domestic Violence Helpline (0808 2000 247)

- Run in partnership with Women's Aid and Refuge.
- Provides information, emotional and practical support to women experiencing domestic abuse and to those seeking help on a woman's behalf.
- Helpline staff are all women, and calls are taken in the strictest of confidence.
- They discuss the available options to enable women to make an informed choice.
- If appropriate, they may refer them to a refuge, outreach services or other sources of help and information.
- The helpline is a member of Language Line and can provide access to an interpreter for non-English speaking callers.
- Helpline staff can also access the Type Talk Service for deaf callers.
- If all lines are busy, there is a voicemail system that enables callers to leave a message, which will be responded to as soon as possible.

FIGURE 1.3 National Domestic Violence Helpline

Further reading

- Women's Aid website. www.womensaid.org.uk (accessed 20 November 2010).
- Home Office. *Tackling Domestic Violence: the role of health professionals.* 2nd ed. London: Home Office; 2004. Available at: http://rds.homeoffice.gov.uk/rds/pdfs04/dpr32.pdf (accessed 9 Janurary 2011).
- British Medical Association (BMA). *Domestic Abuse: a report from the BMA Board of Science.* London: BMA; 2007. Available at: www.bma/org/uk/images/Domestic%20Abuse_tcm41-183509.pdf (accessed 9 January 2011).

Station 1.4

Actor's notes

Background

- You are Mark Thompson, a 29-year-old Caucasian investment banker.

Opening statement

- 'Hello doctor. I'm here to get an HIV test.'

History

- You had unprotected sex four weeks ago after meeting someone for the first time at a party.

Ideas, concerns and expectations

- You have had unprotected sexual intercourse (UPSI) several times over the last six months. The last occasion was four weeks ago.
- Yesterday, you spoke to a friend who told you that your ex-partner in New York tested positive for human immunodeficiency virus (HIV) a few months ago.
- You are worried that he may have passed HIV on to you.
- You feel extremely foolish for not using a condom over the last six months and are scared you may have picked up HIV.
- You do not want your colleagues to know you are gay, or that you have asked for an HIV test because some of them are homophobic, and you are concerned you will lose your job if they found out.
- You are expecting to be offered a blood test by the GP today.
- You are busy with work and will be travelling to Germany tomorrow for one week. You definitely want the test and the result before you fly tomorrow afternoon.

Further history candidate may elicit

- You moved to the UK six months ago from New York for work, and expect to stay another year.
- The episode of UPSI four weeks ago was with another man and you do not know anything about him. He was Caucasian. You did not notice any tattoos on him and do not know if he is an intravenous drug user (IVDU). You gave and received anal sex with him.
- You had some casual relationships with women as a teenager, and lost your virginity age 17. You realised you were gay when you were 19 years old. Since then, you have had sexual relations only with men. Initially, you had some casual relationships with men, and always used a condom. In the past, you have given and received oral sex.
- You have had one long-term relationship with a man, which lasted four years. This relationship ended six months ago when you moved to the UK for work. A few months into this relationship, you and your partner had a sexual health check-up. Both of you tested

negative for HIV and other sexually transmitted infections (STIs) so you both stopped using condoms. You were faithful in this relationship and did not cheat on your partner. To your knowledge, your partner was faithful too. However, you are now worried he may have cheated on you when you were together and so picked up HIV and passed it on to you.

- Since coming to the UK, you have entered a social scene where many men do not use condoms.
- You have had UPSI in three or four casual flings with men in the UK over the last six months.
- Some of the men were from the African and Asian subcontinent. You do not know anything about them in terms of their HIV risk factors.
- Most of episodes of casual sex involved alcohol and drugs.
- You have never used post-exposure prophylaxis (PEP) after the episodes of UPSI.

Medical history
- You had an HIV test four years ago, which was negative. You have not had another test since then.
- You have no long-term health conditions and have never had any sexually transmitted disease (STD).
- You have not had any flu-like symptoms in the last few months.

Drug history
- Nil.

Family history
- Your parents and younger sister live in New York and are well.
- They are unaware that you are gay and you are not planning on telling them in the near future.

Social history
- You do not smoke. You drink cocktails when you go out with friends, particularly at gay clubs.
- You have used cocaine and ecstasy since coming to the UK, usually at parties or clubs.
- You have never used intravenous drugs or heroin.
- You enjoy your work as an investment banker in the city.
- You moved to the UK with work six months ago and will be returning to New York in one year.
- Your partner in New York was upset that you chose to leave the USA, and you both decided to go on a 'break'.

Approach to scenario
- You are a well-dressed, articulate man.
- You are worried you may have contracted HIV from your ex-partner or from one of the recent casual flings.
- You feel stupid because you have not used condoms recently.
- You are upset to hear your ex-partner has HIV, but also angry that he may have cheated on you.
- You are worried about him but are not sure if you should contact him, since you have not spoken in six months.
- You find it difficult to disclose details about your sex life. However, if the doctor comes across as being non-judgemental and understanding, you reveal you are gay and have had several episodes of unprotected sex over the last few months, involving alcohol and drugs.
- You are particularly concerned that your work not be informed about this consultation, the HIV test request or the results.

- You want to have the test and result today. Since you have been in the UK for only six months, you do not know where you can have the test.
- You are happy to have the test at the GP surgery, but if the doctor tells you it cannot be done at the surgery, you are happy to attend another clinic to have the test, or will pay to have it done privately.

Information gathering
Presenting complaint
- Explore why he wants an HIV test.
- Explore the episode of unprotected sex last night.
  — Man or woman.
  — Number of partners involved.
  — Check if anal +/– oral sex were involved.
  — Confirm if he gave +/– received anal/oral sex, or both.
  — Risk factors of partner (IVDU, tattoos and ethnicity).
  — Confirm if either he or partner used a condom.
  — Ask about use of alcohol and drugs.
- Ask about current or recent symptoms.
  — Sero-conversion illness (fever, sore throat, etc.).
  — Urethral discharge.
  — Penile itching.
  — Oral symptoms.
  — Anal symptoms.

Sexual history
a *Partners*
- Number of sexual partners.
- Sex with prostitutes or sex-workers.
- Confirm if partners are male, female or both.
- Partner's risk factors (IVDU, ethnicity, history of STDs).

b *Sexual practices*
- Use of condoms and history of unprotected sex.
- Type of sexual activity (vaginal, anal, oral).

c *Past history of STDs*
- Ask about previous screening/treatment of STDs.

d *Past history of HIV tests*
- Ask if he has had an HIV test before; if so, confirm result.

e *HIV and hepatitis risk*
- History of hepatitis A or B vaccination.

Medical history
- Any other medical condition.
- History of STI.
- Ask about recent flu-like symptoms.

Family history
- Ask about family support in the UK and USA.
- Ask about any health conditions affecting the family.

Drug history
- Previous use of PEP.
- Hepatitis A or B vaccination.
- Use of recreational and intravenous drugs.

Social history
- Occupation.
- Alcohol, drugs and smoking.
- Enquire about recent move to the UK.

Patient's agenda
- Explore his understanding of HIV disease.
- Explore his understanding of HIV tests.
- Explore the patient's concerns about:
  — the possibility he may have HIV
  — preserving confidentiality from his work
  — having the test and result available today.

Clinical management
1 Pre-test counselling
- Agree that the patient needs an HIV test, and this can be arranged today.
- Explore what he knows about HIV and transmission (UPSI, IVDU, tattoos or body piercing).
- Explain that there is no cure for HIV, but it can be treated through a combination of drugs, and people can stay well for years.
- Reassure him that the test is confidential – you will not inform his work, regardless of the outcome.
- Explain the test involves either a blood sample or finger-prick test.

2 Discuss the consequences of a negative result
- Explain that if the test is negative today, it still needs to be repeated in two months (which is three months after the last episode of UPSI), because some people only test positive three months after the initial exposure.
- Emphasise that if the test is negative today, he must still use condoms for the next two months to prevent potential transmission to other people, and protect himself from HIV transmission.
- If the second test (in two months) is also negative, he can be reassured that he does not have HIV.
- However, a negative test now does not safeguard from developing HIV in the future – underline the importance of condom use, and adjustment of risk factors such as alcohol and drug use.

3 Discuss the consequences of a positive result
- If the test is positive today or in two months, explain that this confirms he has HIV and he can begin treatment for HIV without delay, through consultation with a specialist team.
- Explain that the test cannot help identify if he has contracted HIV from his ex-partner or from one of the men he has had UPSI with in the UK.
- Strongly advise him of the importance of contacting his previous partners to notify them of his HIV status, so they can also be checked.

4 Discuss the options of having an HIV test

- Explain that he could have the test today or when he returns from Europe.
- Explore how he would cope if the test was positive today and had to go on business tomorrow.
- Explain that you can arrange a blood test at the surgery today, but will not get the results today.
- Explain he could have the test and results today if he has the test at:
  — the local genitourinary medicine (GUM) clinic
  — the Terrence Higgins 'Fastest' clinic
  — a private clinic.
- Offer to provide contact details for the GUM/Terrence Higgins/private clinic.

5 Test for other STDs

- Advise him that he should consider being tested for other STDs such as syphilis, hepatitis A and B (by blood test), gonorrhoea (by swabs from rectum, throat and urethra) and Chlamydia (by urine testing or swab from the penis).

6 Reduce risk

- Use condoms at all times.
- Avoid use of drugs and excessive alcohol use.
- Have the hepatitis A and B vaccinations at the surgery, GUM clinic or privately.

7 Follow-up

- Inform him of the Terrence Higgins Trust (www.tht.org.uk) and provide appropriate leaflets.
- Offer him a follow-up appointment to discuss any other issues or the results of the test.

Interpersonal skills

- Sexual history taking can be 'embarrassing' for both the doctor and patient.
- Start the consultation with open questions and try to keep the patient at ease.
  — 'What has happened recently that makes you ask for an HIV test?'
  — 'What do you understand about HIV?'
- When asking more direct questions regarding the sexual history, try to put the patient at ease by explaining why you are asking them these questions.
  — 'I am going to ask you some questions about your sexual health. These questions are very personal, but it is important for me to ask them so I can help you stay healthy and reduce the likelihood of problems in future.'
  — 'I ask these questions to all of my patients regardless of age or marital status. They are just as important as other questions about your physical and mental health.'
  — 'This information is strictly confidential and will not be shared with anyone.'
- Ensure you maintain a non-judgemental, sensitive approach, and reassure the patient that confidentiality will be maintained.

O—⚷ Key summary

- Elicit a clear sexual history and risk assessment for HIV.
- Explore his current understanding of HIV and HIV testing.
- Explore his concerns about maintaining confidentiality.
- Offer pre-test counselling and explain the options available to have the test.
- Discuss the importance of contact tracing if the test is positive.
- Address risk factors and lifestyle changes to reduce HIV risk.

HIV disease
Pathology
- HIV is the precursor to acquired immune deficiency syndrome (AIDS). The retrovirus replicates rapidly in CD4 lymphocytes, and then destroys these cells.
- Initially, the replacement of CD4 lymphocytes matches the destruction of CD4 lymphocytes, but, with time, destruction overtakes replacement, resulting in immunological deficiency and the development of AIDS-defining illness.
- It is transmitted through sexual contact, blood products or via breast milk from an infected mother.

Stages of HIV infection
a Incubation period
- Asymptomatic and lasts two to four weeks.

b Sero-conversion illness
- Patients are initially asymptomatic following infection.
- After two to six weeks there may be a sero-conversion illness for about two weeks.

i Clinical features
- Fever.
- Arthralgia and myalgia.
- Lymphadenopathy.
- Morbilliform skin rash.
- Meningoencephalitis.

ii Investigations
- Reduced lymphocyte count and CD4 count.
- Blood film shows atypical lymphocytes.

iii Diagnosis
- HIV polymerase chain reaction (PCR) test and p24 antigen test are positive in first few weeks.
- HIV antibodies take three months to form, so test three months after suspected HIV exposure.

Note:
- The British Association for Sexual Health and HIV (BASHH, 2008) recommends the use of fourth generation HIV tests in patients who have potentially been exposed to HIV >4 weeks ago.
- These tests involve assays that check for HIV antibodies and p24 antigen simultaneously.
- A negative result at four weeks post-exposure is very reassuring and is highly likely to exclude HIV infection.
- An additional HIV test should be offered to all persons at three months to definitively exclude HIV infection. Patients at lower risk may opt to wait until three months to avoid the need for HIV testing twice.

c Latency stage
- Can last 2 weeks to 20 years, during which patients show few or no symptoms.
- Some conditions are more common, such as shingles and seborrhoeic dermatitis.

d Increased susceptibility to pathogenic organisms
- Tuberculosis (TB).
- Candidiasis (oral and oesophageal).
- Respiratory tract infections.
- GI infections causing diarrhoea (salmonella, shigella).

e AIDS
- The CD4 count is $<200 \times 10^6/L$.
- Patients develop symptoms and signs of various opportunistic infections and tumours (AIDS-defining illnesses) that do not normally affect an immunocompetent person.

Treatment of HIV and AIDS: highly active antiretroviral therapy (HAART)
- There is currently no cure for HIV.
- HAART involves treating patients with ≥ 3 drugs.
- Usually, initial triple therapy is with two nucleoside reverse transcriptase inhibitors (NRTIs) and either a protease inhibitor (PI) or a non-nucleoside reverse transcriptase inhibitor (NNRTI).

Which groups of patients with HIV should receive HAART?
- Patients with:
  - clinical features of HIV, or
  - CD4 count <350 cells/mm^3, or
  - viral load $>30\,000$.

What is post-exposure prophylaxis?
- Antiretroviral triple therapy is available to health workers who have been exposed to blood or other bodily fluids from a known HIV patient or a patient at high risk of HIV.
- It is also prescribed for those who have had unprotected sex in the last 72 hours and are considered to be at high risk of contracting HIV.
- The sooner it is started, the more effective the treatment. However, it is not 100% effective.
- Antiretroviral therapy is given for four weeks. Common side effects include diarrhoea, vomiting and headaches.

Further reading
- Terrence Higgins Trust. Information resources: HIV and AIDS. London: Terrence Higgins Trust; 2011. Available at: www.tht.org.uk/informationresources/hivandaids (accessed 20 November 2010).
- Health Protection Agency. *HIV in the United Kingdom: 2009 report.* London: Health Protection Agency; n.d. Available at: www.hpa.org.uk/web/HPAwebFile/HPAweb_C/1259151891830 (accessed 20 November 2010).
- Pattman R, Snow M, Handy P, *et al.*, editors. *Oxford Handbook of Genitourinary Medicine, HIV and AIDS.* Oxford: Oxford University Press; 2005.
- British HIV Association, British Association for Sexual Health and HIV, British Infection Society. *UK National Guidelines for HIV Testing* 2008. Available at: www.bashh.org/guidelines (accessed 20 November 2010).

Station 1.5

Candidate's notes

Name	Freda Hawthorne
Age	73
Medical history	Hypertension
Medication	Ramipril 5 mg od
Allergies	Nil
Last consultation	Seen two weeks ago by another colleague
	Presented with shoulder pains
	GP suggested bloods and radiographs of the shoulders
	Routine BP check normal
	Advised to take ibuprofen and paracetamol
	To return for results of blood tests and radiographs

Blood results

FBC	= normal
Renal function	= normal
Liver function	= normal
Calcium	= normal
ESR	= 89 mm/h

Radiograph report

No abnormality detected in left or right shoulder. No evidence of osteoarthritis or metastatic disease.

Actor's notes

Background
- You are Freda Hawthorne, a 73-year-old Caucasian lady.
- You are a retired librarian but work one day a week as a volunteer at the local charity shop.

Opening statement
- 'Doctor, I've come for the results of my tests.'

History
- Over the last seven weeks or so, you have noticed that you feel very stiff around both shoulders.
- Two weeks ago you saw another GP who advised you take ibuprofen and paracetamol for the pain.
- The doctor suggested you may have arthritis and advised a blood test and X-rays of your shoulders.
- You have come for the results today.

Ideas, concerns and expectations
- The stiffness in the shoulders is bothering you considerably. Over the last three weeks, you have not worked at the charity shop because you are finding it painful to pick up and display clothes.

- In addition, you have had to stop playing golf because of the stiffness in your shoulders and hips.
- You are concerned that you may have arthritis. You are worried that 'old age is catching up' with you and your mobility will continue to decline with time.
- You would like the doctor to explain the test results and the cause of the pain and stiffness in your shoulders and hips.
- You would also like to discuss treatment options and the complications of this condition. Ideally, you would prefer to use complementary therapies, like acupuncture, rather than steroids, because you have read in a magazine that they can cause diabetes, weight gain and thinning of the bones.

Further history candidate may elicit
- Initially, both your shoulders were painful and stiff. Now, your neck muscles and hips are also painful and stiff. The stiffness is worse in the morning. There is no weakness.
- Over the last week, it has become difficult to turn in bed, and your husband has to occasionally help you get out of your armchair.
- You feel more tired than normal, even though have not changed or increased your daily activities.
- You have taken the ibuprofen and paracetamol regularly for the last two weeks, but the pain has not settled. A friend suggested acupuncture, which she found useful when she had back pain.
- You do not have any back pain, headaches, scalp tenderness, visual disturbances, jaw claudication, weight loss, night sweats or muscle weakness.
- You have no pain or swelling in any joints, e.g. knee, elbow or small joints of the hands and feet.

Medical history
- Hypertension – well controlled for a number of years.

Drug history
- Ramipril 5 mg od.
- Ibuprofen 200 mg tds.
- Paracetamol 1–2 tablets qds.

Social history
- You do not smoke. You drink a glass of wine only on special occasions.
- You live with your husband in a four-bedroom house. You find it painful to walk up the stairs.
- You enjoy keeping active by playing golf three times a week, and going for regular long walks with your husband. You have stopped these activities because of the pain in your hips and shoulders.
- You volunteer one day a week at a charity shop but have not been for the last three weeks.

Family history
- You have two sons and three grandchildren who live nearby. The family are well.
- There is no family history of autoimmune or joint problems.

Approach to scenario
- You are keen to hear the results of the investigations you have had. The previous GP suggested some investigations to rule out osteoarthritis.
- You are frustrated at how your symptoms have affected your lifestyle and feel 'achy and old'.
- You are relieved to hear you do not have osteoarthritis.
- You have not heard of polymyalgia rheumatica (PMR) before and ask the doctor to explain it to you and tell you about any complications.

- If the doctor mentions that PMR is associated with temporal arteritis, which can lead to blindness, you become alarmed, but are reassured if they explain that it is preventable.
- You are not keen on taking steroids because of the potential side effects you have read about in a magazine, and would prefer to try acupuncture.
- If the doctor is able to communicate well with you regarding the cause of your symptoms, the potential complications and the importance of steroids, you agree to the treatment and feel reassured.
- If the doctor does not come across well, you become anxious about the potential side effects of the steroids and suggest you will see another GP for advice, and try acupuncture instead.

Information gathering
Presenting complaint
a Pain and stiffness
- Explore why the patient had the X-rays performed.
- Check how long the symptoms have occurred for.
- Confirm which parts of the body are affected.
- Ask about alleviating and exacerbating factors.
- Ask about use of painkillers and their effects.
- Ask about joint pain or stiffness of the hands and knees.

b Other features
- Tiredness.
- Headaches.
- Visual problems.
- Weight loss.
- Scalp tenderness.
- Jaw claudication.

Medical history
- Any other medical condition.

Family history
- Joint disease.

Drug history
- Current medications and use of painkillers.

Social history
- Alcohol and smoking.
- Previous occupation.
- Social activities.
- Marital status.
- Home circumstances (house/flat/bungalow).

Patient's agenda
- Explore the impact her symptoms have had on her activities.
- Explore her understanding about steroids and acupuncture.

Examination
- Offer to examine the patient's hips and shoulders, check for scalp tenderness and perform fundoscopy.

- 'I'd like to examine your hips and shoulders if that's okay. Also, I'd like to look at the back of your eyes and feel your scalp to check for any other conditions that could be related.'

Examination card

Shoulders	Normal power
	Full range of movement but painful
Hips	Normal power
	Full range of movement but painful
Fundoscopy	Normal
Scalp vessels	No tenderness
	No palpable or enlarged temporal vessels present

Clinical management

1 Discuss the diagnosis of polymyalgia rheumatica

- Explain and reassure the patient that the X-rays of hips and shoulders are normal and do not show any arthritis or bone abnormality.
- Explain that her blood result revealed an elevated erythrocyte sedimentation rate (ESR), which is a marker of inflammation.
- Explain that the combination of a high ESR and symptoms of muscle pain and tenderness of the shoulders, neck and hips suggest she has PMR, which results from inflammation of the muscles.
- Explain that PMR is sometimes associated with temporal arteritis.
- Reassure the patient she does not have any symptoms to suggest temporal arteritis at present.
- Outline the common symptoms of temporal arteritis (headaches, visual disturbances, scalp tenderness and jaw claudication).

2 Discuss complications of polymyalgia rheumatica and temporal arteritis

- Explain that PMR is not a serious condition per se, but can be rather debilitating if untreated.
- Explain that temporal arteritis is a more serious condition, and that it usually presents with localised pain at the temple.
- Mention the main complication of temporal arteritis is visual loss.
- Advise her to attend accident and emergency (A+E) or the surgery immediately if she experiences any visual problems.
- Explain that in both conditions, patients respond well to medication.

3 Explain the management of polymyalgia rheumatica

a Steroid treatment

- Explain that she needs to start on oral steroids.
- Explore her concerns about starting on steroids.
- Discuss the common side effects of (short- and long-term) steroids, but emphasise that the benefits in PMR outweigh these.
- Explain that she should mention that she is on steroids to any other doctor she sees.
- Explain that she must see a doctor if she feels unwell, as signs of infection can be masked by steroids.

b Future treatment

- Explain that if she responds well to steroids, steroid treatment may be continued long/medium-term, reducing the dose over time.
- If she is on long-term steroids, she would be started on a bisphosphonate and calcium supplement for bone protection, which would prevent the bones from thinning.
- In addition, she may be started on a proton pump inhibitor for gastric protection.

4 Discuss acupuncture and follow-up

- Advise her that acupuncture can be useful for a number of conditions but is not a recognised treatment for PMR as there is no scientific evidence to suggest it has any benefit.
- Explain that acupuncture for PMR is not available through the NHS and she would have to pay for this privately.
- Advise her to speak to an acupuncture therapist to find out if it can be a useful treatment in PMR.
- Advise her that if she chooses to take steroids and try acupuncture in addition, she should inform the acupuncture therapist prior to starting.
- Offer her a follow-up appointment in two weeks to review her progress on the steroids.
- Provide her with leaflets on PMR.

Interpersonal skills

- Reassure the patient about her X-ray results early on in the consultation to help develop rapport.
  - 'I am pleased to say the X-rays of your shoulders and hips were normal. They show normal healthy bone. There is no sign of osteoarthritis or "wear and tear", which occurs with degeneration.'
- Recognise the patient's frustration regarding the impact her symptoms have had on her lifestyle.
  - 'I can see you're fed up with all of this. Let's see what we can do to get you back on track.'
- Be sensitive when explaining that blindness is a complication of temporal arteritis.
  - 'Temporal arteritis is a condition that causes inflammation of some of the large blood vessels in your body, especially the ones in your scalp. When these vessels get inflamed, they can cause headaches.
  - 'If the blood vessels to your eyes get inflamed, then your vision can become affected, and there is a risk that you could go blind. So it's very important that you see a doctor immediately if you develop any problems with your eyes, since treatment can save your vision.'
- Encourage the patient to start treatment with steroids by discussing the risks and benefits.
  - 'Steroid therapy will help resolve your symptoms and restore your quality of life.'
  - 'Steroids do have a number of side effects, just like many other drugs. They can cause thinning of the bones, diabetes and weight gain if they are used over a long time and at high dose. However, patients with PMR have low-dose steroids, not high-dose steroids, so reducing the risk of side effects.'
  - 'In addition, there are tablets that we could start to help protect the bones to prevent them from getting thin.'

O⎯ᴴ Key summary
- Explore the impact of the symptoms on the patient's lifestyle.
- Elicit the symptoms of PMR whilst excluding other conditions.
- Enquire about temporal arteritis and exclude an ophthalmological emergency.
- Explain the likely diagnosis of PMR and reassure the patient she does not have osteoarthritis.
- Discuss the treatment options available and advise her to seek medical attention urgently if she develops visual problems.

Polymyalgia rheumatica

- This is a condition that causes inflammation of muscles and is characterised by symmetrical pain and stiffness of the proximal muscle groups (the pectoral and pelvic girdles).
- The condition is most common in women >50 years and is associated with temporal arteritis.

Clinical features

- Pain and stiffness at the shoulders, upper arms, neck and hips.
  - Symptoms worse first thing in the morning.
  - Patients have difficulty turning in bed, rising from a bed or chair, or raising arms shoulder height.
  - True weakness does not occur although power and movement may be limited due to pain and stiffness.
- Systemic symptoms include tiredness, depression, night sweats, fever, appetite and weight loss.
- Symptoms of temporal arteritis may also occur.

Investigations

a Bloods

- Full blood count (FBC) may reveal a normochromic, normocytic anaemia.
- ESR is usually markedly elevated but returns to normal with treatment.
- C-reactive protein (CRP) and alkaline phosphatase (ALP) may be raised but return to normal with treatment.
- Aspartate aminotransferase (AST), alanine aminotransferase (ALT), creatinine kinase (CK), autoimmune screen and calcium levels are normal.

Treatment

a Oral corticosteroid treatment with prednisolone

- Start with 15–20 mg once a day and slowly reduce over one month to 10 mg daily.
- Taper dose thereafter by 1 mg every 4–6 weeks, guided by clinical picture.
- Patients may need steroid treatment for 2 years.

b Other treatments

- Steroid sparing drugs such as methotrexate and azathioprine can be used in patients who require a longer duration of steroids.
- Calcium, vitamin D and bisphosphonates are used to prevent worsening of osteoporosis.
- Proton pump inhibitors provide gastric protection.

Temporal arteritis or giant cell arteritis

- This is a vasculitis effecting medium-size and large arteries.
- It is more common in women than men >50 years.
- The condition primarily affects the aorta and its extracranial branches such as the carotid artery.
- Intracranial arteries are only rarely involved.
- PMR precedes or accompanies temporal arteritis in more than 50% of cases.

Clinical features

- Temporal headache.
- Scalp tenderness.
- Malaise.
- Fever.
- Anorexia and weight loss.
- Jaw claudication.
- Transient visual disturbances.
- Symptoms of PMR.

Note:
- Temporal arteries may be tender, dilated, inflamed, thickened or cordlike. The artery may be pulsatile and bruits may occur if there is partial occlusion.

Complications
- Sudden loss of vision due to ischaemic optic neuropathy or central retinal artery occlusion.
- Angina and MI.
- Aortic arch syndrome.
- Thoracic aorta aneurysm or dissection.
- Intracerebral artery involvement (rare) can cause hemiplegia and epilepsy.

Diagnosis
- The American College of Rheumatology considers that ≥3 of the 5 developed diagnostic criteria must be met to support diagnosis of temporal arteritis.
- The diagnostic criteria are:
  - age 50 years or older
  - new-onset localised headache
  - temporal artery tenderness on palpation or decreased temporal artery pulse
  - ESR of at least 50 mm/h
  - abnormal artery biopsy specimen characterised by mononuclear infiltration or granulomatous inflammation.

Management
a Ophthalmology referral
- Visual disturbance is an emergency and requires immediate referral to ophthalmology.

b Steroid therapy
- Prednisolone 60–80 mg if visual symptoms present; 40–60 mg per day if visual symptoms absent.
- IV methylprednisolone may be necessary in cases of impending vision loss.
- Continue treatment even if loss of vision in one eye, to prevent visual loss in the contralateral eye.
- Steroid treatment is slowly tapered by 5–10 mg every 2 weeks until dose reaches 20 mg per day and then more slowly. The effectiveness of treatment is monitored by the patient's ESR.
- Aspirin 75 mg daily (if no contraindications) is started to manage complications of stroke and MI.
- Proton pump inhibitor for gastric protection.
- Calcium, vitamin D and bisphosphonates for bone protection.

c Other points
- Monitor blood sugar regularly in view of high-dose steroids.
- Maintain a high index of suspicion for infections during courses of high-dose steroid treatment as this may mask symptoms and signs of infection.

Further reading
- Arthritis Research Campaign. *Polymyalgia Rheumatica: an information booklet*. Chesterfield: Arthritis Research Campaign; 2006. Available at: www.arthritisresearchuk.org/files/6032_PMR_06-1_01032010142816.pdf (accessed 20 November 2010).
- Dasgupta, B, Kalke, S. Polymyalgia rheumatica and giant cell arteritis. In Adebajo, AO, Dickson, DJ, editors. *Collected Reports on the Rheumatic Diseases: 2005; series 4 (revised)*. Chesterfield: Arthritis Research Campaign; 2005. Available at: www.arthritisresearchuk.org/files/6602_07032010173942.pdf (accessed 20 November 2010).
- Adebajo A, editor. *ABC of Rheumatology*. 4th ed. Oxford: Wiley-Blackwell; 2009.
- Hakim A, Clunie G, Haq I. *Oxford Handbook of Rheumatology*. 2nd ed. Oxford: Oxford University Press; 2006.

Station 1.6

Actor's notes

Background

- You are John Stroke, a 58-year-old Caucasian bus driver.

Opening statement

- 'Doctor, my wife has asked me to see you today.'

History

- You woke up today and noticed your left arm felt numb. When brushing your teeth, you noticed the left side of your face looked slightly different. You thought this was because you slept awkwardly.
- Whilst you were having breakfast, your left arm felt weak. You struggled to pick up the cup and plate with your left hand, so used your right hand instead. Whilst drinking your tea, you began to drool from the left side of your mouth. Your wife became concerned because she thought the left side of your face looked 'droopy'. She made the appointment for you to see the doctor.
- The weakness in your arm and face improved slowly, and returned to normal after 30 minutes.

Ideas, concerns and expectations

- You think your wife is making an unnecessary fuss because everything has returned to normal.
- You think the weakness in your arm and face are a result of sleeping awkwardly on your left side.
- You expect the doctor to agree that there is nothing seriously wrong with you.
- You are concerned how you will manage financially if you stop working.

Further history candidate may elicit

- You have never had an episode like this before. You have not had a head injury.
- You did not have any problems with dizziness, speech, gait, swallowing or leg weakness.
- You have never had chest pains, palpitations or sudden onset of shortness of breath or dizziness.
- Tonight you are starting one week's night shift as a bus driver.

Medical history and drug history

- Nil.

Family history
- Your father died of a stroke aged 68. Your mother died of a heart attack last year, aged 82.

Social history
- You have been a local bus driver for the last 15 years.
- You smoke 15–20 cigarettes a day and drink 3–4 pints of beer at the weekend.
- You live with your wife, who is a teacher. You have a daughter who is married and lives locally.

Approach to scenario
- You apologise several times during the consultation for 'wasting your time, Doctor'.
- You come across as unconcerned about your symptoms and explain that you only came today because your wife made the appointment.
- If the doctor explains that you may have had a transient ischaemic attack (TIA), or 'mini-stroke', you become concerned, explaining that your father had a serious stroke some years ago and did not recover.
- You want to know what treatment is available to prevent you from having a stroke in the future.
- If the doctor explains that you cannot drive tonight and may have to declare the condition to the Driver and Vehicle Licensing Agency (DVLA) after seeing the hospital specialist, you become upset, and explain that you have been a driver for years and are unlikely to get another job. You are worried how you will pay the bills if you cannot work.
- If the doctor insists you cannot drive, you suggest 'don't write down why I've come to see you today' so there is no record of the TIA in your notes. You also refuse to see the hospital specialist because you are well now, and then do not have to declare the TIA to the DVLA.
- If the doctor is empathic and explains the importance of going to hospital and the need to stop driving, you reluctantly agree to be referred to hospital and agree not to drive until you see the specialist. You agree to inform the DVLA after your hospital appointment, if needed.
- If the doctor does not come across well, you get angry and comment 'You really don't understand what this means for me do you, Doctor?'

Information gathering
Presenting complaint
a Symptoms
- Ask if left- or right-handed.
- Clarify how long the symptoms lasted and if they have resolved.
- Ask about other neurological symptoms:
  — headache
  — syncope
  — confusion
  — slurred speech
  — visual problems (e.g. amaurosis fugax)
  — numbness
  — weakness of legs.
- Ask about cardiac symptoms:
  — chest pain
  — palpitations
  — shortness of breath.
- Ask about previous episodes of cardiac or neurological symptoms.

b Risk factors
- Diabetes.
- Smoking.

41

- Hypertension.
- Hypercholesterolaemia.
- History of stroke or heart disease.
- Family history of stroke or heart disease.

Medical history
- Atrial fibrillation, diabetes and hypertension.

Family history
- Stroke or heart disease.

Drug history
- Current medications.

Social history
- Occupation.
- Smoking and alcohol.
- Home and financial circumstances.

Patient's agenda
- Explore his understanding of TIA and stroke.
- Explore his concerns about losing his driver licence.

Examination
- Offer to perform a cardiovascular and neurological examination, including blood pressure (BP), peripheral pulses and fundoscopy.
- 'If it's okay with you, I will check the nerves to your arms, legs and face, and use a light to look at the back of your eyes. I will listen to your heart, check your pulses and blood pressure.'

Examination card
General examination   Normal speech and gait

Cardiovascular examination

BP	= 135/83 mmHg	Heart rate	= 70/minute and regular
Heart sounds	= normal, no murmurs	JVP	= normal
Carotid sounds	= normal	Peripheral pulses	= normal

Neurological Examination

Upper limbs	= normal	Lower limbs	= normal
Cranial nerves	= normal	Fundoscopy	= normal

Clinical management
1 Explain the diagnosis of transient ischaemic attack
- Reassure the patient that cardiovascular and neurological examinations were normal.
- Explain his symptoms suggest he has had a TIA, or mini-stroke, where symptoms last <24 hours.
- Explore his understanding of the terms 'TIA' and 'stroke'.
- Explain that a TIA occurs when there is a temporary interruption of blood to part of the brain due to a 'blockage' in the carotid arteries or 'blood clots from the heart'.
- Reassure him that he has not had a stroke, where the neurological deficit lasts >24 hours.

- Explain that the risk factors for a TIA include hypertension, smoking, diabetes, hypercholesterolaemia and a family history of stroke.
- Explain that TIAs are a risk factor for stroke and MI and that steps can be taken to reduce this risk substantially to prevent him having a stroke like his father.

2 Discuss the management of transient ischaemic attack

- Using the data you have gathered, score the patient according to the ABCD2 criteria, and recognise the patient has a score of 3, hence must be referred urgently to a hospital specialist.
- Explain he needs to see the hospital specialist within one week for investigations, which could include an electrocardiogram (ECG) 'to look for an abnormal heart rhythm', an MRI brain scan 'to look at the brain' and carotid dopplers to 'look at the blood supply to the brain'.
- Explain that he will also need to have a blood test (including cholesterol and glucose), but this needs to be performed when he is fasting. Since he has had breakfast, the blood test cannot be performed today, but he can return tomorrow to have the blood test at the surgery, or wait and have it at the hospital with the other tests.
- Explain that if the carotid dopplers reveal carotid artery stenosis, surgery is a possibility. Surgery would remove 'the blockage' and so reduce the risk of further TIAs and stroke.
- Explain that he should take aspirin 300 mg immediately, which you will give him before he leaves, since this reduces the risk of further clot formation, and then a lower dose to take daily until the specialist has seen him.
- Discuss that other medication, such as statins to lower cholesterol, may be needed.

3 Discuss the effect of transient ischaemic attack on driving

- Recognise and explain to the patient that the DVLA has clear guidelines about driving after a TIA or stroke. Approach this sensitively with the patient.
  - Advise him to stop driving immediately, because he has had a suspected TIA, and he will need to inform his employer that he cannot work the night shift.
  - Explain that if the specialist confirms he has had a TIA, he has to inform the DVLA.
  - Explain that the DVLA guidelines state that HGV drivers lose their licence for one year after a confirmed TIA or stroke. The licence can be reinstated if he has no subsequent events.
  - If a TIA is confirmed, he cannot drive a car or motorbike for one month, and can only resume driving if he recovers, with no subsequent events.
- Explain that the basis for this is that he is a risk to himself and the public.
- Explain you are obliged to document this consultation, and cannot withhold it from the notes.
- If necessary, advise the patient that you can breach confidentiality if he does not declare his condition to the DVLA.

4 Offer follow-up

- Offer a follow-up appointment to discuss risk-factor modification such as smoking cessation and healthy lifestyle measures. Further discussion about driving and the DVLA can also be considered.
- Explain if he develops weakness or speech problems again, he should seek urgent medical advice.
- Provide leaflets about TIA and stroke.

Interpersonal skills

- This patient is unaware of the seriousness of his symptoms, and expects the doctor to reassure him that he is well. The candidate would be expected to delicately explain that his symptoms warrant investigation and treatment for a potentially life-threatening condition.
  - 'I am pleased that everything seems to have returned to normal. However, the symptoms that you have described to me suggest we need to look into this further.'

— 'I am concerned you may have had a TIA or "mini-stroke". This occurs when a small blood clot becomes stuck in a blood vessel in the brain, so blocking the blood flow and starving the brain of oxygen. The blood clot breaks up, so blood flows normally once more.'

- Declaring the TIA to the DVLA has major implications on this patient's financial circumstances, and the candidate must be empathic to the patient's situation.
  — 'It is important that you are seen within one week by the hospital specialist to reduce the risk of you developing a stroke. However, patients with this condition cannot drive. Is there someone who can take you to hospital? Your wife, or a friend?'
  — 'In the long term, it is important that you tell the DVLA if the specialist confirms that you have had a TIA. Unfortunately, you will lose your HGV licence for a year. You can apply to have it reinstated if you do not develop another TIA or stroke in that time.'
  — 'I can understand why you don't want to tell the DVLA. However, I have to write what we have discussed in your notes because it's important that we keep your records up to date. It's also really important you go to hospital to prevent this from becoming a stroke, which could be life threatening or leave you paralysed.'
  — 'The reason to let the DVLA know is because there is a risk of you losing control of your vehicle if this was to happen again when you are driving. How would you feel if you were seriously hurt, or injured another person?'

⚬━ **Key summary**
- Explain to the patient that he has a potentially serious condition that requires urgent referral to hospital for investigation and management.
- Be familiar with the ABCD2 score for stroke risk, and explain this to the patient.
- Inform the patient about the consequences of TIA/stroke on driving.
- Be aware of the need for immediate treatment with antiplatelet therapy.

Transient ischaemic attack
ABCD2 score
- NICE (2008) recommends that all patients with TIA should be assessed using the ABCD2 score, to identify people at high risk of stroke after a TIA and determine appropriate management.

TABLE 1.7 Using the ABCD2 score

ABBREVIATION	CONDITION	POINT
A – *Age*	Age ≥60 years	1
B – *BP*	BP at presentation ≥140/90 mmHg	1
C – *Clinical features*	Unilateral weakness	2
	Speech disturbance without weakness	1
D – *Duration of symptoms*	≥60 minutes	2
	10–59 minutes	1
	<10 minutes	0
2	Diabetes	1

TABLE 1.8 Interpreting the ABCD2 score

SCORE	RISK	TREATMENT
≥4	High risk	Aspirin 300 mg immediately
		Specialist assessment and investigation within 24 hours of onset of symptoms
		Start secondary prevention as soon as diagnosis is confirmed
<4	Low risk	Aspirin 300 mg immediately
		Specialist assessment as soon as possible, definitely within 1 week
		Start secondary prevention as soon as diagnosis is confirmed

Note:
- A patient with ≥2 TIAs in one week or with a history of atrial fibrillation (AF) or on anticoagulation should be considered at high risk, even if ABCD2 score is <3.

Investigations
- MRI of the brain should be performed urgently if the patient is at high risk (as per the ABCD2 score), or within one week if the patient is at low risk of a stroke.
- Carotid imaging should be performed within one week of onset of symptoms.
- Bloods, including FBC, ESR, renal function, cholesterol and fasting blood glucose.
- ECG and 24-hour tape to check for cardiac arrhythmia, e.g. AF.
- Echocardiogram, especially if AF present, to exclude cardiac thrombus formation.

Reducing risk of stroke
a General measures
- Control of risk factors, e.g. smoking cessation, daily exercise and maintenance of a normal body mass index (BMI).
- Control hypertension with a target BP <130/<80 mmHg.
- Control hyperlipidaemia, aiming for total cholesterol <4.0 and LDL cholesterol <2.0.

b Antiplatelet therapy
- Combination of dipyridamole and aspirin is recommended for two years after TIA or stroke.
- Patients should receive long-term treatment with low-dose aspirin.
- Clopidogrel is recommended for people who are intolerant of low-dose aspirin.
- Anticoagulant therapy is effective in patients in AF.

c Carotid endarterectomy
- Reduces stroke in symptomatic patients with 70–99% stenosis of the internal carotid artery.
- Patients with ≥70–99% stenosis should be offered surgery within two weeks of onset of symptoms in addition to medical treatment.
- Patients with <70% stenosis should not undergo surgery.

Driving and the DVLA guidelines (February 2010)
Note: This excerpt is taken from the *For Medical Practitioners: at a glance guide to the current medical standards of fitness to drive* published by DVLA. Please note that this publication is updated every six months and it is advisable to check the latest version on the DVLA website at www.dvla.gov.uk/medical.aspx This excerpt is protected by Crown Copyright and cannot be reproduced from this publication in any way.

Types of driving licence

TABLE 1.9 Comparison of Group 1 and Group 2 driving licences

GROUP 1	GROUP 2
Cars and motorcycles	Lorries, buses and minibuses
Valid until 70 years of age	Can be issued after 21 years
No upper age limit	Valid until 45 years
Renewable every 3 years after age 70	Renewable every 5 years until age 65, then renewable annually

Neurological conditions

TABLE 1.10 Advice on neurological conditions for Group 1 and Group 2 licences

CONDITION	GROUP 1	GROUP 2
Single TIA or stroke	Must not drive for 1 month May resume driving after this period if clinical recovery is satisfactory No need to inform DVLA unless residual neurological deficit 1 month after episode e.g. • visual field defects • cognitive defects • impaired limb function.	Licence revoked for 1 year following stroke or TIA May resume driving after this period if complete recovery Licensing subject to satisfactory medical reports including exercise ECG
Multiple TIA	Must not drive for 3 months Must notify the DVLA	Licence revoked for 1 year May resume driving after this period if complete recovery Licensing subject to satisfactory medical reports including exercise ECG
Epilepsy	Licence revoked until fit free for 1 year (+/− anticonvulsant medications)	Licence revoked until fit free for 10 years and without anticonvulsant medications
Chronic neurological disorders (e.g. MS, MND, PD)	Can be issued a 1, 2, or 3-year licence providing medical assessment confirms that driving performance is not impaired	Licence revoked if condition is progressing or disabling

Diabetes

TABLE 1.11 Advice on diabetes for Group 1 and Group 2 licences

Requires insulin	Can retain licence **if** can recognise warning symptoms of hypoglycaemia and meet required visual standards Issued 1-, 2- or 3-year licence	Licence revoked May reapply if insulin treatment is discontinued
Diet or tablet controlled	No need to inform DVLA unless complications (e.g. diabetic retinopathy or neuropathy) or insulin needed	As for Group 1

Cardiac conditions

TABLE 1.12 Advice on cardiac conditions for Group 1 and Group 2 licences

Arrhythmias	Stop driving until underlying cause identified and controlled for at least 4 weeks	Driving permitted when arrhythmia is controlled for at least 3 months **and** LV EF >40%
Hypertension	Driving may continue unless treatment causes unacceptable side effects	Disqualified from driving if resting systolic BP >180 mmHg or diastolic BP >100 mmHg Can be permitted when BP controlled **and** providing treatment does not cause side effects that may interfere with driving
Angina	Stop driving when symptoms occur at rest, with emotion, or at the wheel	License revoked if continuing symptoms (treated or untreated) Can be permitted if symptom free for 6 weeks **and** satisfactory exercise ECG
Myocardial infarction	Stop driving for at least 4 weeks	Driving must cease for 6 weeks Relicensing can occur thereafter if satisfactory exercise ECG
Angioplasty	Driving must cease for at least 1 week	Driving must cease for 6 weeks Relicensing can occur thereafter if satisfactory exercise ECG
CABG	Driving must cease for at least 4 weeks	Driving must cease for at least 3 months Can be permitted thereafter if LV EF >40% **and** exercise ECG satisfactory
Heart failure	Driving may continue provided there are no symptoms that could distract the driver's attention	Disqualified from driving if symptomatic Can be permitted if LV EF >40%

Visual conditions

TABLE 1.13 Advice on visual conditions for Group 1 and Group 2 licences

Acuity	Must be able to read a number plate at 20 m (+/− contact lenses or glasses)	Applicant barred if corrected acuity worse than 6/9 in better eye **or** worse than 6/12 in other eye The uncorrected acuity in each eye must be at least 3/60
One eye	Can drive if normal vision in other eye	Licence revoked

Psychiatric conditions

TABLE 1.14 Advice on psychiatric conditions for Group 1 and Group 2 licences

Acute psychotic disorder	Driving must cease during the acute episode Re-licensing can be considered when well for at least 3 months, compliant with treatment, free from adverse effects of medications and subject to a favourable specialist report	As for Group 1 **and** required to be well for 3 years
Dementia	Licence subject to annual review	Licence revoked

Alcohol and drug use

TABLE 1.15 Advice on substance misuse for Group 1 and Group 2 licences

Alcohol misuse	Confirmed by medical inquiry +/− unexplained abnormal blood markers	Confirmed by medical inquiry +/− unexplained abnormal blood markers
	Cease driving until 6 months of controlled drinking/abstinence with normal blood markers	Cease driving until 1 year of controlled drinking/abstinence with normal blood markers
Alcohol dependence	Licence may be returned after 1 year of abstinence **and** normal blood markers	Licence may be returned after 3 years of abstinence **and** normal blood markers
Drug use	**Cannabis, ecstasy, amphetamines, LSD**	**Cannabis, ecstasy, amphetamines, LSD**
	Licence revoked until 6 months of abstinence achieved	Licence revoked until at least 1 year abstinence achieved
	DVLA may require confirmation by an independent report/urine screen	DVLA will require confirmation by an independent report/urine screen
	Opiates or cocaine	**Opiates or cocaine**
	Licence revoked until 1 year of abstinence achieved	Licence revoked until 3 years of abstinence achieved
	DVLA may require confirmation by an independent report/urine screen	DVLA will require confirmation by an independent report/urine screen
	NB: May be licensed if fully compliant with a consultant-led methadone replacement programme depending on a favourable medical report	NB: May be issued with an annual review licence if fully compliant with a consultant-led methadone replacement programme for 3 years **and** favourable random urine tests and assessment

Respiratory conditions

TABLE 1.16 Advice on respiratory conditions for Group 1 and Group 2 licences

Obstructive sleep apnoea	Stop driving until satisfactory control of symptoms, confirmed by a medical review	Stop driving until satisfactory control of symptoms and ongoing compliance with treatment, confirmed by specialist

Further reading

- National Institute for Health and Clinical Excellence. Diagnosis and initial management of acute stroke and transient ischaemic attack: NICE guideline CG68. London: NIHCE; 2008. www.nice.org.uk/nicemedia/live/12018/41331/41331.pdf (accessed 20 November 2010).
- Driver and Vehicle Licensing Agency. '*For Medical Practitioners: at a glance guide to the current medical standards of fitness to drive.*' Go the website for the most recent guidelines. www.dft.gov.uk/dvla/medical.aspx (accessed 20 November 2010).
- Simon C, Everitt H, van Dorp F. *Oxford Handbook of General Practice.* 3rd ed. Oxford: Oxford University Press; 2010.
- Longmore M, Wilkinson I, Davidson E, *et al. Oxford Handbook of Clinical Medicine.* 8th ed. Oxford: Oxford University Press; 2010.

Station 1.7

Actor's notes

Background
- You are Tracy Andrews, a 35-year-old, working as a banker in the city.

Opening statement
- 'I'm sorry to waste your time, Doctor. My dad said I should come in and see you because I've been a bit down lately.'

History
- Two months ago you delivered a baby boy.
- Your pregnancy was uneventful until you went into premature labour spontaneously.
- For the last few weeks, you have been tearful at times and eating much less than you used to.

Ideas, concerns and expectations
- You feel low and unhappy, but think this is normal after having a baby.
- Your main concern is about your baby – he was born prematurely and you are worried about his health and feel guilty that you are struggling to cope.
- You have come to the GP today because your father is worried that you are tearful. You think you are wasting the doctor's time and expect them to reassure you that you are well.

Further history candidate may elicit
- You suddenly went into early labour at 34 weeks and needed to have an emergency caesarean section because of fetal distress. You did not suffer any complications and were discharged from hospital three days later. You named your baby David. He is your first child.
- David was admitted to the special baby unit for two weeks. He had some breathing problems for the first week but then began to improve and came home one week later. He has been followed up by the paediatricians since birth and they are happy with his progress.
- You have been trying to breastfeed but David has not latched onto your breast well, so you are relying more on formula feeds and expressing. You feel you are not bonding well with him.
- Since the birth you have been feeling increasingly alone and low. You often find yourself unable to concentrate on simple tasks, such as watching television. Your sleep patterns are generally poor – primarily because David wakes up intermittently at night. However, when you do have time to lie down, you find it difficult to fall asleep, and sometimes wake up unexpectedly, even when David is asleep.
- You are exhausted and have no energy to play with David or provide him with the stimulation you feel he needs.

- Since the delivery, you have lost a stone in weight, have a poor appetite and are not eating well.
- You have not left David alone and your parents have been available to care a few hours if needed.
- You occasionally feel that life is a struggle and that it would be easier if you did not exist but would never seriously consider ending your life or harming yourself. This is because you would not want to let down your parents or David.
- You have made no previous attempts or plans to self-harm or attempt suicide. You have not had any thoughts of harming David. You have not heard any voices and do not feel paranoid about situations.
- Your father has been concerned about you, saying you have been tearful and very upset. He made the appointment and you agreed reluctantly to come here today.
- You met David's father two years ago. He was married with children. The two of you had an affair for a few months and he promised to leave his wife. When you fell pregnant he ended the relationship with you, but did offer to help support you and the baby financially. You felt devastated. You were eight weeks pregnant at the time and after some thought decided to keep the baby. You told the father that you were not interested in his help or money.
- Your parents are very supportive but you feel guilty asking them for help as they are getting old.

Medical and psychiatric history
- Nil.

Obstetric and gynaecological history
- David is your first child and you have not had any previous pregnancies.
- Cervical smears are up to date and are all negative.
- Your periods have not yet returned.
- You do not have any vaginal discharge.

Drug history and family history
- Nil.

Social history
- You have not had any alcohol since becoming pregnant. Before the pregnancy you drank alcohol only occasionally.
- You are a non-smoker and have never used any recreational drugs.
- You work as a banker in a large city bank and are on maternity leave for six months. You have the option of extending this to a year.
- You live in a large flat in an affluent area and have no financial concerns.
- Your parents live locally. You have a brother who lives in Australia with his wife and children.
- Your parents visit your brother and stay with his family for four months a year.

Approach to scenario
- You feel that you are wasting the doctor's time. You mention this to the doctor repeatedly and are apologetic, saying 'I'm really sorry for taking up your time today'.
- If asked why you feel this way, you tell the doctor that there must be patients who are far sicker than yourself and explain that you only came because of your father's insistence.
- You feel down but your main concern is David because of the problems he has had since birth.
- If the doctor suggests that you are depressed, then at first you will dismiss this and say that 'I'll get over it, it's just a phase'.
- However, if the doctor sensitively pursues this point, by explaining to you why this is the case, as well as taking on board your concerns about your child, then you will accept that you are depressed and accept help if it is offered.

- If the doctor does not come across sympathetically, does not consider concerns about your child or provide a good explanation about why you are depressed, then you will continue to be dismissive of his suggestion.
- You may agree to come back to see the doctor again or, if the consultation is not going well, say 'I'll think about coming back, but I just don't have the time at the moment'.

Information gathering
Presenting complaint
- Ask why she feels down and when this started.

a Depression
- Ask about:
  — weight loss
  — loss of appetite
  — sleep pattern
  — early morning wakening
  — tearfulness
  — feelings of guilt
  — negative views of self, world and the future.

b Suicide risk assessment
- Enquire about suicidal ideation, e.g. thoughts, plans and intent.
- Enquire about deliberate self-harm.
- Enquire about thoughts of harming the baby.

c Psychotic symptoms
- Ask about any psychotic phenomena, e.g.
  — hearing voices
  — paranoid ideation
  — delusions of grandeur.

d Baby
- Discuss the issues around the premature birth.
- Ask about any complications to the baby.
- Enquire if breast or bottle fed.
- Ask how often baby is feeding.
- Discuss the baby's daily routines, e.g. sleeping and washing.
- Ask about any help available to her to look after the baby.

Medical history
- Anaemia and thyroid disorders.

Obstetric and gynaecological history
- Postoperative complications.
- History of miscarriage and fertility treatments.

Psychiatric history
- Mental illness, e.g. depression or schizophrenia.
- Suicide attempts and deliberate self-harm.

Family history
- Psychiatric history.
- Postnatal depression.

Drug history
- Previous use of antidepressants.
- Current medications that could interfere with breastfeeding.

Social history
- Smoking, drug and alcohol history.
- Marital status.
- Occupational history.
- Housing and financial problems.
- Support networks, e.g. family and friends.

Patient's agenda
- Explore her understanding about what might be wrong.
- Explore her concerns regarding her baby.
- Explore her views on treatment.

Examination
- Offer to examine BP, pulse, weight, abdominal scar and check for signs of anaemia.
- Perform a patient health questionnaire (PHQ9) survey.
- 'Can I check your blood pressure and your weight, and examine your tummy and scar to make sure you are recovering well from the surgery?'

Examination card	
Vital signs	BP = 124/72 mmHg
	Pulse = 62/minute and regular
	No signs of anaemia
Abdominal examination	The scar is healing well
	There is mild tenderness over the scar with no guarding or rebound tenderness
	Bowel sounds are present
PHQ9 score	12/30

Clinical management
1 Discuss the patient's problems
- Explain that the symptoms are due to postnatal depression.
- Emphasise that this is common and affects 10% of mothers.
- Explain that this can be managed by:
  — lifestyle measures
  — improving the support she receives
  — counselling and cognitive therapies
  — antidepressants.

2 Discuss lifestyle measures
- Offer advice about exercise and taking time out for herself – this could be achieved by arranging babysitters or by liaising with her parents.
- Encourage her to talk through her problems and draw on support from family and friends.
- Provide information about self-help groups for single parents and parents of premature babies.
- Suggest obtaining domestic help, e.g. cleaners or a live-in nanny.
- Advise her that you will speak to the health visitor, who will be in touch to see how she is progressing.

3 Discuss counselling services

- Encourage her to engage with psychological therapies, for example, cognitive behavioural therapy (CBT) or simple counselling.

4 Discuss drug treatments

- Advise her that guidelines suggest she does not require antidepressants at this stage but they could be considered in future.
- Explain that other measures are considered first-line since antidepressants should be avoided in breastfed and premature infants.

Note:

- If you are not sure about the best course of action, suggest that you will liaise with the local mental health team or obstetrician for advice.

5 Offer blood tests

- Suggest carrying out blood tests, particularly to check for anaemia and thyroid status.

6 Address her other concerns

- Reassure her that many babies are born prematurely and develop normally, emphasising that the paediatricians are happy with her baby's progress.
- Encourage her to continue trying to breastfeed, explaining the benefits, e.g. nutritional advantages for baby, improvements in bonding, etc.

7 Offer follow-up

- Offer to see her with other family members, e.g. her father.
- Offer to review her baby for further reassurance.
- Follow up in one week. Make the appointment for her then and there.
- Provide her with information about postnatal depression, e.g. online resources and leaflets.

Interpersonal skills

- Reassure the patient early that she is not wasting your time.
  - 'Please don't feel you are wasting my time. What makes you feel that way?'
  - 'So, what is worrying your dad?'
- Elicit the patient's symptoms through open questions; many of the features of depression are best sought by a patient-centred approach.
  - 'Tell me some more about the low mood you have been experiencing.'
  - 'How are you managing to look after David given your low energy levels?'
- Use relevant cues to explore the psychosocial factors that may be contributing to her low mood.
  - 'You mentioned that your partner left when you were eight weeks pregnant. That must have been terrible for you – how did you cope?'
  - 'So David was born prematurely? Tell me about what happened?'
  - 'It must have been upsetting for you to go through all of that by yourself?'
- Sensitively approach the subject of her feeling she would be better off not existing. Gently persevere on this point to assess her suicide risk, whilst maintaining a caring approach.
  - 'So you have felt you'd be better off not existing? . . . (pause) . . . What sort of thoughts have you had?'
  - 'Is it all getting too much for you at the moment?'
- If the patient is surprised at your diagnosis of depression, allow her the opportunity to reflect on this, ensuring your explanations are simple and easy to follow.
  - 'I think you may have depression related to your pregnancy. This is a common problem and understandable given the set backs that have happened.'
  - 'There are a few reasons why I think you have depression. The low mood and tearfulness

would fit, but also the weight loss and the negative thoughts you have had . . . (pause) . . . these all point towards this as the likely cause.'

- Work with the patient in negotiating a management plan, taking into account any individual considerations.
  — 'I wonder if we ought to try a special form of counselling? It might help to work through things. What do you think?'
  — 'If you feel you are too busy for that, there are self-help treatments that you could start straight away?'
- Check with the patient that she is clear about the management plan, particularly about safety netting.
  — 'I know we have discussed a lot and it must be hard for you to digest. What will you tell your father that we have talked about?'
  — 'Can I check – what will you do if you start feeling much worse?'
- Close the consultation by making sure the patient is happy and that all her concerns are addressed.
  — 'Are there any other questions or worries before you leave?'
  — 'Do remember to access the support groups we talked about.'
  — 'I will see David and you next week.'

⚬— Key summary
- Take a detailed history of her low mood.
- Ensure the patient does not present a risk to herself or the baby.
- Be aware of the NICE guidelines for postnatal depression.
- Involve other allied professionals in managing the depression, e.g. health visitor, counsellor, support groups.
- Arrange early follow-up.

Mental illness in the puerperium
Be aware of the main types of mental illness occurring in the puerperium.
- **'Baby blues'** usually occurs in the first 10 days after delivery. It is common and involves tearfulness and low mood. It is usually self-limiting and often resolves within a few days.
- **Postnatal depression** occurs a few weeks after birth and peaks at around three months. Mothers often put off presenting to doctors because they feel they have failed their child by not being able to cope.
- **Puerperal psychosis** is a rare illness. It is characterised by features of depression, as well as psychotic symptoms, and thoughts of harming the baby. This requires urgent inpatient admission to a mother–baby unit.

Postnatal depression
- Presents in approximately 10% of mothers.
- Symptoms often begin a few weeks after birth and usually peak at around three months postpartum.
- Mothers often under-report symptoms due to feelings of failure to cope.
- Management according to NICE guidelines is as follows:
  — In mild to moderate depression encourage self-help methods, simple counselling or cognitive therapies.
  — In those with severe depression, antidepressants and mental health referral should be considered.

- The choice of antidepressant in breastfeeding mothers with severe depression should take the following into account:
  - In those with infants that are unwell, premature or low birth weight prescription of antidepressants should be considered with caution.
  - Certain tricyclic antidepressants (TCAs) are known to have lower risks to the baby in breast-feeding mothers, e.g. amitriptyline, imipramine and nortriptyline.
  - Fluoxetine is considered to be the safest selective serotonin reuptake inhibitor (SSRI) of choice.
  - Bear in mind that all antidepressants can be toxic and lead to withdrawal effects in neonates . These effects are usually mild and pass.
  - Always weigh up the potential risks and benefits when considering antidepressant prescribing and take advice from local mental health or obstetric services if not sure.

Further reading

- National Institute for Health and Clinical Excellence. Antenatal and Postnatal Mental Health: NICE guideline 45. London: NIHCE; 2007. www.nice.org.uk/guidance/CG45 (accessed 21 November 2010).
- Collier J, Longmore M, Turmezei T, *et al. Oxford Handbook of Clinical Specialties.* 8th ed. Oxford: Oxford University Press; 2009.
- Musters C, McDonald E, Jones I. Management of postnatal depression. *BMJ.* 2008; **337:** a736.
- Single parents' websites: www.gingerbread.org.uk and www.lone-parents.org.uk (accessed 21 May 2010).
- Premature babies' website: www.forparentsbyparents.com (accessed 21 May 2010).

Station 1.8

Actor's notes

Background
- You are Dipti Patel, a 29-year-old solicitor, working for a large city firm.

Opening statement
- 'Hello Doctor, I had a bad episode with my heart recently. I am really worried and need it to be put right so I can go back to work.'

History
- Two weeks ago you were in a meeting at work and experienced palpitations for 20 minutes.
- You had to leave and took the rest of the day off.
- This was an important meeting with a big client for a contract your company is trying to secure.
- You have taken the last two weeks off from work as part of annual leave.

Ideas, concerns and expectations
- You have had palpitations before. You want to know what is wrong and how they can be treated.
- You are worried because your father had a heart attack aged 55 and wonder if these palpitations indicate a heart attack or something similar.
- After the latest episode during the meeting, you are wondering if this might happen again, and if so, how this will affect your work.
- There are redundancies looming at work, and you worry that the company may end your contract because of poor health.

Further history candidate may elicit
- You have experienced similar episodes for the past three months, each lasting 1–4 minutes. They have been increasing in frequency over the past fortnight. You have not seen a doctor before.
- During the last episode at work, you felt light-headed and were unable to continue the meeting.
- This frightened you, so you decided to book a routine appointment to see a doctor.
- If asked to tap out the rhythm, it is fast and regular.
- You experienced no chest pain and no other symptoms of note.
- You have also lost two stone in weight over the past four months, but you put it down to attending the gym four to five times per week and using the treadmill and swimming pool.
- You become hot, sweaty and jittery very easily. Stress makes this worse.
- Your appetite has increased and you are surprised that you are losing weight.
- Your bowels are opening more frequently and are looser than usual.

- If asked about any other symptoms, you can say 'No, although my boyfriend says that I do seem to have a slightly short fuse at present.'
- You have been leading a large project at work for the past several weeks and have had to work long hours and weekends. You originally thought your symptoms were a result of overwork and stress.
- You are upset that you had to leave the meeting before being able to close the deal with the client. You have since heard that the client decided against entering into the contract. You feel responsible for this.
- You feel bad that you do not see family and friends as much as you would like to nowadays.

Medical history
- Nil.

Drug history
- Contraceptive pill, as directed (prescribed by local family planning clinic).

Social history
- You are a non-smoker and drink alcohol only occasionally.
- You are of Indian origin, having been born and raised in Manchester. You have lived there all your life.
- You live alone in a flat. You met your boyfriend one year ago and have a good relationship.
- Your work is stressful and you have a poor relationship with your boss. He seems to interact well with the men in the office but distances himself from females.
- You have not discussed the latest incident with him so far.

Family history
- Your father had a heart bypass operation in his early 50s. He is relatively well and is 67 years old.
- Your mother is 64 and well. You have one younger brother who is at university.
- Your maternal grandmother suffered from hypothyroidism.
- Your maternal aunt is currently taking thyroxine – you vaguely remember your mother telling you that this happened after she took a chemical, which she had to go into hospital for.

Approach to scenario
- You are determined to know what is wrong and feel you cannot afford to take time off work.
- You have a sense of urgency and you really want to get to the bottom of what is wrong.
- If you feel the doctor will not provide you with fast answers and solutions to the problem, you become increasingly frustrated and anxious (and will let it show).
- You strongly suspect that the palpitations are related to stress and are interested to hear any suggestions about how to tackle this problem.
- You are also particularly worried about the family history of heart disease and are worried these palpitations could be a similar problem to your father's illness. It is really important to you to seek clarification on this point.
- If you feel the doctor is sympathetic and addresses your concerns, you will be happy to carry out their suggested management plan.
- If the doctor does not provide a satisfactory explanation about what is wrong, nor agrees to make a referral, you will tell the doctor that 'I can't afford to let this linger on'.
- If the doctor discusses treatments with you, you will wish to explore things further, asking 'What if that doesn't work?' several times. If radioiodine is mentioned as a treatment, you become visibly disturbed and shocked, saying, 'Are you telling me they are going to make me take a radioactive substance?'
- However, if the doctor remains calm, explains to you the circumstances when radioiodine is used and explains that the dose is safe, you will feel reassured.

- If the doctor does not come across well, you resort to asking more questions and, if necessary, ask to see another GP.

Information gathering
Presenting complaint
a Palpitations
- Duration.
- Severity.
- Frequency.
- Previous episodes.
- Alleviating factors.
- Nature of the palpitations (regular or irregular).

b Triggers
- Alcohol.
- Caffeine.
- Stress.
- Relationship to any specific time or activities, e.g. sport.

c Associated symptoms
- Ask about cardiac symptoms:
  — chest pains
  — dizziness
  — shortness of breath.
- Ask about hyperthyroid symptoms:
  — sweating
  — tremor
  — heat intolerance
  — loose bowel motions
  — increased appetite
  — weight loss.
- Ask about anxiety-related symptoms:
  — mood
  — sweaty palms
  — concentration
  — sleep pattern
  — pins and needles
  — 'Do your friends think you are an anxious person?'

d Cardiac risk factors
- Smoking.
- Hypertension.
- Diabetes.
- Hypercholesterolaemia.
- Family history of heart disease and arrhythmias.

Medical history
- Palpitations and heart disease, e.g. Wolff–Parkinson–White syndrome (WPW).

Drug history
- Use of any sympathomimetics, e.g. salbutamol inhalers.

Family history
- Ischaemic heart disease or arrhythmias.

Social history
- Smoking and alcohol.
- Recreational drug use, e.g. amphetamines.
- Occupational history and sick leave.
- Relationships.
- Financial situation.

Patient's agenda
- Ask about any underlying fears about her heart.
- Explore her understanding of what might be wrong.
- Explore her reasons for requesting referral.
- Explore the impact of symptoms on her life.

Examination
- Offer to examine the patient.
- 'I would like to examine your pulse, blood pressure and heart sounds if that's okay.'

Examination card	
General examination	Agitated at rest
	Sweaty palms
	No neck swelling
	Normal eyes and eye movements
Cardiovascular examination	BP = 115/68 mmHg
	Pulse = 105/minute and regular
	JVP = normal
	Heart rate = normal sounds and no murmurs

Clinical management
1 Explain the likely diagnosis of hyperthyroidism
- Reassure the patient that the palpitations do not represent a heart attack and that her heart sounds are normal.
- Explain that her symptoms suggest the cause of her palpitations is an overactive thyroid gland. This is supported by her symptoms of palpitations, looser stools and weight loss, along with the examination findings of sweaty palms and high heart rate.
- Explain that hyperthyroidism results in excess production of thyroid hormone, which increases the metabolic rate, and so leads to symptoms such as tachycardia, heat intolerance and agitation.
- Advise her that hyperthyroidism needs to be excluded, and that stress may have an impact.

2 Focus on lifestyle factors
- Take this opportunity to advise on dealing with any work-related stress, e.g. relaxation, more time off work, speaking to her boss about her latest illness.
- Offer a sick note.

3 Offer a management plan
a Immediate management
- Suggest a blood test to check her thyroid function and to look at cardiac risk factors, e.g. fasting glucose and lipid profile.
- Suggest an ECG to check for any underlying electrical abnormalities.
- Explain that you need to refer her to an endocrinologist for suspected hyperthyroidism.
- Suggest starting a course of β-blockers, which would help treat her symptoms, including the palpitations, tremor and anxiety.
- Explain that this medication works by blocking the effects of the thyroid hormone and so reduces heart rate.

b Further management
- Explain that she will need further treatment to reduce the level of thyroid hormone.
- Advise her that tablets, usually carbimazole, can reduce the production of thyroid hormone.
- These need to be taken daily for 12–18 months.
- If this is unsuccessful, another course of antithyroid medication can be tried.
- Alternatively, radioactive iodine or surgery may be needed.

4 Arrange follow-up
- Offer her information leaflets.
- Arrange to see or telephone the patient with the results.
- Explain that you will be referring her to an endocrinologist.
- Advise her to seek urgent medical attention if she has any prolonged spells of palpitations (>10 minutes), is light-headed or develops chest pain.

Interpersonal skills
- The patient has had time to think about what might be going on. It is a good idea to start by asking open questions and following a patient-centred approach to the consultation.
  - 'Tell me about what happened.'
  - 'How did the episode at work affect you?'
- Explore relevant cues to identify her general concerns.
  - 'Tell me more about your father's heart problems.'
  - 'You mentioned that you're worried about redundancies at work. Tell me more.'
- After a series of open questions, use some closed questions to elicit features of thyroid disease or anxiety disorders.
  - 'Has your weight changed recently?'
  - 'Did you develop chest pain with the palpitations?'
  - 'Tap out the rhythm of the palpitations for me if you can.'
  - 'Do large crowds bring on the symptoms?'
- Coming into the consultation the patient is clear about what she would like. Address this head on, by addressing her ideas, concerns and expectations.
  - 'What ideas do you have about what might have happened?'
- Share your thoughts about what you think might be going on, keeping the explanations in lay terms. Check for patient understanding as you go along.
  - 'I think you have a condition where the thyroid gland is overactive. Do you know what the thyroid gland does?'
  - 'This is usually due to something called Graves' disease, but there are other possible causes. If it is Graves' disease, this is where the body's own immune system causes the thyroid gland to produce too much thyroid hormone.'
- Share management options.
  - 'How would you feel about having some blood tests to check your thyroid gland?'
  - 'Clearly this is a stressful time for you, do you feel counselling may help?'
- Avoid alarming the patient when explaining treatments for hyperthyroidism.

- Keep the answers simple and avoid overloading her.
- For example, mentioning the word 'radioactive' may shock her, so try to avoid its use.
  — 'There are very effective drugs to treat hyperthyroidism. Patients will often be given a 12- to 18-month course.'
  — 'If this does not work, then a further course of the drug may be needed.'
  — 'Alternatively, a special drink or capsule can be given that blocks the hormone within the gland. Surgery can be an option to physically remove part of the thyroid gland.'
- If the patient is keen to pursue the issues in further depth, then discuss the use of radioactive iodine separately, to avoid alarming her.
  — 'The capsule has a special chemical known as radioiodine.'
  — 'The dose of radioactivity is very low and not dangerous to your overall health.'
- Address the health beliefs and worries picked up in the history.
  — 'I can understand that you are worried about your heart because of what happened to your father. However, it seems very unlikely that your symptoms are related to an underlying heart problem.'
- Help the patient feel that everything possible is being done to help her.
  — 'I agree we need to find out what is wrong. As I say, it is very likely you have an overactive thyroid. Here is a blood and ECG form. You can get these tests done today.'
  — 'I'll make an urgent referral to an endocrine doctor. And as soon as the results of the blood tests are back I would like to speak to you on the phone to see if there's anything else we need to do. How does that all sound?'

Key summary
- Recognise the features of hyperthyroidism.
- Communicate to the patient why they have palpitations.
- Reassure them about their concerns of having heart disease.
- Ensure the patient is referred to an endocrinologist whilst you await results of blood tests.

Hyperthyroidism

Causes of hyperthyroidism

TABLE 1.17 Primary and secondary causes of hyperthyroidism

PRIMARY	SECONDARY
Graves' disease	TSH-secreting pituitary adenoma
Toxic adenoma	Excessive release of TRH from hypothalamus
Multinodular goitre	Hydatidiform mole
Postpartum thyroiditis	Choriocarcinoma
De Quervain's thyroiditis	Struma ovarii
Excess thyroxine replacement	

Complications of hyperthyroidism

- AF.
- Heart failure.
- Proximal myopathy.
- Alopecia.
- Osteoporosis.

Graves' disease

a Definition

- Graves' disease is an autoimmune condition where thyroid stimulating hormone (TSH)-receptor antibodies stimulate the thyroid gland by activating the TSH receptor.

b Epidemiology

- Graves' disease is the commonest cause of hyperthyroidism.
- It affects females more frequently than males at a ratio of 5:1.

c Clinical features

TABLE 1.18 Clinical features of hyperthyroidism

SYMPTOMS	SIGNS
Weight loss	Fine tremor
Heat intolerance	Sweaty palms
Sweating	Palmar erythema
Insomnia	Tachycardia
Irritability and nervousness	Onycholysis
Increased appetite	Eye signs:
Fatigue	• lid lag
Muscle weakness	• lid retraction
Palpitations	• diplopia
Diarrhoea	• ophthalmoplegia
Oligomenorrhoea	• exophthalmos.*
Shortness of breath	Thyroid acropachy*
	Pretibial myxoedema*

* Specific to Graves' disease only. Other symptoms and signs present in all other causes of hyperthyroidism too.

Management of hyperthyroidism (and Graves' disease)

a Symptomatic treatment

- β-blockers as a symptomatic treatment.

b Antithyroid medication

- Carbimazole impairs production of thyroid hormone. Usually administered as a 12–18 months' course of treatment to render the patient euthyroid.
- Fifty per cent of patients require no further treatment, but fifty per cent of patients relapse.
- Those who relapse can be managed by a further course of antithyroid medication, radioiodine or surgery.
- Advise patients to inform their doctor immediately of a sore throat, due to the risk of drug-induced agranulocytosis.

c Radioactive iodine

- This involves taking a drink or swallowing a capsule containing radioactive iodine. It acts by destroying some of the thyroid tissue and decreasing thyroid hormone levels.
- The dose of radioactivity to the rest of the body is very low and not dangerous.
- Most patients go on to become hypothyroid and require thyroxine replacement.
- Patients should avoid becoming pregnant for at least six months, and should avoid prolonged contact with others for two to four weeks.

d Surgery

- Can be either partial or total thyroidectomy.
- Surgery is used much less commonly nowadays.

e Other

- Patients with eye signs should be referred to an ophthalmologist.

Further reading

- Turner H, Wass J. *Oxford Handbook of Endocrinology and Diabetes*. 2nd ed. Oxford: Oxford University Press; 2009.
- Society for Endocrinology. *Thyroid Resources*. Bristol: Society for Endocrinology; various dates. Available at: www.endocrinology.org/education/category.aspx?catid=11 (accessed 21 November 2010).
- Holt R, Hanley N. *Essential Endocrinology and Diabetes*. 5th ed. Oxford: Blackwell Publishing; 2007.

Station 1.9

Candidate's notes

Name	Jennifer Taylor
Age	33
Medical history	Nil relevant
Medication	Nil
Last consultation	Uncomplicated gastroenteritis a year ago
Other information	Up to date with smears (all normal)

Actor's notes
Background
- You are Jennifer Taylor, a 33-year-old part-time dinner lady.

Opening statement
- 'Hello Doctor, I'd like to be referred for sterilisation please.'

History
- You have decided after two children that you have completed your family.
- A month ago you decided you wanted to have a sterilisation and so booked this appointment.

Ideas, concerns and expectations
- You have had some marital difficulties and are scared that if you have any more children, your marriage may not survive.
- You heard that sterilisation would be the best form of permanent contraception.
- You are worried about what the procedure entails. You remember an aunt had the procedure and she did not have any complications.
- You are concerned about how much time you would have to take off from work as your sick leave entitlement is very limited.

Further history candidate may elicit
- You have tried using condoms and the contraceptive pill in the past, but found it difficult to remember to take the pills every day. You often forget to use condoms 'in the heat of the moment'.
- A year ago you discovered your husband was having an affair with someone he worked with at his taxi company.
- You became suspicious and thought he was having an affair because he did not seem interested in having sex with you and would come home late from work. You eventually confronted him and it transpired that he had been having the affair for a year.
- Your husband regretted the affair and soon after your discovery he left the woman, but this has left you feeling insecure about your relationship. You spent the first few months arguing and slept in different rooms.
- Your relationship with your husband became strained following the birth of your second child because you both had less time to spend together and stopped communicating well.
- Having a second child stretched you financially and you do not think you can afford to have a third child. You are worried that a third child may put a strain on your marriage and that next time your husband might leave you.
- The two of you have made efforts within the past year to improve the marriage for the sake

of your children. In the past two months you have started sleeping in the same bed and have recently resumed sexual relations. You currently use condoms.

- Your husband has been your only sexual partner for the past 17 years. You have never been for a sexual health screen. As far as you know, your husband has never had a sexual health check-up.
- Your husband is aware of your decision to have sterilisation. He is keen to have another child at some stage and would rather you keep your options open.

Obstetric and gynaecological history
- You have a daughter aged seven, and a son aged two. They were born naturally.
- Your periods are regular and not painful or heavy. You have no gynaecological problems.
- Your smear tests have always been negative. The last one was a year ago.

Medical history
- Nil.

Drug history
- You are not currently on any regular medications.

Social history
- You drink approximately six units of alcohol per week and have never smoked.
- Your partner works as a taxi driver. He has to work many night shifts, which can be difficult as some weeks he hardly gets to spend much time with the children or yourself.
- Finances are particularly tight with credit card debts and a mortgage.
- You work part time and spend the rest of your time as a housewife.
- At times, you find it difficult to manage looking after your two children.

Family history
- Nil relevant.

Approach to scenario
- You feel that you don't know very much about the range of family planning methods available.
- You are reluctant to consider other contraceptive methods, such as the coil.
- However, if the doctor presents constructive and reasonable arguments for these you will be prepared to enquire further about them.
- You will begin to shift your position about wanting sterilisation in the following circumstances:
    — If the doctor mentions there are methods as effective as sterilisation.
    — If the doctor informs you that sterilisation should be considered irreversible.
    — If the doctor explores your reasons for no longer wishing to have children and addresses marital difficulties, you will start to think you may want children again in the future.
- You have not heard of long-acting reversible contraception (LARC), but have heard about the coil.
- You had not considered these options, but if the doctor suggests them, you will say that the idea of having a coil inserted does not appeal to you as you heard it can cause infections.
- However, if all the options are presented to you in a way that you understand, you decide against having a sterilisation and wish to come back and see the doctor to discuss alternative methods further.
- Out of all the LARC methods mentioned, you are most interested in the coil.
- If the doctor is not sensitive in exploring your reasons for the request, or fails to explain the alternatives well, you become exasperated and say 'If I have another child, my husband will leave me!' You will pursue your request for sterilisation and will not be happy if this is not followed.

Information gathering
Presenting complaint
- Ask about reasons for requesting sterilisation.
- Check if she has discussed this with her partner.
- Check if she already has children.
- Ask if she feels she has completed her family.
- Establish her understanding of alternative methods such as:
  — vasectomy
  — contraceptive pill
  — LARC methods such as the coil.

Sexual history
- Enquire about her current sexual partner and other recent partners.
- Ask about current contraception, including use of condoms.
- Enquire about past sexual health screens.
- Check for history of STIs.

Medical history
- Surgical history and complications.
- Specific contraindications to other forms of contraception, e.g.
  — stroke
  — liver disease
  — migraine with aura
  — thromboembolic disease.

Obstetric and gynaecological history
- Past pregnancies.
- Contraceptive history.

Drug history
- Any regular medications.
- Drug allergies.

Family history
- Relevant to contraception, e.g. breast cancer or thromboembolism.

Social history
- Smoking and alcohol.
- Home and family circumstances.
- Marital issues.
- Occupational history.
- Financial issues.

Patient agenda
- Explore her understanding about sterilisation.
- Identify reasons why she does not wish to have further children.
- Explore marital issues and how much support there is from the partner.
- Explore social issues, including her financial situation.

Clinical management
1 Explanation about sterilisation
- Carefully explain the procedure, complications, failure rates and take questions.
- Explain that the procedure is carried out under a general anaesthetic.

- Explore what support she has as childcare arrangements would need to be made.
- Tell her that the procedure is considered irreversible. Although in some cases it can be reversed, this unlikely to be available through the NHS.
- Explain that most patients can return to work within a week.

2 Explanation about family planning methods
- Consider the different forms of contraception and tailor the explanation according to her understanding:
  — barrier protection – male and female condoms, vaginal ring, contraceptive patch
  — contraceptive pill – combined pill and mini-pill
  — contraceptive patches
  — LARC:
     (i) intrauterine devices
     (ii) intrauterine system (IUS)
     (iii) injectable contraceptives
     (iv) progestogen-only subdermal implants.
  — mention vasectomy as an option for husband.
- Emphasise to her that some of these methods, e.g. intrauterine contraceptive device (IUCD), are as effective as female sterilisation.

3 Explore general health advice
- Explain that female sterilisation does not protect against STIs – only condoms can be used for this.
- Given the husband's recent affair, suggest the couple have a sexual health screen.

4 Explore the psychosocial difficulties
- Advise her to speak to her husband further about their expectations towards further children.
- Propose marital counselling to help explore any marital tension (e.g. through the Relate organisation).
- Suggest she speaks to Citizens Advice bureau about any financial difficulties.

5 Finalise a plan and discuss follow-up
- Allow her the opportunity to reconsider her options and return with her husband.
- Offer contact details for the local family planning clinic.
- Offer written information in the form of leaflets and fact sheets.
- If relevant, explain the referral procedure for sterilisation.

Interpersonal skills
- Ask open questions when eliciting her reasons for wanting a sterilisation.
  — 'Tell me about your reasons for wishing to have a sterilisation.'
- Be flexible in your discussion, allowing the patient to ask other questions, but at the same time guiding her back to the subject if it is important.
  — 'We spoke about coils a moment ago. Have you thought about coils as an alternative to sterilisation?'
- Picking up on the patient's cues will help to elicit her concerns in greater depth.
  — 'You mentioned that you are having some financial difficulties. Tell me some more about this.'
  — 'This procedure works by blocking off the tubes that carry your eggs from your ovaries to the womb. This is how it prevents pregnancy.'
  — 'You mentioned that you are worried about what another child would do to your marriage. How do you feel another child might affect things?'
- Keep to lay terms when explaining how the various family planning methods work.
  — 'The copper coil is a small piece of copper-coated plastic that is placed in the womb. It mainly works by preventing the egg and sperm meeting each other.'

- Whilst taking the history, be mindful of whether the patient fully understands the implications of having a sterilisation, and has capacity to make such a decision. She should also be aware of the advantages and disadvantages involved. Also ensure that there has been no coercion.
  — 'Have you considered the downsides of having a sterilisation?'
  — 'Just so I understand – is female sterilisation your preferred option, or is it something that your husband feels is the best choice?'
- Show empathy whilst guiding the patient through making her decisions.
  — 'The circumstances you describe must be very difficult for your husband and yourself. I can understand you feeling that you do not want more children. Sterilisation is one way to achieve this. Are you aware that sterilisation is not the only method, though?'
  — 'Do you know there are also other equally effective methods?'
  — 'What other methods are you familiar with?'
- Arrive at a shared management plan of action, by showing that you are flexible but also offering her the opportunity to consider alternatives. Do not be afraid to let her know if you feel that sterilisation would not be in her best interests.
  — 'Obviously this is very much a personal decision for you. Having discussed possible alternatives, do you still feel a sterilisation would be the best option?'
  — 'After thinking this through some more and discussing it further with your husband, we could arrange for a sterilisation. However, I do wonder if there are better options out there. Do you still feel the same as when you did before you came to see me?'
  — 'Perhaps you would like to come back and see me with your husband before making a final decision?'

🔑 Key summary
- Explore her reasons for requesting sterilisation.
- Ensure she recognises that the procedure should be considered irreversible.
- Provide information about alternative family planning methods.
- Address any underlying psychosocial issues leading to this decision.

Sterilisation
Female sterilisation
- This is usually performed as a laparoscopic procedure.
- The fallopian tubes are occluded (most commonly using Filshie Clips), which prevents the sperm reaching the egg. It is often carried out as a day case under general anaesthetic (GA).
- Risks include:
  — 1:200 risk of pregnancy
  — small increased risk of ectopic pregnancy – patients should be advised to perform a pregnancy test if they miss a period
  — operative and anaesthetic risks.
- Other considerations:
  — Reversibility rates vary. The procedure is to be considered irreversible when explaining it to the patient.
  — Patients should use contraception until the onset of the first period postoperatively. The first few periods may be heavier than usual.
  — Most patients recover within a few days and are back to work in approximately a week.
  — Regret rate is increased:
    (i) if the procedure is carried out at birth
    (ii) in women <30 years
    (iii) in those without children.
  — One to two per cent of patients eventually request reversal of the procedure.

- If any of the following factors are present, then try to discourage the patient from having a sterilisation:
  — no children
  — those currently pregnant
  — those <25 years of age
  — response to a relationship breakdown
  — any suggestion of coercion.

Vasectomy
- The vas deferens is occluded, usually under local anaesthetic as a day-case procedure.
- There is a 1:2000 risk of pregnancy, which is 10× less than with female sterilisation.
- Like female sterilisation, the procedure should be considered irreversible.
- Any attempts at reversal are unlikely to be available through the NHS.
- There are generally fewer complications than with female sterilisation.
- The main complications include pain, bleeding and infection.
- Most patients are back to work within a few days and return to normal function within a fortnight.
- Patients should use contraception until there are two semen specimens demonstrating absent sperm (taken at least eight weeks post procedure and two to four weeks apart).

LARC
- One of the main advantages over sterilisation methods is that these methods can be reversed if patients change their mind.

Injectable progestogen, e.g. Depo Provera
- This is administered as a deep intramuscular injection every 12 weeks.
- Unlike the pill, it does not rely on the patient having to remember to take it every day.
- It works by rendering the patient anovulant.
- The main side effects are menstrual irregularity and weight gain.
- There is evidence of a possible increased risk of osteoporosis, deranged lipid profile and arterial effects.
- Alternative contraception should be used for the first seven days after the injection (unless it is given within the first five days of menses).
- It is hard to predict the time taken for fertility to return to normal after stopping the injections.

Implant
- A small flexible rod containing progesterone is placed intradermally and is effective for three years.
- Like the injectable progesterone, it works mainly by inducing anovulation.
- It can be used after birth, miscarriage or abortion.
- The main side effects are skin changes such as acne, irregular periods, breast tenderness, mood changes and a small risk of infection at the site of insertion.
- Fertility returns to normal almost immediately following removal.
- Unless the implant is fitted within the first five days of a period, the patient will need to use alternative contraceptive methods for the first seven days after implantation.

IUCD
- Most are effective until menopause in those aged >40.
- They can be removed at any time if pregnancy is desired.
- The IUCD is highly effective with a low infection risk.
- There are two types of IUCD, the copper intrauterine device (IUD) and the progestogen IUS.

TABLE 1.19 Comparison between copper IUD and progestogen IUS

	COPPER IUD	PROGESTOGEN IUS
Mode of action	Prevents fertilisation and implantation Reduces sperm survival and motility	Levonorgestrel is released Prevents ovulation-induced endometrial proliferation and thins cervical mucus
Main advantages	Highly effective (both 99.8%) Both as effective as female sterilisation Can be used from 4 weeks postpartum or within 15 minutes of delivering the placenta Safe to use following TOP Safe to breast feed Easily removed	
	Very safe and lasts 5–10 years Useful as emergency contraception up to 5 days following intercourse or ovulation	Has a 5-year licence Can also be used to manage menorrhagia and dysmenorrhoea Useful for PMS and perimenopausal symptoms Confers endometrial protection with HRT
Adverse effects	Risk of infection (rare nowadays) Very low risks of perforation, expulsion and ectopic pregnancy	
	May make periods heavier and more painful Allergy to copper	Menstrual irregularity Bloating Breast tenderness Acne Mood disturbance
5-year failure rate	2/100	1/100

Further reading

- National Institute of Health and Clinical Excellence. Long-acting Reversible Contraception: NICE guideline 30. London: NIHCE; 2005. http://guidance.nice.org.uk/CG30 (accessed 21 November 2010).
- Collins S, Arulkumaran S, Hayes K, *et al. Oxford Handbook of Obstetrics and Gynaecology.* 2nd ed. Oxford; Oxford University Press; 2008.
- Royal College of Obstetricians and Gynaecologists (RCOG). *Male and Female Sterilisation: evidence-based clinical guideline 4.* London: RCOG; 2004. Available at: www.rcog.org.uk/womens-health/clinical-guidance/male-and-female-sterilisation (accessed 21 November 2010).

Station 1.10

Actor's notes

Background
* You are Michelle Clegg, a 25-year-old primary school teacher.

Opening statement
* 'Hi Doctor, I'm getting these tummy pains and they are starting to worry me.'

History
* You have been getting a lot of abdominal cramp-like pains recently.
* The pain has been getting more frequent and severe over the past few days.

Ideas, concerns and expectations
* You are upset because the symptoms are affecting your work. Your colleagues have worked out that something is wrong.
* You want to be referred to see a specialist because you are worried about having colon cancer.
* Your 72-year-old grandmother was diagnosed with colon cancer last year. She has had part of her bowel removed and now has a colostomy bag.

Further history candidate may elicit
* The pain started about 18 months ago and occurs every few weeks.
* When it starts, it occurs every few hours and takes several days to resolve.
* The pain is usually located centrally but it can move about.
* Each episode lasts from half a minute up to 2–3 minutes.
* You sometimes try taking ibuprofen or paracetamol, which has limited benefit.
* Your abdomen often becomes bloated and distended.
* Your bowels alternate between constipation and having loose stools. The loose stools lead to you visiting the toilet more frequently to open your bowels.
* You occasionally have nausea and indigestion, but no vomiting.
* There has been no blood, mucus or pus in the stools and the colour is normal.
* You have had no change in appetite or loss of weight.
* You used to eat lots of junk food, but since the symptoms began your diet has been healthier.
* You are non-vegetarian and do not skip meals.
* You have kept a diary of when the symptoms come on and show this to the doctor.
* The pain seems to come on by eating heavy meals or when you are stressed or have had less sleep.
* Once a week you will go out with friends at work and have a curry or Chinese meal – this makes the symptoms worse.
* You find working as a schoolteacher quite stressful, particularly trying to keep the children in order. You qualified as a teacher two years ago and now teach six- to seven-year-olds.

- You lead a busy active family and social life, making lots of effort to see your family and friends.
- Finances are quite tight – you are on a basic income but have high expenses, such as renting an expensive flat.
- You answer 'no' to any other questions about physical and psychological symptoms.

Medical history
- Nil.

Drug history
- Ibuprofen and paracetamol prn for abdominal pain.

Social history
- You occasionally drink alcohol when you go out with your friends, but never to excess.
- You enjoy exercise and go jogging three to four times a week.
- You are a non-smoker. You are single and live on your own.

Family history
- Your grandmother was diagnosed with colon cancer last year.
- Your parents and older brother are well.

Approach to scenario
- At the start of the consultation, you are noticeably worried about your symptoms. Throughout the consultation, you will come back to asking the doctor if they think this is something serious.
- You are worried about the possibility of having bowel cancer and repeatedly ask to be referred to a specialist.
- You have always been a worrier and often focus on small details.
- If the doctor says anything that makes you concerned, you become visibly more anxious and start asking questions to reflect your anxiety.
- When answering a question you will offer a great deal of detail in your answers. If the doctor attempts to cut you off, you will continue talking and complete what you were saying. You will often interrupt the doctor.
- If the doctor listens, does not antagonise you, and takes the time to explain what they think is wrong, you will be prepared to consider the diagnosis of irritable bowel syndrome (IBS).
- Furthermore, if you feel something is being done to investigate your symptoms, you will be willing to revisit the possibility of a referral in the future.
- If the doctor does not come across well, does not hear what you have to say, does not provide a reasonable explanation about what is wrong or reassure you about cancer, then you will not accept IBS as a possibility and leave disappointed.

Information gathering
Presenting complaint
a Pain
- Site.
- Radiation.
- Frequency, e.g. daily, weekly, monthly.
- Nature of the pain, e.g. crampy, sharp, burning.
- Alleviating and exacerbating factors, e.g. diet, stress.

b Bowel habit
- Constipation.
- Diarrhoea.
- Alternating constipation and diarrhoea.

- Consistency of motions.
- Colour of stool.
- Presence of mucus, pus or blood in stool.

c Other symptoms
- Nausea and vomiting.
- Abdominal bloating.
- Systemic features, e.g. weight loss and loss of appetite.

d Lifestyle
- Ask about diet and eating patterns.
- Check for features of anxiety and depression.

Medical history
- IBS.
- Inflammatory bowel disease (IBD).

Drug history
- Analgesics, e.g. NSAIDs and codeine-based products.
- Laxatives.
- Over-the-counter remedies.

Family history
- IBS, IBD or carcinoma.

Social history
- Alcohol and smoking.
- Occupation.
- Financial circumstances.
- Marital status and dependents.
- Social support, e.g. family and friends.

Patient's agenda
- Explore her understanding of bowel cancer.
- Explore the psychosocial factors that may be impacting on her symptoms.
- Explore her expectations of investigations and referral.

Examination
- Offer to examine her abdomen, weight, vital signs and to perform a rectal examination.
- 'I would like to examine your abdomen, check your blood pressure, weight and temperature, and also examine your back passage if that's okay?'

Examination card	
General examination	Temperature = 36.5 °C
	Pulse = 80/minute and regular
	BP = 124/72 mmHg
	BMI = 24.0
Abdominal examination	No jaundice, anaemia, clubbing or lymphadenopathy
	Soft and non-tender and no organomegaly
	Mildly distended with no shifting dullness
	Bowel sounds present and normal sounding

Clinical management

1 Explain the likely diagnosis of irritable bowel syndrome
- Explain that the most likely cause for her symptoms is IBS.
- Reassure her that examination revealed mild abdominal distension and no mass.
- Reassure her that she does not have symptoms to suggest bowel cancer, coeliac disease or inflammatory bowel disease (IBD).
- Address the patient's concerns, particularly her worries about bowel cancer, explaining that her family history of bowel cancer is less likely to be significant given her grandmother's age.

2 Offer conservative management options
- Discuss dietary measures, e.g.
  — regular meals
  — avoid heavy meals
  — limit high-fibre foods
  — try oats and linseeds for symptoms of bloating.
- Advise on regular exercise and relaxation.
- Consider referral to a dietician.
- Discuss any stress and help the patient work through this.

3 Offer other treatments for irritable bowel syndrome symptoms
- Suggest antispasmodics, e.g. hyoscine, mebeverine or peppermint oil.
- Suggest CBT, explaining that it is effective in IBS.
- Explain that if these treatments are unsuccessful other treatments, e.g. TCAs and SSRIs, are available, but not considered at this early stage.

4 Perform blood tests
- Offer a blood test to check for coeliac disease.
- Suggest you can check for other markers, e.g. FBC and liver function tests (LFTs), to ensure that there is no other abnormality contributing to her symptoms.

5 Discuss referral
- Advise her that IBS can be managed in primary care.
- Offer to see her with the results of the blood tests and make a decision then.

6 Offer to follow up
- Offer the opportunity for the patient to come back to review the blood tests or any medications prescribed.

Interpersonal skills
- Be guided by the patient's opening statement to help pick up the consultation.
  — 'I'm sorry to hear about the abdominal pains. Tell me about them.'
- If the patient is worried by her symptoms, use the opportunity to explore her ideas and concerns further through open questions.
  — 'I can see you are quite worried by these symptoms. Do you want to discuss this some more?'
  — 'So what did you have in mind about what's causing the pain?'
- Avoid showing you are upset or offended if the patient interrupts you. This would make the situation worse. Instead, adopt a calm demeanour and show your interest through non-verbal cues (such as open body language, eye contact).
- Provide the patient with positive feedback using reassuring verbal sounds. Often this approach will provide you with valuable information, including the patient's ideas, concerns and expectations.

- If the patient continues interrupting, keep the consultation patient centred, making a mental note of any salient features mentioned that you can come back to when there are silences.
  - 'You mentioned a moment ago that your grandmother had cancer. Tell me about your grandmother.'
- Explain carefully your reasons for performing any tests.
  - 'I think we also need to perform some blood tests . . . (silence) . . . Would you be okay with that?'
  - 'The reason for doing these is that we should check if there is anything else, such as a condition called coeliac disease. It is unlikely, but it could explain the symptoms you have been having.'
  - 'I want to reassure you that cancer is unlikely given your age. I know your grandmother suffered from bowel cancer, but it is unlikely to be the cause of your symptoms.'
  - 'We will check the liver and look for anaemia. These are signs that can come from bowel cancer.'
- Keep your explanations about the possible diagnosis in simple, lay terms; often reflecting back the language the patient uses can help.
  - 'The symptoms most resemble a condition called irritable bowel syndrome. In this condition the gut can become overactive, causing pain and loose stools.'
- Be sensitive in dealing with the request for referral; show you are on side and be prepared to negotiate.
  - 'I can understand your worry about bowel cancer . . . (silence) . . . How about we do some blood tests and I prescribe you something for the cramps?'
  - 'CBT has been shown to be effective in treating IBS symptoms. It often helps patients cope with the stress that can contribute to IBS. That's something we could try first along with the medication we discussed. How does that sound?'
  - 'One option would be to review the results with you and then consider referral at that stage. How does that sound?'

Key summary

- Take a focussed history, paying attention to red flags.
- Address the patient's concerns about colon cancer.
- Be aware of the investigations to perform in a case of suspected IBS.
- Explain the management of IBS.
- Remain calm when dealing with a patient who continually interrupts.

NICE guidelines for management of irritable bowel syndrome

(Reproduced with permission of NICE.)

Diagnostic criteria

Diagnosis is based on initial presentation and positive diagnostic criteria for IBS.

a Initial presentation

- IBS should be considered if a patient presents with any of the following symptoms for ≥6 months:
  - abdominal pain or discomfort
  - bloating
  - change in bowel habit.

b Positive diagnostic criteria for IBS

- If the patient presents with any of the criteria above, consider IBS **only** if the person has *abdominal pain* or *discomfort* that is:
  - relieved by defaecation **or**

— associated with altered bowel frequency or stool form
— **and** at least two of the following:
    (i) altered stool passage (straining, urgency, incomplete evacuation)
    (ii) abdominal bloating, distension, tension or hardness
    (iii) symptoms made worse by eating
    (iv) passage of mucus.
- Lethargy, nausea, backache and bladder symptoms may be used to support the diagnosis of IBS.

Investigations
- Patients meeting the diagnostic criteria for IBS should have the following blood tests:
  — FBC
  — ESR and CRP
  — coeliac disease testing (endomysial and tissue transglutaminase antibodies).
- NICE advises there is no indication to carry out further tests, e.g. USS, sigmoidoscopy, colonoscopy, stool culture, faecal occult blood or thyroid function.

Management
- Patients with IBS should be provided information to explain the importance of self-help, for example:
  — general lifestyle advice
  — physical activity
  — dietary advice
  — symptom-targeted medication.
- Review fibre intake, usually reducing it, while monitoring its effect on symptoms.
  — Discourage patients from insoluble fibre, e.g. bran.
  — If an increase in dietary fibre is advised, suggest soluble fibre, e.g. ispaghula powder or oats.
- Advise how to adjust laxative or antimotility doses according to clinical response. The dose should be titrated according to stool consistency, aiming to achieve a soft, well-formed stool.
- Consider TCAs as second-line treatment if laxatives, loperamide or antispasmodics have not helped. TCAs are primarily used for treatment of depression but are only recommended here for their analgesic effect. Treatment should be started at a low dose (5–10 mg equivalent of amitriptyline), which should be taken once at night and reviewed regularly. The dose may be increased, but does not usually need to exceed 30 mg.

Criteria for referral of irritable bowel syndrome patients to secondary care
- Unexplained weight loss.
- Family history of colon cancer.
- Patients >60 years of age with a change of bowel habit for more than six weeks.
- Rectal bleeding.
- Anaemia, rectal or abdominal masses or raised inflammatory markers.

Further reading
- National Institute for Health and Clinical Excellence. Irritable Bowel Syndrome in Adults: diagnosis and management of irritable bowel syndrome in primary care; NICE guideline 61. London: NIHCE; 2008. http://guidance.nice.org.uk/CG61 (accessed 21 November 2010).
- Bloom S, Webster G. *Oxford Handbook of Gastroenterology and Hepatology*. Oxford: Oxford University Press; 2006.
- Spiller R, Aziz Q, Creed F, *et al*. Guidelines on the irritable bowel syndrome: mechanisms and practical management. *Gut*. 2007; **56**: 1770–98. Available at: http://gut.bmj.com/content/56/12/1770.full.pdf (accessed 10 January 2010).

Station 1.11

Actor's notes

Background
- You are Jenny Kapoor, a 32-year-old housewife.

Opening statement
- 'Hi, thanks for calling me back, Doctor, I am so worried about Rahul – he has a high temperature.'

History
- Rahul has had a fever for the past two days.
- You have used a thermometer to measure his temperature, which ranges from 37.5–39 °C, worse mainly at night.
- He started having a dry cough and runny nose last night.

Ideas, concerns and expectations
- You think Rahul picked up this fever from a toddler playgroup, which he joined a week ago.
- Some of the other children in the group have come down with colds over the past few days.
- You do not understand why the fever has not settled after two days of regular paracetamol.
- You are worried about meningitis, particularly as you have heard a lot in the media about how quickly it can affect young children.
- You are tired and wonder what the doctor can suggest to treat the illness as soon as possible.

Further history candidate may elicit
- Rahul is irritable, drinking less than normal and is less playful than usual.
- He has been sleeping more than usual since yesterday.
- In the past 24 hours, his nappies have been less wet than normal. You have changed his nappies four times.
- Rahul has developed a rash in the past 4 hours. The rash is over most of the body. There are lots of little 'spots'. He is not scratching them.
- If the doctor discusses the 'glass test', you have never heard of this. If asked, you will carry out the glass test but will need to ask a lot of questions to clarify the doctor's instructions. The glass test will show that the rash clears when passing the glass over them.
- Rahul has had no vomiting, diarrhoea or any other physical symptoms.

- You also have a five-year-old boy, called Sachin. He has spina bifida and is significantly disabled.
- You are his main carer, which has been more stressful after having a second child.
- Your husband is currently in New York on business for three weeks. You have little external help.
- In the past two days, you have barely slept. You wish your husband was at home.
- One of the mothers from Rahul's toddler group might be willing to come and look after Sachin, but you try not to impose.
- Sachin attends a local special needs school for children with disabilities and is under the care of specialists.
- Carers attend the house every day to help provide you with some respite.

Medical history
- Nil.

Drugs and vaccination history
- Regular paracetamol for children, for the past two days.
- Ibuprofen for children, started today.
- Up to date with vaccinations.

Birth and development history
- Rahul was born at term by normal vaginal delivery.
- He has had no significant problems since birth and seems to be developing well.

Family history
- Rahul has a five-year-old brother called Sachin who has spina bifida.
- Other family members are well.

Social history
- You are married to the child's father.
- You used to work in the city as a solicitor but stopped working when you had children.
- Your parents and siblings live in London and you have very little social support where you live.
- Your husband works as a sports journalist and spends a lot of time travelling around the world.

Approach to scenario
- You are worried about Rahul's symptoms.
- You feel stressed at having to look after two children on your own.
- As a result, you are reluctant to leave the house and would prefer that the doctor visits.
- Since the rash came on a few hours ago, you have started to worry this could be meningitis.
- You want to know if Rahul needs antibiotics and want to know how often to give the paracetamol and ibuprofen.
- If the doctor suggests coming in to the surgery you feel that this is very impractical.
- It would mean bringing both children with you, which would be very difficult, given Sachin's problems. There is nobody to look after Sachin if you left him at home.
- If the doctor is caring and sympathetic and points out the potential seriousness of the situation, then you will be prepared to be more open to other options, such as asking your friend to look after Sachin for a while or getting help from a practice receptionist.
- If the doctor does not communicate well or does not provide good reasons why they cannot visit, you will say that you will call for an ambulance.
- If the doctor tries to reassure you about the condition, but is not able to communicate effectively, then you say 'I'm really worried this is meningitis'.

Information gathering
Presenting complaint
- Clarify what is wrong.
- Check if the mother has measured the temperature.
- Ask what the temperature readings have been.
- Enquire about measures to reduce temperature:
  — tepid sponging
  — paracetamol
  — ibuprofen.
- Ask about associated focal symptoms:
  — GI symptoms, e.g. vomiting and diarrhoea
  — upper respiratory tract, e.g. runny nose and cough
  — chest symptoms, e.g. sputum production and wheeze.
- Enquire about the rash:
  — onset
  — brief description
  — scratching
  — ask the mother to perform the glass test.
- Ask about non-specific symptoms:
  — oral intake and feeding patterns
  — alertness and playfulness
  — lethargy
  — irritability +/– crying
  — frequency of nappy changing and wet nappies.
- Ask about any potential triggers:
  — unwell contacts
  — recent travel
  — attendance at any toddler groups.

Medical history
- Febrile illnesses.
- Birth history and general development to date.

Family history
- Familial conditions.
- Siblings and father.

Drug history
- Current medications.
- Vaccination status.

Social history
- Occupation of parents.
- Carers, e.g. father and grandparents.
- Other sources of support.

Patient's agenda
- Explore the mother's concerns about the fever.
- Explore her understanding of meningitis.
- Enquire how this illness is effecting the mother and the family.

Clinical management

1 Offer a likely explanation

- Explain that you think this is likely to be a viral upper respiratory tract infection (URTI) with rash.
- Inform her that given the rash, fever and increased sleeping, it would be sensible to assess the child as soon as possible.
- Share any concerns you may have about the child's condition, e.g. dehydration.
- Explain that meningitis does need to be ruled out by examining the child.
- Answer any questions the mother may have, e.g. about antibiotics, explaining that in this case it is difficult to make a complete assessment without also examining Rahul.

2 Discuss managing the condition

- Provide useful suggestions for treating the condition, such as:
  — increasing fluid intake for dehydration
  — taking regular paracetamol and ibuprofen
  — fanning and removing clothing for temperature control.
- When discussing medication, include explanations about dosage and frequency.

3 Consider the wider needs of mother and family

- Advise the mother to make a routine appointment herself to come in to discuss the general ongoing issues and stress, which have become apparent in the consultation.

4 Management plan and safety netting

- Given the fever and rash in a young child, the best possible outcome would be to review the child as soon as possible.
- This could be achieved in various ways, but possible outcomes could include the following.

a *Arranging an immediate home visit*

- This would be least preferable as you have a full clinic of emergency patients who would be kept waiting.

b *Organising her friend to look after Sachin whilst bringing Rahul to the surgery*

- If this is not possible, explore the feasibility of her coming to the surgery and having one of your receptionists assist in supervising the older child while Rahul is being assessed.

c *Take the child straight to hospital*

- The child could be taken to hospital in an ambulance (you could offer to call to arrange this) or in a taxi, but this may present the same problems for the mother in terms of how Sachin is to be looked after.

Interpersonal skills

- Telephone consultation is a very different way of interacting with patients. You only have the verbal part of communication.
- Connect with the mother by introducing yourself and maintaining a friendly voice with an open approach from the outset.
  — 'Hello Mrs Kapoor, my name is Dr X. I am one of the GPs here at the practice.'
  — 'I am sorry to hear about Rahul. So tell me some more about what's wrong.'
- Demonstrate that you are actively listening by saying reassuring things or by making reassuring sounds.
  — 'Yes . . . um . . . uh-huh . . . I see, tell me more.'

- When offering explanations, regularly check her understanding – this applies particularly to the glass test, which will help you determine how serious the rash is.
  — 'Place a glass on its side over a collection of rashes . . . (pause) . . . have you done that? Any questions so far? . . . Okay, now slowly roll the glass over the rashes. As you do so, I want you to see if the rashes clear . . . (pause) . . . How is that so far? Is there anything you'd like me to explain again?'
- Be open and honest with the patient when explaining your provisional diagnosis. Be prepared to highlight the limitations of a telephone consultation.
  — 'The rash clearing with the glass test is reassuring. However, what is difficult to reassure you about over the telephone is the fact that Rahul is passing less urine and is less alert than usual. A simple physical examination would be able to clarify for us if he needs antibiotics and tell us how dehydrated he might be.'
- Explore the mother's underlying concerns and worries through a combination of active listening, open questions and demonstrating an interest in her problems.
  — 'Are there any reasons why you can't come up to the practice?'
  — 'Tell me some more about the friend you mentioned. Do you think she be would be willing to look after Sachin while you come to see me?'
  — 'You said you're worried about meningitis. Have you any experience with this illness?'
- If you feel the mother is making an unrealistic request, try to keep her on side by offering reasonable alternatives.
  — 'I understand that you would like a home visit now, but that is going to be very difficult to organise. I am in an emergency clinic and have lots of patients waiting to be seen. The soonest I could come out would be in 2–3 hours. Obviously that's too long and we should arrange for Rahul to be seen sooner than that.'
  — 'If we see Rahul here at the practice, I can offer to see him soon after you get here.'
- This could potentially be a difficult consultation in terms of reaching a mutually agreed plan of action. Be prepared to keep negotiating, but guide the discussion towards a constructive outcome.
- Tell the mother that your priority is the clinical care of the child and highlight the importance of avoiding delays.
  — 'How is Rahul right now, Mrs Kapoor?'
  — 'Okay, I do understand getting here with both your children is going to be difficult. How about I ask one of the receptionists to give you a hand as soon as you get here?'
  — 'I appreciate coming to see me here will be difficult. But, given the new rash, it is important that Rahul is seen by a doctor as soon as possible. Do you have any thoughts about how we could arrange that?'
- Before terminating the consultation, summarise and ensure the mother is happy with the plan. Provide pauses as you speak to check on understanding.
  — 'So, just to clarify what we have agreed; you agree to come to see me (silence) . . . When you arrive the receptionist will come and help bring Sachin into the building and supervise him while you are here. How does that sound?'

O⟲ Key summary
- Recognise the importance of the symptoms, paying particular attention to any red flags.
- Address the mother's concerns about meningitis.
- Negotiate to ensure the child is seen as quickly as possible.
- Recognise, and do not be afraid to communicate, the limitations of a telephone consultation.

Telephone consultations

- Roger Neighbour's consultation model is one way of approaching telephone consultations. It is outlined below.

Connecting

- Prior to calling the patient, check the notes for personal details, medical history, drug history and look back at recent visits.
- When the patient picks up the telephone, introduce yourself by stating your name, position and where you are calling from.
- Clarify who you are speaking to. If a third party, be aware of confidentiality issues.
- Explore the reasons for the request to call, take a focussed history, adopting a patient-centred style. Be prepared to move towards closed questions when appropriate.
- Ask about the patient's ideas, concerns and expectations.

Summarising

- Summarise the salient features in the history.
- Negotiate an agreed plan of action and summarise.

Handing over

- Clarify patient understanding.
- Ensure the patient agrees with the plan.

Safety netting

- Advise the patient on warning signs to look out for.
- Offer clear instructions about what to do if there are any concerning features.
- Agree on a follow-up plan or how to access medical care, e.g. A+E, out of hours.
- Close the consultation amicably.

Housekeeping

- Ensure you feel ready to deal with the next patient.
- If appropriate, take a few moments to clear your head, particularly after a stressful consultation.
- Reflect on PUNs and DENs.

Further reading

- Neighbour R. *The Inner Consultation: how to develop an effective and intuitive consulting style.* Oxford: Radcliffe Publishing; 2004.
- Patient UK. *Telephone Consultations.* Patient UK; 2009. Available at: www.patient.co.uk/doctor/Telephone-Consultations.htm (accessed 21 November 2010).
- National Institute for Health and Clinical Excellence. Feverish Illness in Children: assessment and initial management in children younger than 5 years; NICE guideline 47. London: NIHCE; 2007. http://guidance.nice.org.uk/CG47 (accessed 21 November 2010).

Station 1.12

Actor's notes

Background

- You are Simone Berlusconi, a 28-year-old actress.

Opening statement

- 'I would like to be referred to the local homeopathic hospital.'

History

- One month ago you saw the GP because of a lump in your neck that had been present for three months. You became concerned because the lump was becoming larger in size and you lost one stone in weight over six weeks.
- The GP referred you urgently to the hospital where you had a number of investigations and were diagnosed with Hodgkin's lymphoma (HL), and advised to start chemotherapy and steroids within the next week.
- You are due to go to the hospital in a few days for a procedure to insert a special kind of tube into your neck vein so that you can receive the drugs.

Ideas, concerns and expectations

- You are worried that the procedure to your neck will be dangerous and painful.
- You read about the side effects of chemotherapy, particularly hair loss and infertility. You are keen to try homeopathy as an alternative to chemotherapy to avoid the side effects.
- You have come to the GP today to ask for a referral to the homeopathic specialist.

Further history candidate may elicit

- After being diagnosed with HL, you have tirelessly researched HL and read a lot of information on the internet about chemotherapy, steroids and the available treatment options.
- You were alarmed to read that chemotherapy could affect your fertility. You have not yet started your family but want to in the next few years. You have been with your boyfriend for one year and are living with him. You are keen to have children in the future.
- You are also scared about losing your hair. The thought of wearing a wig is extremely distressing.
- In addition, you do not wish to have a tube inserted into your neck. You have looked this up on the internet, and are scared of something being inserted deep into your neck. The blood tests at the hospital were painful, and you are worried that having this tube will be even more painful.
- You are concerned about the side effects of taking steroids. Several family members have

type II diabetes and you have read that steroids can cause this and other conditions such as high BP.

- The specialist explained that you have an 'aggressive' type of lymphoma in the neck. It has spread to a few glands but not around the body. The specialist explained there is a good chance the cancer will respond well to the chemotherapy and steroids.
- Whilst on the internet, you read a lot about alternative therapies. You found that many patients have had positive results with homeopathy for a range of medical conditions, including cancer.
- You believe that homeopathy can help cure your condition whilst avoiding many of the side effects that chemotherapy would entail.
- You are still working even though your boyfriend suggested you take a break.
- Your close family and boyfriend are worried about you and all feel you should listen to what the doctors say. You, however, do not agree with this and feel certain that medical science does not always get it right.

Medical history
- Nil.

Drug history
- Nil.

Social history
- You drink on occasions. You do not smoke.
- You work as an actress in the theatre, with daily performances, which involve long hours.
- You are reluctant to take any sick leave as you are one of the main cast members in the play and do not want to let anyone down. You have not told work about what has happened yet.
- Your parents live locally and are well. You told them you have HL and they have been very supportive. You have no siblings.

Family history
- Nil relevant.

Approach to scenario
- Going into the consultation, your main agenda is to get a referral to a homeopathy specialist. If the doctor declines to make this referral, you will inform them that you have looked at the British Homeopathy Association's website and are entitled to see a homeopathy specialist through the NHS.
- You go into the consultation anxious and worried about your condition. If the consultation is not going your way, you will become fidgety and upset.
- You are particularly worried about the risk of infertility from chemotherapy.
- You have faith in homeopathy as an option.
- You are not convinced that traditional treatments are the only methods available.
- If the doctor explains the limitations of homeopathy well, you start to accept these.
- If the doctor is sympathetic, communicates well and addresses your main concerns, you will be prepared to engage with chemotherapy and steroids. This would be on the proviso that you are referred for homeopathy – you will accept paying for a private referral if needed.
- If the doctor does not communicate well, cannot sufficiently reassure you about conventional treatments or agree to homeopathy referral, then you will not agree to having chemotherapy or steroid treatment.
- Depending how you are feeling at this stage, you will either say you do not want these treatments altogether or you might agree to think about things and return another time.

Information gathering

Presenting complaint

- Clarify she understands the diagnosis and recommended treatment.
- Clarify the patient's reasons for requesting homeopathy.
- Clarify details of the outpatient visits at the hospital.

Medical history

- Previous cancers or other significant illnesses.

Family history

- Particularly of any cancers.

Drug history

- Previous use of homeopathy.
- Contraception.
- Any medications she may be currently taking.

Social history

- Marital status and children.
- Occupation and work policy on sick leave.
- Support from family and friends.
- Smoking and alcohol use.

Patient agenda

- Explore her understanding of HL and homeopathy.
- Explore her concerns about chemotherapy.
- Discuss how she is coping at present.

Clinical management

1 Discuss homeopathy as a potential treatment for Hodgkin's lymphoma

- Explore her understanding of HL and homeopathy, emphasising that in her case HL is curable with chemotherapy.
- Explain the likely natural history of HL if left untreated – the tumour will increase in size and spread through the bloodstream to other organs, which will be fatal.
- Explain that there is no evidence to suggest that homeopathy alone is a curative treatment in HL.
- Advise it may be possible to use homeopathy in combination with conventional chemotherapy.

2 Inform the patient about the benefits of conventional treatments

- Explain that chemotherapy helps to reduce the size of the tumour and stops the cancer cells from spreading around the body.
- Treatment can be curative and allow the patient to have a normal life expectancy thereafter.
- Emphasise that time is of the essence – the longer the cancer is left untreated, the more likely it is to spread. If the cancer spreads to other parts of the body, she may not survive.

3 Address the patient's concerns about conventional treatments

- Discuss the common side effects of chemotherapy and steroid treatment, particularly addressing the ones that concern her most.

a Fertility

- Explain that her eggs could be removed and stored by the fertility specialists. If she became infertile from chemotherapy, she could use her stored eggs to conceive using in-vitro fertilisation (IVF) treatment.

- Offer to refer her to the fertility specialists urgently for further discussion.
- Explain that egg collection could take several weeks, which would delay treatment.
- Advise her to discuss this further with her specialist.

b Alopecia
- Inform her that many people go on to wear wigs, hats and scarves.
- Explain this is temporary and that hair will grow back a few months after stopping treatment.

c Nausea and vomiting
- Reassure her that there are a number of medications to help control these symptoms.

d Other
- Discuss the side effects of steroids, informing her that complications such as hypertension and type II diabetes are less common with the short-term steroid treatment she would require.
- Reassure her that her BP and blood sugar will be monitored to manage these complications if they develop.
- Explore her concerns about line insertion for chemotherapy, reassuring her that this will be performed under local anaesthetic and used to deliver chemotherapy **and** take blood samples. Therefore, she will not need repeated blood tests.

4 Discuss referral to a homeopathic specialist
- Advise her that you can refer her to a homeopathist, but she would have to wait several weeks to be seen, and so there would be a delay in her receiving treatment.
- Explain that even if you make the referral, the local primary care trust (PCT) may not agree to fund homeopathic treatment due to limited NHS funding in the UK.
- Explain that she could see a homeopathic specialist privately to prevent any delay.
- Suggest a homeopathy referral alongside conventional treatment as a compromise.

5 Other issues and follow-up
- Offer a sick note for work and advise her to discuss her condition with her employer.
- Advise her to return for follow-up to review her progress or, if she wants, to reconsider her options.

Interpersonal skills
- The presenting complaint is not a symptom, but a request for an unconventional treatment for HL.
- Do not be thrown by this, and do not decline her request outright.
- Adopt open questions in a friendly manner to gather information.
  — 'How do you feel homeopathy will help?'
  — 'What worries you so much about having chemotherapy?'
- Show compassion and empathy at her recent diagnosis.
  — 'All of this has happened so recently. It must all have come as such a shock.'
- Take her request for homeopathy seriously, even if you do not personally agree, and avoid being negative.
  — 'Complementary treatments have an important role to play in a range of medical conditions. What information have you come across about their benefits in HL?'
- Be open and honest about any limitations in your own knowledge about HL and homeopathy.
  — 'I must admit, my own knowledge of homeopathy is limited. With all the reading you have done, I am sure you will know more than me on the subject!'

- Adopt active listening skills, paying particular attention to verbal and non-verbal cues throughout and using these to help guide her through the consultation.
  — 'Tell me some more about the concerns you have about chemotherapy.'
- Be encouraging and show an interest in the patient's research into the condition.
  — 'It is very positive that you have looked into the condition and homeopathy as much as you have. Tell me some more about what you've read.'
- Be clear and straightforward when explaining the risks involved in not treating her condition.
  — 'If we don't treat the lymphoma with chemotherapy and steroids, the cancer will continue to grow in size. It will also start spreading and this could be fatal.'
- Ensure you deal with the patient's main concerns about infertility.
  — 'It is perfectly understandable that you are worried about this. The difficulty is that if we wait for treatments to stimulate your ovaries to produce eggs to use for storage, this could take several weeks. As I mentioned, in this time the cancer would spread more and this could be fatal. That unfortunately is the choice we would be making.'
  — 'Would it help if I speak to your specialist today and also a fertility specialist to see if there is any other way around this problem?'
- Be prepared to negotiate and compromise when trying to persuade her to accept chemotherapy. Allow the patient to interject and ask questions.
  — 'If I make a private referral to a homeopathy specialist and make the arrangements for you to deal with the issues of future fertility, would you then be willing to have the recommended treatments?'
- Be positive in trying to persuade the patient to engage with the hospital's recommendations.
  — 'This is a life-saving treatment. Success rates are very high and there would be a very good chance of you going back to a totally normal quality of life with a normal life expectancy.'
- If you feel you are struggling to negotiate with the patient, try asking a question about her point of view or offering to involve others she might trust.
  — 'What do you understand will happen if you do not have chemotherapy?'
  — 'How about you come back and see me with your boyfriend?'

O╌ Key summary
- Explore her reasons for requesting homeopathy.
- Address the concerns about chemotherapy and steroids, especially about fertility risk.
- Negotiate by emphasising the importance of pursuing conventional treatments, but also explain the issues surrounding homeopathy.
- Ensure the patient understands the overall issues.

Homeopathy

- Homeopathy is based on the theory that 'like cures like'.
- Remedies are used in small amounts to treat symptoms that they would actually cause if used in large amounts.
- To achieve this effect, the homeopathic substance is highly diluted.
- In homeopathic theory, the more diluted the substance, the greater its potency.
- Most remedies originate from plants. Sometimes animal sources or chemicals are used.
- Evidence for its benefits is currently inconclusive, but there have been studies that have found an overall benefit for certain specific medical problems, e.g.:
  — childhood diarrhoea
  — hay fever
  — postoperative ileus
  — respiratory tract infection
  — vertigo
  — influenza.

- Homeopathy's main practical use is for self-limiting conditions.
- It is a slow form of treatment, with homeopathic theory stating that for each year of symptoms, the patient will require a month of treatment.
- There is no evidence that homeopathy can cure cancer.
- It should not be used to treat harmful diseases where there is not enough evidence to support its benefits.
- Remedies that are diluted more than 30 times are unlikely to cause any side effects or interact with traditional treatments.
- Doctors can refer for homeopathic treatment within the NHS, but this can be subject to local budget and resource constraints. There are four NHS homeopathic hospitals in the UK. These are in London, Liverpool, Bristol and Glasgow.
- For further information, visit www.britishhomeopathic.org and www.homeopathy-soh.org (accessed 21 November 2010).

Further reading

- Useful internet resources for homeopathy: www.homeopathy-soh.org/ and www.britishhomeopathic.org/ (accessed 21 November 2010).
- Ernst E, Pittler MH, Wider MB, *et al. Oxford Handbook of Complementary Medicine.* Oxford: Oxford University Press; 2008.
- Provan D, editor. *ABC of Clinical Haematology.* 3rd ed. Oxford: Blackwell Publishing; 2007.

Station 1.13

Actor's notes

Background
- You are Peter Baker, a 55-year-old businessman.

Opening statement
- 'I think I've developed another chest infection, Doctor. Can I get some more antibiotics please?'

History
- For the past seven days you have been coughing more.
- This started with a cold that began last week.

Ideas, concerns and expectations
- You are concerned that you keep developing chest infections.
- Your father died one year ago from lung cancer – you are worried that this may be the reason you keep having chest infections.
- Your wife is worried that you smoke and will develop lung cancer 'like your father'.
- You are keen to stop smoking, and have spoken to the pharmacist who advised you to see your GP.
- You have come to see the doctor today for antibiotics to clear the chest infection, discuss how to stop smoking and have a chest X-ray (CXR) to rule out cancer.

Further history candidate may elicit
- In the last week, you have been coughing up copious amounts of green sputum but no blood. In between flare ups, you usually cough clear sputum on most mornings.
- The current flare up has not significantly affected your breathing and you are trying your best to carry on as normal.
- You have been using your Ventolin inhaler more in the past week.
- You were diagnosed with COPD four years ago after you saw the doctor for shortness of breath, which occurred after walking several hundred yards on a flat surface.
- Since diagnosis, your shortness of breath has worsened, and nowadays you become short of breath after walking 50–60 yards on a flat surface or walking up a flight of stairs.

- You were prescribed two inhalers. You use the Tiotropium inhaler regularly and do not forget to use it. You have used the Ventolin® inhaler more frequently in the past few weeks, particularly during this latest flare up.
- Over the last year you have seen the doctor several times for chest infections. Each time, the doctor gave you a course of antibiotics, which cleared the infection.
- You have experienced no weight loss and you can answer 'no' if asked about other symptoms.
- You remember having a CXR at the time of diagnosis that was normal.
- You have never been admitted to hospital.
- Your father was a lifelong smoker. He smoked 30 cigarettes a day. He was in good health until he developed lung cancer at the age of 77. The cancer was inoperable and he passed away peacefully four months after his diagnosis.
- You smoke 20 cigarettes a day and when stressed or under pressure you smoke more.
- Following your father's death your wife has been pushing you to stop smoking.
- Over time you have become worried about developing lung cancer and have tried to stop smoking several times in the last year. You have tried chewing Nicorette gum with no success.
- You asked the pharmacist for some advice but he was very busy and suggested you see the GP or come back another time.
- The longest you have not smoked for is a week. Eventually you develop intense cravings.
- You have never tried any formal smoking cessation services.
- You saw the practice nurse a few months ago to have your annual check-up.

Medical history
- COPD.

Drug history
- Salbutamol inhaler 100 mcg one to two puffs as required.
- Tiotropium inhalation powder inhaler 18 mcg daily.
- No drug allergies.

Social history
- You have smoked 20 cigarettes per day since age 18.
- You drink approximately 10 units of alcohol per week.
- Your business involves importing crockery products from China and so you often have to travel.
- You have worked in this business for the past 25 years.
- You have three children. Two are working and the other is at university.

Family history
- Your father died of lung cancer last year, aged 77.
- Your mother is well and lives alone.
- You have two younger brothers who are well.

Approach to scenario
- You come across as feeling frustrated about your current illness and concerned about having another chest infection.
- Given your father's recent illness, you are worried you may also have lung cancer.
- You will only raise these concerns if prompted by the doctor.
- If the doctor does not address your concerns, you become visibly upset and keep your answers to a minimum.
- You do not like to complain or bother anyone, and are not sure how to raise the issues of wanting a CXR or to stop smoking.
- If the doctor makes you feel at ease, explores your concerns and asks if there is anything else you would like help with, you request a CXR and ask for help with smoking cessation.

- If the doctor discusses possible methods to stop smoking and emphasises the benefits of stopping smoking, you agree to try taking a tablet, if this is suggested.
- If the doctor is not caring, or does not effectively communicate what is wrong, you will be reluctant to raise your concerns about lung cancer.
- If the doctor does not ask you if there is anything you would like, you will not request a CXR or ask for help with smoking cessation.

Information gathering
Presenting complaint
- Establish the patient's reasons for requesting antibiotics.
- Ask about chest symptoms:
  — cough
  — haemoptysis
  — shortness of breath
  — exercise tolerance
  — sputum production, e.g. frequency and colour.
- Ask about the natural history of his COPD:
  — chest infections
  — hospital admissions.
- Check smoking history:
  — pack years
  — age of onset
  — attempts to stop and methods used.

Medical history
- Asthma or other respiratory conditions.
- Heart failure.

Drug history
- Use of inhalers and concordance.
- Drug allergies.

Family history
- Asthma, bronchitis, lung cancer.

Social history
- Alcohol history.
- Marital status.
- Financial issues.
- Occupational history and occupational factors associated with lung disease.

Patient's agenda
- Explore the impact of this latest illness on his daily life.
- Explore his concerns about his chest symptoms.
- Explore his understanding of COPD and lung cancer.
- Explore his understanding of ways to stop smoking.

Examination
- Offer to perform a cardiovascular, respiratory and ear, nose and throat (ENT) examination.
- Check his oxygen saturation, vital signs, peak flow and BMI.
- 'I would like to examine your chest and perform some other basic checks, if that's okay.'

Examination card

General Examination	BP = 130/80 mmHg
	Pulse = 90/minute and regular
	Temperature = 37.2 °C
	BMI = 25.5
	Oxygen saturation = 96%
	No lymph nodes palpable in the neck
ENT examination	Unremarkable
Respiratory examination	No peripheral or central cyanosis
	No signs of respiratory distress
	Peak flow = 250 L/min (best value 260 L/min)
	Mildly breathless following the examination
	Chest examination reveals crackles at the right base
	There are no signs of cardiac failure

Clinical management

1 Discuss the diagnosis

- Explain that in view of his symptoms and findings on clinical examination, he would appear to have an exacerbation of COPD and a right-sided chest infection.
- Explain to the patient that his spirometry tests three months ago demonstrated moderate impairment of lung function. This would account for the limited exercise distance. Steps to help control the COPD might help slow the progression of the disease.
- Counsel him about the nature of the condition and that stopping smoking is likely to help.

2 Offer treatments for chronic obstructive pulmonary disease

- Explain the purpose of antibiotics to treat the chest infection.
- Offer amoxicillin 500 mg tds for one week.
- The patient does not require steroids at the present time because the breathlessness is not interfering with activities of daily living (although it has gradually deteriorated over time).
- Advise adding in a combined long-acting β_2 agonist (LABA) and an inhaled corticosteroid (ICS) since he is having frequent exacerbations (according to NICE guidelines – *see* pages 95–6 for further details).
- Discuss inhaler techniques and concordance.
- Offer referral for pulmonary rehabilitation, e.g. by referring to a community respiratory team.

3 Discuss smoking status and management

- Ascertain his understanding about smoking and assess where he is in the cycle of change (*see* page 95).
- Emphasise the risks of smoking in terms of impact on COPD and how it may lead to lung cancer.
- Discuss the option of stopping abruptly versus gradually reducing the number of cigarettes he smokes.
- Suggest and discuss the treatments to help stop smoking, highlighting that a combination of pharmacotherapy and non-pharmacotherapy tends to offer the best outcomes.
- Outline potential side effects where relevant. Examples of treatments include:
  — nicotine replacement, e.g. patches and gum
  — bupropion
  — varenicline
  — non-pharmacological therapies, e.g. behavioural support.
- Offer a referral to smoking cessation services at the practice or pharmacy.
- Provide details of self-help groups, e.g. NHS Smokefree (http://smokefree.nhs.uk) and Quit With Help (http://quitwithhelp.co.uk).

4 Consider investigations
- Discuss option of a CXR.
- Reassure him that there are no signs to indicate any lung cancer, but in view of his recent recurrent chest infections, and given the last CXR was four years ago, it would be reasonable to perform this investigation.
- Offer routine blood tests to check that he is not anaemic.
- Consider repeating spirometry tests when his condition is stable.

5 Arrange follow-up
- Advise him to return if his shortness of breath worsens or if the chest infection does not clear with the antibiotics.
- Offer a follow-up appointment to monitor response to inhalers, see if he has stopped smoking and discuss the results of the investigations.
- Offer information leaflets on COPD.

Interpersonal skills
- Establish rapport with the patient at the start of the consultation by addressing his opening statement.
  - 'Tell me about the chest infection you feel you've come down with.'
  - 'So tell me your reasons for requesting antibiotics?'
- Be attentive to non-verbal and verbal cues, as well as adopting a combination of open questions and active silence to identify any hidden agendas.
  - 'Are there any other reasons you would like a CXR? ... (silence) ...'
  - 'You seem worried about something? Is there something else you would like to discuss?'
- Adopt a caring and sympathetic approach, particularly if anything upsets the patient.
  - 'I'm sorry to hear about the loss of your father ... (silence) ... tell me about your worries.'
  - 'I take it the chest infections are starting to get you down?'
- Be supportive to the patient without offering false hope.
  - 'It is really good that you are seriously considering stopping smoking. It is a very hard thing to do. I know you have tried before. But there are some very effective treatments that can be used and we can get you to see a specialist smoking advisor.'
- Offer shared management options, addressing his concerns and expectations as you do so.
  - 'I think antibiotics may be helpful because you have signs of an infection in the lower right side of your chest. They will help you feel much better.'
  - 'Introducing this new inhaler should help to limit the attacks of chest infections you are worried about. Is this something you'd be willing to try?'
  - 'One option would be to leave this but there is a good chance it could get worse. What are your thoughts about that?'
- It is important to ensure that the patient understands that smoking cessation is done according to the principles of the cycle of change. Adopt an empathic, patient-centred approach, exploring the patient's feelings about stopping smoking.
  - 'Have you often thought about quitting?'
  - 'What thoughts have you had about quitting?'
  - 'Do you feel there are any barriers at the moment to stopping?'

O—u Key summary
- Consider hidden agendas whilst taking a focussed history.
- Recognise the NICE guidelines for COPD.
- Address smoking cessation and be aware of the main treatments.
- If the patient is responsive, outline the main treatments for smoking cessation.

Smoking cessation

- Patients motivated to stop smoking should receive support from a smoking clinic.

Bupropion (Zyban®)

- This is an atypical antidepressant. Its mechanism in smoking cessation is poorly understood.
- It decreases nicotine cravings and withdrawal effects.
- The Committee on Safety of Medicines (CSM) advises that bupropion is contraindicated in:
  — epilepsy (risk of seizures)
  — eating disorders
  — tumours of the central nervous system (CNS).

Nicotine replacement therapy (NRT)

- NRT is available to use as:
  — patches
  — inhalers
  — nasal spray
  — gum
  — sublingual tablet and lozenge.
- NRT is safe in most patients. Like bupropion, it also helps reduce the craving patients experience when they stop smoking.
- It should be used with caution in patients with a history of significant cardiovascular disease.

Varenicline   Chenlit

- This is a selective nicotine receptor partial agonist.
- It should be used in conjunction with behavioural therapy.
- There have been reports of suicidal thoughts and actions in those taking this drug, so it should be used with caution where there is a history of mental health problems.
- Pregnancy is also a contraindication.

NICE guidelines for smoking cessation

- NICE (2008) have recommended the use of bupropion, NRT or varenicline to those who intend to stop smoking and commit to a target stop date. The choice among these medications should be decided on the basis of:
  — the patient's motivation
  — available support and counselling
  — medical factors
  — patient preference.
- NICE advocates the use of a combination of services, including behavioural counselling, drug therapies or a combination of the two. This should involve several service providers, including pharmacists, midwives, health visitors and GPs.
- There is evidence to support the use of the following methods for smoking cessation, given in Table 1.20.

TABLE 1.20 Pharmacological versus non-pharmacological therapies in smoking cessation

PHARMACOTHERAPIES	NON-PHARMACOTHERAPIES
NRT	Brief intervention
Varenicline	Behavioural one-to-one counselling
Bupropion	Group therapy
	Telephone support
	Media campaigns
	Self-help methods, e.g. online materials

Transtheoretical model

- This is also known as the 'stages of change' model.
- The model can be applied when approaching the subject of smoking cessation with a patient.
- According to the model, a patient has to go through six key stages if they are going to change their behaviour (smoking is used as an example to explain the stages, but it could refer equally to any other lifestyle behaviour):
    1 **Precontemplation** – the patient does not intend to stop smoking within the next six months.
    2 **Contemplation** – the patient intends to stop smoking within the next six months.
    3 **Preparation** – the patient is planning to take action in the next month.
    4 **Action** – the patient has made positive alterations in smoking habits within the last six months, e.g. has stopped smoking.
    5 **Maintenance** – the patient is taking steps to maintain the modified behaviour.
    6 **Termination** – the patient returns to smoking again.
- Identifying which stage a patient is at is important in helping them consider or take seriously your request to stop smoking. There is evidence that attempts to modify behaviour should be matched to the stage a patient is at in the cycle of change.

Management of chronic obstructive pulmonary disease

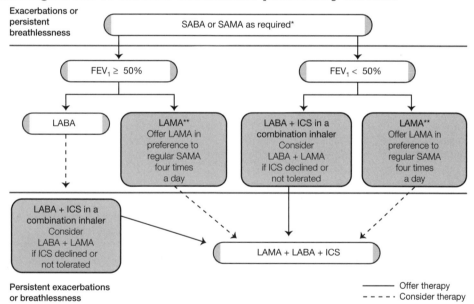

- Choose a drug based on the person's symptomatic response and preference, the drug's side effects, potential to reduce exacerbations and cost.
- Do not use oral corticosteroid reversibility tests to identify patients who will benefit from inhaled corticosteroids.
- Be aware of the potential risk of developing side effects (including non-fatal pneumonia) in people with COPD treated with inhaled corticosteroids and be prepared to discuss this with patients.

* SABA as required may continue at all stages; ** Discontinue SAMA.

SABA, short-acting beta$_2$ agonist; SAMA, short-acting muscarinic antagonist.

FIGURE 1.4 Management of COPD: inhaled therapy

(Reproduced with permission of National Institute of Health and Clinical Excellence.)

National Institute of Health and Clinical Excellence. Chronic Obstructive Pulmonary Disease: NICE guideline 101. London: NIHCE; 2010. http://guidance.nice.org.uk/CG101 (accessed 21 November 2010).

TABLE 1.21 Managing symptoms and conditions in stable COPD

ASSESS SYMPTOMS OR CONDITION AND MANAGE AS DESCRIBED BELOW

Breathlessness and exacerbations	• Manage breathlessness and exercise limitation with inhaled therapy • For exacerbations or persistent breathlessness: — use long-acting bronchodilators or LABA + ICS — consider adding theophylline if still symptomatic • Offer pulmonary rehabilitation to all suitable people • Refer patients who are breathless, have a single large bulla on a CT scan and an FEV_1 less than 50% predicted for consideration of bullectomy • Refer people with severe COPD for consideration of lung volume reduction surgery if they remain breathless with marked restrictions of their activities of daily living, despite maximal medical therapy (including rehabilitation), and meet all of the following: — FEV_1 greater than 20% predicted — $Paco_2$ less than 7.3 kPa — upper lobe predominant emphysema — T_LCO greater than 20% predicted • Consider referring people with severe COPD for assessment for lung transplantation if they remain breathless with marked restrictions of their activities of daily living despite maximal medical therapy. Considerations include: — age — FEV_1 — $Paco_2$ — homogeneously distributed emphysema on CT scan — elevated pulmonary artery pressures with progressive deterioration — comorbidities — local surgical protocols
Frequent exacerbations	• Optimise inhaled therapy • Offer vaccinations and prophylaxis • Give self-management advice • Consider osteoporosis prophylaxis for people requiring frequent oral corticosteroids
Cor pulmonale	• Consider in people who have peripheral oedema, a raised venous pressure, a systolic parasternal heave, a loud pulmonary second heart sound • Exclude other causes of peripheral oedema • Perform pulse oximetry, ECG and echocardiogram if features of cor pulmonale
Cor pulmonale (*cont.*)	• Assess need for LTOT • Treat oedema with diuretic • Angiotensin converting enzyme inhibitors, calcium channel blockers, alpha blockers are not recommended • Digoxin may be used where there is atrial fibrillation
Respiratory failure	• Assess for appropriate oxygen • Consider referral for assessment for long-term domiciliary NIV therapy
Abnormal BMI	• Refer for dietetic advice • Offer nutritional supplements if the BMI is low • Pay attention to weight changes in older patients (especially >3 kg)

(continued)

ASSESS SYMPTOMS OR CONDITION AND MANAGE AS DESCRIBED BELOW

Chronic productive cough	• Consider mucolytic therapy
Anxiety and depression	• Screen for anxiety and depression using validated tools in people who: — are hypoxic — are severely breathless or — have recently been seen or treated at a hospital for an exacerbation
Alpha-1 antitrypsin deficiency	• Offer referral to a specialist centre to discuss the clinical management of this condition • Alpha-1 antitrypsin replacement therapy is not recommended
Palliative setting	• Opioids should be used when appropriate for the palliations of breathlessness in people with end-stage COPD unresponsive to other medical therapy • Use benzodiazepines, tricyclic antidepressants, major tranquillisers and oxygen to treat breathlessness • Provide access to multidisciplinary palliative care teams and hospices

(Reproduced with permission of National Institute of Health and Clinical Excellence.)

National Institute of Health and Clinical Excellence. Chronic Obstructive Pulmonary Disease: NICE guideline 101. London: NIHCE; 2010. http://guidance.nice.org.uk/CG101 (accessed 21 November 2010).

Further reading

- National Institute of Health and Clinical Excellence. Chronic Obstructive Pulmonary Disease: NICE guideline 101. London: NIHCE; 2010. http://guidance.nice.org.uk/CG101 (accessed 21 November 2010).
- National Institute for Health and Clinical Excellence. Smoking Cessation Services: NICE public health guidance 10. London NIHCE; 2008. http://guidance.nice.org.uk/PH10 (accessed 21 November 2010).
- National Institute of Health and Clinical Excellence. Depression with a Chronic Physical Health Problem: NICE guideline 91. London: NIHCE; 2009. http://guidance.nice.org.uk/CG91 (accessed 11 December 2010).
- Wikipedia. *Transtheoretical Model.* Available at: www.wikipedia.org/wiki/Transtheoretical_model (accessed 11 December 2010).

Circuit 2

Station 2.1

Candidate's notes

Name	Mark Flutter-Heart
Age	59
Medical history	Hypertension
Medication	Sotalol 5 mg od
	Metformin 500 mg tds
	Ramipril 5 mg od
	Warfarin as per INR
Allergies	Nil
Last consultation	Five months ago with UTRI

St Wonderful Hospital
St Wonderful Road
St Wonderful
ST1 WOND

DISCHARGE SUMMARY FOR MARK FLUTTER-HEART

Dear GP

Diagnosis
- Admitted with newly diagnosed AF.

Investigations
- Troponin negative.
- Other bloods normal, including cholesterol, renal and thyroid function.
- Echocardiogram showed a slightly enlarged LA but normal LV and valvular function.

Drugs on discharge
- Sotalol 80 mg bd.
- Ramipril 5 mg od.
- Warfarin as per INR (target range 2–3). Referred to anticoagulation clinic.

Management plan
- He has been given an appointment for DC cardioversion in four weeks.
- Please maintain his INR between 2.0 and 3.0 so we can proceed with DC cardioversion.

Review date
- Cardiology clinic four weeks after DC cardioversion to discuss if he needs to continue on long-term sotalol and warfarin.

Yours sincerely
Dr C Ardiologist

Actor's notes

Background
- You are Mark Flutter-Heart, a 59-year-old architect.

Opening statement
- 'Doctor, I want to speak to you today about my heart.'

History
- Last week, you developed sudden onset of palpitations whilst you were walking your dog.
- You went to casualty and were told you had a fast, irregular heartbeat. You were started on a tablet to make your heart beat at a 'normal rate' and another tablet to 'thin the blood'.
- On the day of discharge from hospital, the doctor informed you that you would be booked in for 'a procedure to the heart' in one month to try to make your heart beat 'regularly' again.
- He was about to explain what this involved but was called away in an emergency.

Ideas, concerns and expectations
- You do not understand why your heartbeat became 'irregular' because you lead a healthy lifestyle.
- You do not understand why you need the 'blood thinning' drug, or how long you need to take it for.
- You are not keen on having regular blood tests for the 'blood thinning' drug and wonder if there is an alternative drug whereby you do not need to have regular blood tests.
- You were alarmed to read on the internet that the 'blood thinning' drug is used to poison rats, and causes death through internal bleeding. You are concerned that it may cause internal bleeding in you.
- You do not understand what the 'procedure to the heart' involves, and become concerned about the effects of electrical shocks on the heart, and are worried that this will do further damage.
- You have come to the GP today to ask why your heartbeat is irregular, discuss the medications you have been given and ask about the procedure you are due to have.

Further history candidate may elicit
- You had palpitations for one week before you went into hospital. These were occurring daily, at any time, for 30–45 minutes, and were associated with shortness of breath.
- The episodes resolved spontaneously and were not associated with chest pain or syncope. You do not recall any obvious precipitating events.
- You did not see a doctor initially because you thought the palpitations would settle down.
- At the weekend, the palpitations continued for 2–3 hours. You were walking your dog at the time and noticed that you became quite breathless. You went home and rested, but the palpitations and shortness of breath continued, so you went to hospital where the doctors told you that your heartbeat was 'fast and irregular'. You had a 'heart scan' and was told it was 'okay'.
- The doctors started you on a tablet to 'control' the heart rate, and another 'blood thinning' drug that will require you to have regular blood tests, but did not explain why you needed this drug.
- You were advised to see your GP for regular blood tests because you were on the 'blood thinning' drug. However, you found the blood tests in hospital very painful, so do not want them regularly.
- The hospital doctor mentioned he had booked you in for 'a procedure' to help the heart rhythm become regular again. The doctor was going to explain what was involved but had to leave to attend an emergency.
- You came home a few days ago and read on the internet that the 'blood thinning' drug is used as a rat poison, which you found alarming. You are unsure whether to take it.

Medical history
- Diabetes.
- Hypertension.

Drug history
- Sotalol 80 mg bd.
- Metformin 500 mg tds.
- Ramipril 5 mg od.
- Warfarin 3 mg od.

Family history
- Nil.

Social history
- You do not smoke. You drink one to two glasses of wine on most days.
- You live with your wife. You have one son who is at university.

Approach to scenario
- You are worried about your heart and ask the doctor 'Will I die soon?'
- You ask the doctor why you developed this heart condition.
- You are keen to understand why you need the 'blood thinning' drug, and how long you will need it for.
- You explain to the doctor that you want to stop it because you do not want to have regular blood tests and because you are concerned it can cause internal bleeding.
- You tell the doctor 'I don't want to die like a rat'.
- You ask the doctor about the 'procedure to the heart' and become concerned about the effects of electrical shocks on the heart, and are worried that this will do further damage.
- If the doctor explains that the benefits of direct current (DC) cardioversion and warfarin outweigh the risks, you agree to have the procedure and remain on the drug for now.
- However, if the doctor is unable to communicate the benefits of the procedure or warfarin adequately, you become upset and say 'I don't understand why the hospital doctors are trying to poison me and electrocute me to death!'

Information gathering
Presenting complaint
a Palpitations
- Ask how long ago the palpitations started and what he was doing at the time.
- Frequency of palpitations, e.g. daily, weekly, monthly.
- How long each episode lasted.
- Precipitating factors, e.g. alcohol, caffeine, stress.
- Associated symptoms:
  — syncope
  — chest pain
  — dizziness
  — shortness of breath.

b Risk factors
- Diabetes.
- Alcohol.
- Smoking.
- Hypertension.
- Hypercholesterolaemia.
- Past history of heart disease or MI.
- Family history of heart disease or MI.

c Hospital admission
- Ask about investigations and treatment whilst in hospital.
- Explore what information he was given.

Medical history
- Diabetes.
- Hypertension.

Family history
- AF or other heart disease.

Drug history
- Confirm medications.
- Check compliance with medications.

Social history
- Occupation.
- Smoking and alcohol.
- Home circumstances.

Patient's agenda
- Explore his understanding of AF.
- Explore his concerns about treatment with warfarin and DC cardioversion.

Examination
- Offer to examine the heart and lungs, and check his BP.
- 'If it's okay with you, I'll just listen to your heart and lungs and check your blood pressure.'

Examination card	
General examination	Looks slim and appears well
Cardiovascular examination	BP = 130/79 mmHg
	Heart rate = 70/minute and irregular
	JVP = normal
	Heart sounds = normal; no murmur
	Ankle oedema = not present
Respiratory examination	RR = normal
	Chest = clear; no crackles present

Clinical management
1 Explain the diagnosis of atrial fibrillation
- Explain that he has AF, which results from a cardiac conduction defect that causes a fast, irregular heart rate.
- As a result, the heart is less efficient and pumps smaller volumes of blood at a quicker rate, which can cause chest pain, dizziness and shortness of breath.
- Explain that this condition is a common complication of hypertension.
- Reassure him it is a common condition and can be successfully controlled.

2 Discuss the complications of atrial fibrillation
- Explain that the main complication of AF is an increased risk of thromboembolic stroke.
- Explain that AF causes turbulent blood flow in the cardiac chambers, which can lead

to thrombus formation. Emboli can travel to the vessels supplying the brain, leading to ischaemia and stroke.

3 Data interpretation

- Using the data available, and the information from the discharge summary, calculate his $CHADS_2$ score (*see* page 108) and recognise and explain he is at high risk of having a stroke because he has diabetes **and** hypertension.

4 Discuss the importance of anticoagulation

- Underline the importance of warfarin in lowering the risk of stroke by reducing the risk of developing blood clots.
- Explain that he needs to be on warfarin for at least four weeks before and after the DC cardioversion to reduce the risk of thromboembolic stroke following the procedure.
- Explain that he will be reviewed by the heart specialist after the procedure to determine if he needs to continue warfarin long term, but this is likely.
- Counsel the patient about use of warfarin:
  — Explain that warfarin is associated with an increased risk of bleeding but this is minimised by monitoring the international normalised ratio (INR) and ensuring it is within a safe range.
  — Explain that monitoring requires finger-prick testing and not repeated blood tests.
  — Explain that many drugs interact with warfarin, enhancing or reducing the anticoagulant effect; therefore he must inform doctors or pharmacists he is taking warfarin before starting any other medication, such as NSAIDs.

5 Explain the treatment of atrial fibrillation

- Explain treatments can control the heart rate at a normal level or try to restore a normal rhythm.

a Rate control

- Explain the purpose of sotalol is to control the rate of his heartbeat and so prevent symptoms such as palpitations, shortness of breath and dizziness.
- Explain that his heart will still beat irregularly, but at a normal rate.

b Rhythm control

- Explain DC cardioversion can restore the heart back to sinus rhythm. This involves:
  — general anaesthetic or sedation with benzodiazepines
  — application of gel pads to the chest wall
  — delivery of an electrical shock, or multiple shocks, to the heart.
- Explain that the benefit of DC cardioversion is to restore the heart to sinus rhythm. This will reduce symptoms and the risk of stroke, and if successful in the long term anticoagulation and rate-control drugs may not be needed.
- Explain the risks of DC cardioversion:
  — local burns to the skin (gel pads used to reduce risk)
  — fifty per cent of people will revert to AF within one year of treatment
  — an increased risk of thromboembolic disease, hence anticoagulation with warfarin is needed four weeks prior and four weeks following the procedure.

6 Follow-up

- Offer a follow-up appointment.
- Advise him he will be reviewed by the cardiology team to discuss this further.
- Provide him with information leaflets on AF.

Interpersonal skills

- During this station, the candidate would be expected to use good communication skills to explain the diagnosis of AF and discuss the management plan that the cardiology team have suggested.
- It is important to provide explanations in lay terms and clarify terms with the patient.
  - 'The reason your heart has become irregular and was beating fast is because you have developed a condition called atrial fibrillation. Have you heard of it before?'
  - 'This is a common condition and occurs for a number of reasons. One of the most common reasons, and the likely reason in your case, is high blood pressure. This puts a strain on the heart, and the electrical activity becomes affected, resulting in a fast and irregular pulse.'
- The candidate should be able to discuss the benefits and risks associated with anticoagulation and DC cardioversion, whilst providing the patient with adequate reassurance where appropriate.
  - 'AF increases the risk of stroke or "brain injury". This is because an irregular heartbeat leads to abnormal blood flow in the heart, which can result in a blood clot forming. If this travels to the brain and blocks a blood vessel, it can cause a stroke.'
  - 'The drug that thins your blood prevents you from developing blood clots, and so considerably reduces the risk of you having a stroke.'
  - 'Although it increases the risk of bleeding, we would monitor the thinness of your blood regularly. This can be annoying, but once you are stable on it, you may only need to be tested every few weeks.'
  - 'You are right – warfarin can be found in rat poison, but I assure you it is not used for the same reason by doctors!'
  - 'To try and make your heart beat regularly again, there is a procedure called DC cardioversion, which the heart specialists suggested. Did they explain to you anything about it? . . . (silence) . . . Have you heard of it before?'
  - 'The procedure involves giving you an anaesthetic or drug to sedate you, so you are not awake during the process. The doctors put some gel pads on your chest, and then use a machine to give an electrical shock to the heart. Sometimes more than one shock is needed.'
  - 'The purpose of this procedure is to make the electrical current in the heart work properly again. If successful, you may not need to take any drugs for the heart and this will prevent a stroke in future.'
  - 'I appreciate it sounds scary, but it is a very common procedure, and aims to improve the functioning of the heart. The main issue is that it is not always successful.'

O—⊷ Key summary
- Be familiar with NICE guidelines for AF, including risk stratification for anticoagulation or antiplatelet therapy.
- Explore the patient's concerns about AF, anticoagulation and cardioversion.
- Counsel the patient about anticoagulation treatment.
- Be able to explain the benefits and risks of procedures, such as cardioversion, in lay terms.
- Provide adequate reassurance where appropriate.

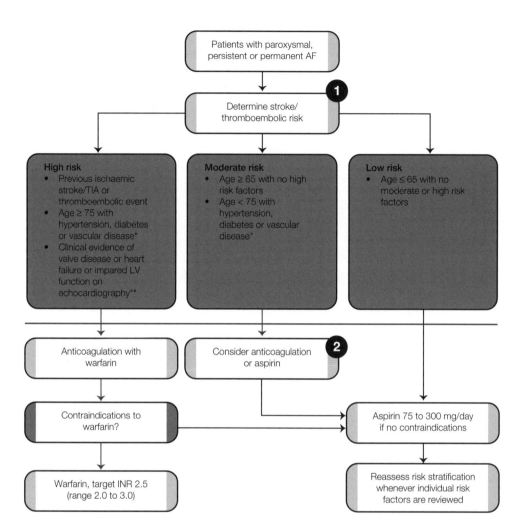

1 Note that risk factors are not mutually exclusive, and are additive to each other in producing a composite risk. Since the incidence of stroke and thromboembolic events in patients with thyrotoxicosis appears similar to that in patients with other aetiologies of AF, antithrombotic treatments should be chosen based on the presence of validated stroke risk factors.

2 Owing to lack of sufficient clear-cut evidence, treatment may be decided on an individual basis, and the physician must balance the risks and benefits of warfarin versus aspirin. As stroke risk factors are cumulative, warfarin may, for example, be used in the presence of two or more moderate stroke risk factors. Referral and echocardiography may help in cases of uncertainty.

* Coronary artery disease or peripheral artery disease.

** an echocardiogram is not needed for routine assessment, but refines clincial risk stratification in the case of moderate or severe LV dysfunction and valve disease.

FIGURE 2.1 Algorithm for stroke risk stratification

(Reproduced with permission of National Institute of Health and Clinical Excellence.)

National Institute for Health and Clinical Excellence. Atrial Fibrillation: NICE guideline CG36. London: NIHCE; 2006. www.nice.org.uk/nicemedia/live/10982/30052/30052.pdf (accessed 22 November 2010).

Anticoagulation in atrial fibrillation

Definitions

- **Acute onset AF** occurs when AF develops suddenly.
- **Paroxysmal AF** describes intermittent episodes of AF that resolve without any treatment.
- **Persistent AF** describes AF for >7 days that is unlikely to revert back to sinus rhythm without treatment by electrical or pharmacological cardioversion.
- **Permanent AF** means that the AF has been present long term. In these patients, rate control is used to ensure normal heart rate, but the rhythm remains irregular.
- This section focuses on the management of persistent AF as suggested by NICE (2006).
- Please consult NICE guidelines (2006) for the management of AF (*see* Further reading below).

CHADS$_2$ score

Indication

- To assess the risk of stroke in patients with AF (use with NICE flow chart, Figure 2.1).

TABLE 2.1 CHADS$_2$ score and risk of stroke

ABBREVIATION	CONDITION	POINT
C	Congestive heart failure	1
H	Hypertension: BP consistently >140/90 mmHg or treated hypertension on medication	1
A	Age >75 years	1
D	Diabetes mellitus	1
S$_2$	Prior stroke or TIA	2

Interpretation

- Add the points that correspond to the conditions that a patient has, to calculate the CHADS$_2$ score.
  - CHADS$_2$ score ≥2:   warfarin with INR 2.0 to 3.0.
  - CHADS$_2$ score 1:   warfarin (INR 2.0 to 3.0) or aspirin.
  - CHADS$_2$ score 0:   aspirin.

Anticoagulation and DC cardioversion

- Before cardioversion, maintain INR at 2.5 (range 2.0 to 3.0) with warfarin for at least three weeks.
- After successful cardioversion, maintain INR at 2.5 (range 2.0 to 3.0) with warfarin for at least four weeks, and consider stopping anticoagulation after review with patient and specialist.
- Continue anticoagulation **long term** in patients with a high risk of AF recurrence (AF present for >12 months, history of failed cardioversion attempts, mitral valve disease, left ventricle [LV] dysfunction or dilated left atrium [LA]) or where it is recommended by the stroke risk stratification algorithm (*see* Figure 2.1, page 107).
- Aspirin can be used **long term** in patients with low or moderate risk of stroke (*see* Figure 2.1, page 107).

Further reading

- Atrial Fibrillation Association website. www.atrialfibrillation.org.uk (accessed 22 November 2010).
- National Institute for Health and Clinical Excellence. Atrial Fibrillation: NICE guideline CG36. London: NIHCE; 2006. www.nice.org.uk/CG36 (accessed 22 November 2010).
- Simon C, Everitt H, van Dorp F. *Oxford Handbook of General Practice.* 3rd ed. Oxford: Oxford University Press; 2010.
- Longmore M, Wilkinson I, Davidson E, *et al. Oxford Handbook of Clinical Medicine.* 8th ed. Oxford: Oxford University Press; 2010.

Station 2.2

Actor's notes

Background

- You are Kali Bal, a 25-year-old Asian fashion model.

Opening statement

- 'Doctor, my hair is falling out!'

History

- Over the last three weeks you have noticed your hair is thinning and you are losing more hair than normal.
- When you wash your hair, the sink gets clogged up with the hair that is falling out. You have also noticed hair on your pillow when you wake up, and a lot of hair in the hairbrush you are using.

Ideas, concerns and expectations

- You are devastated to see your hair falling out. You are worried about the impact this will have on your career as a model.
- You cannot understand why your hair is falling out because your entire family have long hair and you think you have 'very good hair genes'.
- You wonder if the hair loss is a result of a new dye the hairdresser used on your hair for highlights.
- Your agent told you about another model who started to lose her hair in patches and eventually had to leave the fashion industry because she had large patches of baldness. He advised you to see the doctor as soon as possible.
- This frightened you and you decided to see the GP for a referral to a specialist to prevent further hair loss.

Further history candidate may elicit

- You have been a freelance model for four months. Over this time, your popularity as a model has risen. You model for magazines and at fashion events. You love the 'buzz' you get when you are on the catwalk.
- However, you work long hours because you often need to attend evening fashion shows or parties. As a result, you are not sleeping much and have been skipping meals. You have lost 3 kg in weight over the last few months. You are vegetarian. You live on Red Bull and coffee. Some days you only have time to eat a snack bar.
- You enjoy your work, but are feeling tired. You put this down to long hours and stress of the job.
- Last week, your agent contacted you because a top Asian fashion company is looking to

recruit a new female model. You have been invited to a photo shoot in two weeks, along with other models, where the company will select the successful candidate. You really want this job and want to look your best at the photo shoot.

- However, for the last three weeks, your hair has been falling out. This seemed to start soon after you went to the hairdresser – she used a new dye on your hair for highlights. The hair loss has continued for about four weeks and you are worried that it will not stop.
- You spoke to your sister who suggested you change your shampoo and conditioner. You have subsequently changed shampoo and conditioner three times, but this has not helped. Your mother suggested using hair oil but you are worried it may exacerbate the hair loss.
- When you spoke to your agent on the telephone about the photo shoot next week, you mentioned your hair was falling out, and that you thought it was due to the highlights.
- Your agent suggested it was probably not the chemicals since they would have worn off by now.
- However, he mentioned that another model who worked for him a few years ago suddenly started to lose her hair. She did not see the GP immediately because she thought it would get better. By the time she saw the GP, she had developed patches of baldness and had to see a specialist. Eventually, she left the fashion industry because she could not hide the bald patches.
- This terrified you, so you decided to see the GP to get a referral to a specialist for further treatment so you do not lose any more hair before the photo shoot in two weeks.
- You are not depressed, do not binge eat or vomit and have no other symptoms.

Medical history
- Nil.

Obstetric and gynaecological history
- Regular monthly periods.
- Period last four days.
- Period not heavy.
- No children.

Drug history
- Nil.

Social history
- You do not smoke. You drink alcohol occasionally at some of the fashion events.
- You have the 'odd snort of cocaine' at some of the parties you attend.
- You live by yourself in a flat and are currently single. Your parents and older sister live locally.

Family history
- Nil relevant.
- No family history of hair loss or hair disorders.

Approach to scenario
- You feel embarrassed speaking to the doctor about your hair loss.
- You want an explanation of why this is happening and 'want to get to the root of the problem'.
- You come across as very anxious about the hair and ask 'I won't go bald, will I, Doctor?'
- You are keen for the doctor to prescribe some kind of treatment today, and want a referral to a specialist to have some tests to determine the reason for the hair loss.
- You want some advice on which hair products to use and which ones to avoid, any dietary changes that you should make, and how the hair loss can be controlled.
- You mention your use of recreational drugs only if the doctor directly asks you. If the doctor

suggests you should avoid using cocaine, you agree, explaining you only use it occasionally and will not use it in future.

- If the doctor is caring, sympathetic and offers you a potential explanation for the hair loss and blood test, you will agree to holding off the referral for now.
- If the doctor does not come across well, you demand a referral to a specialist and refuse to leave until the doctor agrees to refer you. If the doctor refuses, you suggest you will make a complaint.

Information gathering
Presenting complaint
a Hair loss
- Ask when the hair loss started.
- Ask how much hair is being lost.
- Check if she has tried any treatments, and if so, what.

b Conditions related to hair loss
i Hyper- and hypothyroidism
- Weight change.
- Palpitations.
- Intolerance to hot or cold.
- Change in bowel habit.

ii Hypoparathyroidism
- Loss of libido.
- Erectile dysfunction (ED) in men.
- Reduced need to shave face in men.

iii Iron deficiency
- Tiredness.
- Shortness of breath.
- Explore causes of iron deficiency, e.g.
  — menorrhagia
  — haematemesis +/– melaena
  — vegetarian diet or change in diet leading to deficient state.

iv Stress
- Crash diets.
- Recent surgery.
- Prolonged illness.
- Recent life events causing emotional stress.

v Eating disorders
- Binge eating.
- Self-induced vomiting.
- Use of laxatives or diuretics.
- Excessive exercise.

Medical history
- Particularly endocrine or autoimmune disorders.

Family history
- Autoimmune disease.
- Premature balding.

Drug history
- Current medications.

Social history
- Current occupation.
- Marital status.
- Life stresses, e.g. financial.
- Enquire about alcohol, smoking and use of recreational drugs.

Patient's agenda
- Explore her concerns about losing her hair.
- Explore her thoughts as to why this is happening.
- Explore what management options she would like to consider.

Examination
- Offer to examine the patient's scalp.
- 'Is it okay if I check your hair?'

Examination card

General examination	Looks pale
	BMI = 20 kg/m^2
	Clinically euthyroid
	Face and eyebrows appear normal
Scalp examination	Non-scarring diffuse loss of hair

Clinical management

1 Discuss hair loss with the patient
- Reassure the patient that hair loss is common and there are many reasons for it.
- Explore her understanding about hair loss and the possible reasons for it.
- Reassure the patient that the hair loss appears to be minimal.
- Explain that there are different patterns of hair loss that suggest the possible causes.
- Explain that she has diffuse hair loss, rather than loss of patches of hair, and there is no associated scar formation.
- Discuss the possible causes, e.g. stress, iron +/– zinc deficiency or endocrine disorders.
- Reassure her that by treating the underlying problem, her hair should continue to grow normally.

2 Discuss the management of hair loss
- Suggest that a blood test would be useful to check for anaemia, iron deficiency and endocrine disorders such as thyroid dysfunction.
- Suggest that emotional and physical stress can exacerbate hair loss, so taking time out to relax and developing relaxation techniques would be helpful.
- Advise her that recreational drugs such as cocaine can also cause or contribute to the loss of hair.
- Encourage her to avoid using recreational drugs, explaining that they can cause other more serious health issues.
- Explain it is important to eat regularly and take multivitamin tablets to ensure there is no dietary deficiency of vitamins or minerals.
- Advise her to eat more green vegetables since they have higher sources of iron.
- Advise her that, at this stage, the cause of the hair loss needs to be determined prior to starting treatment.

- Negotiate with the patient to hold off a specialist referral, reassuring her that a referral to a dermatologist could be considered if the blood test does not reveal any abnormality and the hair loss continues.

3 Offer follow-up
- Offer her leaflets on hair loss.
- Offer her a follow-up appointment for review once blood results are available.

Interpersonal skills
- Show the patient you care from the outset, in an attempt to create a good rapport. A good way to do this is to respond to the patient's opening statement by reflecting the problem back.
  — 'I'm very sorry that your hair is falling out. That must be quite distressing for you?'
- During this station, the candidate would need to recognise the potential causes of hair loss through a combination of history taking and interpretation of the examination findings. Adopt a combination of open and closed questions to achieve this.
  — 'Tell me some more about the hair loss.'
  — 'What sort of diet do you have? Are you vegetarian?'
- The candidate would also be expected to exclude an eating disorder in view of the poor diet, weight loss and occupation.
- Conditions affecting appearance can cause significant distress and embarrassment to an individual. Elicit any concerns the patient may have.
  — 'Did you have any ideas about why this might be happening?'
  — 'Tell me more about your reasons for thinking there might be a connection between the hair loss and hair dye.'
- By discussing this sensitively with the patient and showing an understanding of her concern, the candidate can negotiate to hold off referral and treatment at the present time. Try and offer shared management options as much as possible.
  — 'This is obviously bothering you considerably. Tell me more.'
  — 'Hair loss is a common problem for men and women. There is often an underlying cause. In your case, it seems the likely cause of your hair loss could be stress or not eating well, which could cause deficiencies in minerals like iron. How do you feel about having a blood test to check your iron levels and some of your hormones in the first instance?'
  — 'You mentioned you use cocaine. Do you use any other recreational drugs?'
- Explore the impact of the hair loss on the patient's personal and work life. Being attentive to verbal and non-verbal cues will help to identify any relevant psychosocial factors.
  — 'I get the impression the photo shoot in two weeks is quite important for your career . . . (silence) . . . Tell me more about it.'
  — 'You mentioned the story that your agent told you. Has that upset you?'
  — 'I can see this problem is getting you down . . . (silence).'
- When dealing with the patient's request for referral, be sensitive to this demand, but at the same time be prepared to negotiate.
  — 'We can investigate hair loss here at the surgery. We can even start most treatments, for example, if you are deficient in iron. How about we start this process, check the blood tests and review with you with the results in a week or two?'

O⊷ Key summary
- Communicate sensitively with the patient.
- Explore her concerns about hair loss.
- Explain the likely causes of hair loss in her case.
- Negotiate to hold off both drug treatment and dermatology referral at present.

Hair loss

TABLE 2.2 Different types of hair loss and causes

TYPE	EXAMPLES
Diffuse, non-scarring	• Male pattern/androgenic • Endocrine disorders — hypothyroidism — hyperthyroidism — hypopituitarism — hypoadrenalism • Mineral deficiencies — iron deficiency — zinc deficiency • Emotional or physical stress — stress — malnutrition — ill health — surgery — pregnancy and postpartum • Drug-induced — cytotoxics — heparin — warfarin — carbimazole
Localised, non-scarring	• Trauma • Ringworm • Alopecia areata
Localised, scarring	• Burns • Morphoea • Lupus erythematosus • Radiation • Lichen planus • Fungal infection (kerion) • Shingles of first trigeminal dermatome

Diffuse, non-scarring
• Patients notice excessive numbers of hairs on the pillow, brush or comb, and after washing their hair. The scalp shows a diffuse reduction in hair density.

Male pattern/androgenic baldness
• This is a common cause of hair loss, usually in men but can also be in females due to polycystic ovary syndrome (PCOS) or after the menopause.
• It tends to cluster in families, and often other relatives are affected.
• Individuals have increased levels of the hormone dihydrotestosterone (DHT), which affects the hair follicles and so prevents normal hair growth.
• In men, bitemporal hair recession followed by a bald crown is the usual pattern.
• Drug treatments include:
  (a) **Minoxidil:**
  — Is available as a topical or 'rub on' preparation and must be applied to the scalp daily.
  — Can take six months before any benefit is seen.

— Side effects include mild scalp irritation.
— Effect is temporary – once stopped, hair loss returns to previous levels.
— Is available over the counter and can be bought without a prescription.
(b) **Finasteride:**
— Inhibits the formation of the hormone DHT, so stops hair loss and stimulates growth.
— Is available in tablet form, and it can take six months before any benefit is seen.
— Side effects include reduced libido and ED.
— Effect is temporary – once stopped, hair loss returns to previous levels.
— Is only available on private prescription.
- Hair transplantation or other surgical options are available but are only available privately.

Localised, non-scarring
Alopecia areata
- Associated with autoimmune disorders. Causes sharply defined non-inflamed bald patches.
- 'Exclamation-mark' hairs, which taper as they approach the scalp, are seen.
- The eyebrows and beard can also be affected. Nail pitting occurs in 10% of patients.
- Can lead to alopecia totalis (loss of all scalp hair) or alopecia universalis (loss of all body hair).
- Regrowth with white hairs can occur.
- Treatment depends on the extent:
    — Localised loss can be treated with intralesional steroid.
    — Extensive loss can be managed with PUVA, but often wigs are needed.

Further reading
- Simon C, Everitt H, van Dorp F. *Oxford Handbook of General Practice.* 3rd ed. Oxford: Oxford University Press; 2010.
- Buxton PK, Morris-Jones R. *ABC of Dermatology.* 5th ed. Oxford: Wiley-Blackwell; 2009.
- Gawkrodger D. *Dermatology: an illustrated colour text.* 4th ed. Oxford: Churchill Livingstone; 2007.

Station 2.3

Actor's notes

Background

- You are Ahmed Masud, a 37-year-old gentleman of Bangladeshi origin who works as a chef.

Opening statement

- 'Doctor, what do I do? – I have an upset tummy!'

History

- You have had diarrhoea for two days, and opened your bowels seven or eight times each day.
- The stool is very watery in nature. There is no blood.
- You vomited a few times yesterday – there was no blood. You have not vomited today.

Ideas, concerns and expectations

- You have never had diarrhoea as severe as on this occasion, and wonder how long it will be before it stops.
- You think it is the result of eating something at your friend's wedding the day before.
- You want to get better soon because you have to get back to work at your restaurant. Without you, the business is struggling – the restaurant is your livelihood.
- You are particularly concerned because, in five days time, you have a big party of guests who have booked the entire restaurant. You need to be well by then to help cater for the event.
- If you do not get better, you will have to cancel the event and your business will suffer.
- You expect the doctor to prescribe some antibiotics to help stop the diarrhoea.

Further history candidate may elicit

- You have some generalised abdominal pain, which is cramp-like in nature. This settles after you have opened your bowels. The pain is not localised to your right lower abdomen.
- You feel slightly feverish and very run down. You have not measured your temperature.
- You are managing to drink fluids but have not eaten since yesterday – eating seems to make the diarrhoea worse. You are drinking mainly water.
- You have had no recent foreign travel and have not eaten products past their sell-by date.
- You attended your friend's wedding three days ago by yourself. Your wife looked after the children. The diarrhoea started the day after the wedding.
- You have no other symptoms and no other member of the family is affected at present.
- You reveal you work as a chef in your restaurant only if the candidate asks about your occupation.

Medical and drug history

- Nil.
- You are not on any regular medication and have not taken anything for your current symptoms.

Social history

- You do not smoke or drink alcohol. You live with your wife in a small house with four children.
- You are originally from Bangladesh. You have not seen the rest of your family in Bangladesh for two years since starting your business in the UK.

Family history

- The family are well. No other members have diarrhoea or vomiting.

Approach to scenario

- You are keen to go back to work as soon as the diarrhoea is 'manageable'.
- You become upset if the doctor suggests that you need to stay off work until the diarrhoea settles completely or until test results are available.
- You ask for antibiotics two to three times to help you get better quickly, and seem surprised if the doctor does not want to prescribe them for you.
- If the doctor explains **clearly** why you should not return to work until you are completely fit, and why antibiotics are not needed, you understand and agree with the suggested management plan.
- If the doctor appears unsympathetic and does not explain clearly, you get angry and demand to speak to another doctor who will give you the antibiotics so you can get better soon.
- You are willing to take the doctor's advice about how to manage your symptoms.

Information gathering
Presenting complaint

- Ask about the diarrhoea:
  — onset
  — frequency
  — presence of blood, and if so, how much.
- Ask about associated symptoms:
  — haematemesis
  — vomiting, and if so, how often
  — fever, and if so, ask if he has measured his temperature.
- Ask about abdominal pain:
  — location
  — nature
  — radiation
  — alleviating and exacerbating factors.
- Ask if he is able to keep down fluids, and if he is eating.
- Enquire about eating foods that have gone past their sell-by date.

Medical history

- GI disease.

Family history

- Ask if other members of the family are affected.
- GI disease.

Drug history
- Medications used, e.g. loperamide and oral rehydration salts.

Social history
- Occupation.
- Recent foreign travel.
- Enquire about alcohol and smoking.
- Social events, e.g. barbeques or weddings where he has eaten.

Patient's agenda
- Explore his ideas about why he has developed diarrhoea.
- Explore his concerns about why he wants to return to work quickly.
- Explore the impact on his financial situation of time off work.

Clinical management
1 Explain the diagnosis
- Explain that the diarrhoea and vomiting have resulted either from an infection, which may be a virus, or something he ate at his friend's wedding.

2 Explain general principles of treatment

a Rehydration and diet
- Advise him to drink plenty of fluids and add rehydration salts, such as Dioralyte® or Rehidrat®, to the fluids.
- Explain that proprietary oral rehydration salts can be obtained over the counter without the need for a prescription.
- Explain that he can try having soups or eating small amounts of bread and pasta.

b Antimotility drugs
- Explain that he can use antimotility drugs, such as loperamide, to help reduce the frequency of the diarrhoea. This is also available over the counter without a prescription.
- Explain that this does not help clear the infection and can cause constipation.

c Hygiene
- Advise him to wash his hands thoroughly after going to the toilet and before eating, to prevent spread to his family and re-contaminating himself.

3 Discuss investigations and role of antibiotics
- Explain that in most cases, antibiotics are not needed, and the diarrhoea is self-limiting.
- However, in some cases, diarrhoea can continue and may require a course of antibiotics to clear.
- To determine if he needs antibiotics, a stool sample is needed, which is sent to the laboratory and analysed. The results take two or three days to return.
- Ask him to bring a stool sample to the surgery today or tomorrow – his wife could collect a specimen bottle.

4 Discuss fitness to work
- Outline how important it is, since he is a chef, for him to stay off work until he is fully recovered, highlighting:
  — If he returns to work too early, he could spread the infection to colleagues and customers.
  — Explain this would be far more detrimental to his business than having to potentially cancel the event in five days.

— Explain that legally regulations state that he can only return to work 48 hours after the diarrhoea +/− vomiting has completely resolved.
— If he returns to work whilst he is still infectious and others contract the infection, this could have health and safety implications, and his business maybe forced to close.
— Emphasise that if the stool sample reveals he has a more severe infection, he may need further time off work, and treatment with antibiotics.

5 Follow-up
- Advise him to telephone the surgery 48–72 hours after the stool sample has been sent, to verify the results and get further advice as to whether he can return to work.
- Explain that he can book an appointment to see a doctor for a face-to-face consultation, if symptoms worsen or his abdominal pain changes.
- Advise him to attend casualty or telephone for further advice if he is struggling to keep down fluids or is becoming dehydrated, with reduced urine output.

Interpersonal skills
- This is a telephone consultation, and you must be aware that non-verbal cues will be missed.
- Please refer to Station 1.11 regarding telephone consultations and the use of Roger Neighbour's consultation model.
- During this consultation, it is particularly important to check the patient's understanding of what has been discussed, including how to manage the diarrhoea, when to seek further medical help and also to emphasise the regulations of fitness to work for food handlers.
- It is important to be sympathetic to the patient's situation, understanding that his restaurant is his livelihood, yet be able to explain why he cannot return to work until he is medically fit.
  — 'I understand why you want to go back to work as soon as possible. However, please make sure you only go back after speaking to a doctor to check it is okay for you to return to work. This is so that you do not spread the infection to your colleagues or your customers. I am sure you would not want others to pick up this infection.'
  — 'There are some strict guidelines for when people working with food can go back to work after infections like you have. If you were to return to work too early, and this infection spread, your restaurant may be shut down.'

⚬⟟ Key summary
- Discuss the cause of diarrhoea and appropriate management.
- Emphasise the importance of *Food Handlers: fitness to work* (2009) guidelines.
- Recognise the need for clear communication and instructions during telephone consultations.

Gastroenteritis
- Most cases are viral.
- Clinical features include fever, diarrhoea and vomiting of acute onset.

When to refer to hospital
- Significant dehydration.
- Unable to tolerate fluids orally.
- Immunocompromised or on long-term steroids.
- Chronic diarrhoea (defined as loose stools for >4 weeks) should be referred as an outpatient.

Food Standards Agency
- Any person must be excluded from food-handling duties and food-handling areas if they have diarrhoea +/− vomiting and/or if they have an area of infected skin that cannot be covered.

- Food-handling duties include directly handling open food or touching surfaces that will come into direct contact with food such as food packaging and food equipment. Food-handling areas are defined as areas where these activities take place.
- Staff handling food or working in a food-handling area must report these symptoms to management immediately.

Diarrhoea and vomiting

(The following guidance is from the Food Standards Agency publication: *Food Handlers: fitness to work* [2009].)

- If a member of staff has had only a single bout of vomiting or one loose stool without fever, and has not had any further symptoms in 24 hours, they can return to work. However, extra care should be taken over personal hygiene practices on return to work, especially hand washing.
- If staff have more than one bout of diarrhoea +/– vomiting, managers must exclude them from working with or around open food, normally for 48 hours from when symptoms stop naturally.
- If a stool sample detects one of the pathogens listed below, the '48-hour exclusion rule' is sufficient.

TABLE 2.3 Examples of pathogens where the 48-hour exclusion rule is sufficient

Salmonella (except *Salmonella typhi* and *Salmonella paratyphi* A, B or C)
Campylobacter
Vibrio (except *Vibrio cholerae* 01 and 0139)
Yersinia
Bacillus
Staphylococcus aureus
Clostridium perfringens
Protozoa, e.g. *Cryptosporidium*, *Giardia lamblia* (except *Entamoeba histolytica*)
Shigella sonnei (but not *Shigella dysenteriae*, *flexneri* and *boydii*)
Worms (except threadworm and *Taenia solium*)

- However, if the pathogen causing diarrhoea +/– vomiting is listed below, specific advice should be followed, as highlighted in the table:

TABLE 2.4 Guidelines for diarrhoea caused by specific pathogens

Salmonella typhi *Salmonella paratyphi* **A, B or C** **(Enteric fever)**	• Transmission through the faecal-oral route • Notifiable diseases • More common in developing countries and hence in patients with a history of foreign travel • May be prolonged, intermittent excretion of bacteria after symptoms stop – patients can be carriers for ≥3 months, resulting in a long exclusion period from food handling • Antibiotic management, often with ciprofloxacin or norfloxacin, should be discussed with microbiology
E. coli	• Can return to work after two consecutive negative stool samples, the second sample being taken 48 hours after the symptoms have stopped naturally
Norovirus	• Transmitted easily through faecal-oral route and also by droplet spread • Therefore, symptomatic food handlers are excluded from the entire business site, not just food-handling duties and areas • Once excluded, they should remain away from work for 48 hours from when symptoms stop
Hepatitis A	• Rare in the UK. Causes jaundice • Food handlers should remain off work for 7 days after the onset of jaundice +/– other symptom
Entamoeba histolytica **(Amoebic dysentery)**	• In addition to the normal 48-hour exclusion, a single negative stool sample taken at least a week after the end of treatment
Shigella dysenteriae, *flexneri,* **and** *boydii*	• Rare in the UK • In addition to the normal 48-hour exclusion, need two consecutive negative stool samples taken at intervals of at least 48 hours
Threadworm and *Taenia solium*	• Exclude from direct handling and serving of open ready-to-eat foods until the infected person is treated
Vibrio cholerae **01 and** **0139**	• Rare in the UK • Excluded for 48 hours after symptoms have resolved and need two consecutive negative stool samples taken at intervals of at least 24 hours

Infected or injured skin

- Damaged skin or sores caused by injury or disease (e.g. boils and septic cuts) can become infected with bacteria such as *Staphylococcus aureus*, which can cause food poisoning.
- Symptoms of infection include scaling, weeping or discharge from lesions.
- It is usually acceptable to continue working with food as long as the infected area is completely covered, e.g. by use of a distinctively coloured, waterproof dressing.
- If an infected lesion cannot be effectively covered then the person should be excluded from any work likely to lead to the contamination of food.
- Lesions not possible to cover adequately include weeping eyes, ears, mouth and gums.

Further reading

- Food Standards Agency. *Food Handlers: fitness to work*. London: Food Standards Agency; 2009. Available at: www.food.gov.uk/multimedia/pdfs/publication/fitnesstoworkguide09v3. pdf (accessed 20 November 2010).
- World Gastroenterology Organisation. *World Gastroenterology Organisation Practice Guideline: acute diarrhea*. Milwaukee, WI: World Gastroenterology Organisation; 2008. Available at: www.worldgastroenterology.org/assets/downloads/en/pdf/guidelines/01_acute_ diarrhea.pdf (accessed 20 November 2010).

Station 2.4

Actor's notes

Background
- You are Janet Smith, a 25-year-old legal secretary.

Opening statement
- 'Hi Doctor. My father has Huntington's disease and I wonder if I should be tested.'

History
- Your 45-year-old father was diagnosed with Huntington's disease (HD) two weeks ago. Over the last year, he developed some uncontrollable movements of his arms. He is becoming clumsy and forgetful. Your mother was worried so arranged to see the GP who organised a referral to the hospital. He had a brain scan and some other tests (you are not sure which ones), and was told that he has HD.
- You looked at several websites about HD because you have never heard of it before.

Ideas, concerns and expectations
- You are worried about how the condition will affect your father and wonder if it will affect you.
- You are about to get married and are scared your partner may cancel the wedding if you have HD.
- You are also worried about passing on the condition to your children.
- You are unsure what to declare to the life insurance and mortgage company.
- You have come to the GP to find out more about HD – how it progresses, if you could develop the condition, what the test involves and whether you should have it.

Further history candidate may elicit
- You are currently fit and well with no symptoms. You are not depressed.
- Your mother is the main carer for your father. They work together in their newsagent shop.
- Your father is fully mobile and largely independent, eating and washing himself. However, he is frequently dropping things, has had a few falls, is becoming forgetful and has involuntary arm movements.
- You discussed your father's diagnosis with your partner. He suggested you should make a decision as to whether you want to have the test or not. You live together in a rented flat and plan to buy a flat together after marriage.
- You are using oral contraception at present and aim to stop when you get married as you and your partner are keen to start a family soon.

Drug history
- Microgynon 30 as prescribed.

Social history
- You do not smoke but drink alcohol on special occasions.
- You live with your partner and have been with him for five years. He works as an accountant.

Family history
- Your father is the only person in the family with HD. He was adopted so does not know if his parents or siblings were affected. Your brother, sister and mother are all well.

Approach to scenario
- You come across as being quite scared about the change in your father, and worried he will get worse.
- You are terrified about developing HD as you have read on the internet that it can be 'awful' and feel anxious about how your partner may react.
- At the beginning, you are not sure whether to have the test and ask the doctor 'What would you do?'
- However, if the doctor discusses the test with you and explains the pros and cons fully, you decide to take some time to think before having the test.
- If the doctor does not come across well, you get upset and say 'You don't care, do you?'
- You are happy to come back to see the doctor if they do not have all the information at hand, and will agree to see a genetic specialist, if suggested by the doctor, to discuss this further.

Information gathering
Presenting complaint
- Ask how her father was diagnosed with the disease.
- Discuss her reasons for wanting the test.
- Explore what she knows about the test.
- Check if she is being forced to have the test.
- Check if she understands how the disease is transmitted.
- Check whether she has any current symptoms.

Medical history
- Any other medical condition.

Family history
- Ask about children, siblings, cousins, aunts, uncles or grandparents.

Drug history
- Check if the patient is on any contraception at present.

Social history
- Alcohol and smoking.
- Marital status.
- Occupation.
- Family support.

Patient's agenda
- Explore her understanding about HD and the test available.
- Explore her concerns about her father's diagnosis:
  — her father's health
  — the possibility she may have the disease
  — transmission to her children
  — potential effect on her social and financial life.

Clinical management

1 Discuss Huntington's disease with the patient

- Briefly explain the clinical manifestations of HD.
- Explain that prevention, cure or specific treatments are not currently available **but** may be available in the future.
- Explain that the prognosis of the disease is variable.
- Explain that the risk of her having the disease is 50%.

2 Discuss the test with the patient

- Advise the patient that she does not have to take the test, and should not feel pressurised into making a decision.
- Explain that the test requires a blood sample to check for the genetic mutation causing the disease.
- Explain that the test is not 100% accurate, and if she is found to have HD, the exact age of onset or severity of the disease cannot be predicted.
- Offer referral to the local genetics team for the blood test.

3 Discuss the consequences of the results

- If negative, explain that the patient does not have the disease and cannot pass the disease on to her children.
- If positive, explain this means that she will develop the disease further on in life.
- Explore the psychological impact of a positive test on the patient, her partner and family.
- Discuss the social consequences of a positive test on future employment and life insurance, explaining she will need to declare the results when applying for future jobs or life insurance.
- Explain that if she tests positive, she could consider selective embryo transfer or adoption so that she does not pass on the condition to her child.
- Explain that antenatal diagnosis with choriocentesis and amniocentesis are also available, which can determine if the baby is a carrier for HD. If so, a termination of pregnancy could be considered.

4 Discuss the alternatives available

- Do not take the test.
- Discuss with family/partner/friends and then return to be referred for the test.
- Refer patient to a specialist today to discuss further and have the test.

5 Provide further information

- Provide her with information leaflets on HD.
- Inform her of the Huntington's Disease Association (www.hda.org.uk) and offer information leaflets.
- Encourage her to discuss this with her family and partner.
- Offer her a follow-up appointment to discuss any other issues or arrange a referral.

Interpersonal skills

- Use a range of open questions.
  - 'What do you understand about Huntington's disease, also called HD?'
  - 'How did you feel when you found out your father was diagnosed with HD?'
- Recognise the patient's concerns about being affected with Huntington's disease:
  - 'I understand you are worried about developing HD. What are your main concerns?'
  - 'I appreciate you are concerned at how your partner may react if the test is positive. Have you shared your fears with him?'
- Communicate risk in lay terms.
  - 'The risk of you developing the disease is 50% or 1 in 2. If your father had 100 children, then 50 would develop the condition and 50 would be unaffected. I cannot tell you which group you would fit into.'

- Discuss the test with the patient.
  - 'This test, like any test, is not 100% accurate. If you test negative, it would be very reassuring for you, and you would not pass on the condition to your children.'
  - 'However, if it is positive, you will have to live with the knowledge that you will develop the condition at some stage later on in life. Unfortunately we cannot tell you exactly when the condition would affect you, or if it will be mild or severe.'
  - 'Have you thought how you would react if you knew the test was positive?'
- Discuss the possibility of transmitting HD to her children.
  - 'If you have HD, there is a 50% chance that you would transmit it to your children. So if you had 100 children, 50 would be affected and 50 would not be affected.'
  - 'Some people who have a positive test choose never to have children. Others have children because they know that there is a good chance the child will never develop HD, and if they do, they would have years of normal life before developing the disease.'
  - 'Nowadays, you can have IVF, which is a fertility treatment available even if your fertility is normal. A specialist takes out your eggs and analyses them. The eggs that do not carry HD are then fertilised with your partner's sperm and implanted back in you. That way, even if you have HD, your child will not.'
  - 'If you get pregnant naturally, there are some special tests, called choriocentesis and amniocentesis, which involve taking a sample of tissue or fluid from around the baby. These tests can tell you if your baby has HD. If positive, then some couples may think about terminating the pregnancy.'
- If you do not know much about HD, explain this to the patient.
  - 'Unfortunately I do not know very much about this rare condition. However, I can look it up and speak with my colleagues later today, and either call you or see you again.'
- Negotiate a shared management plan with the patient, aiming for her to explore her options fully, and being open to a referral depending on her request.

> ⊙━ **Key summary**
> - Elicit her current understanding of HD.
> - Explore her concerns about developing the disease herself, and passing it on to her children.
> - Communicate risk to the patient and discuss the pros and cons of genetic testing.
> - Offer support to the patient in terms of follow-up, information and support groups.

Huntington's disease
Pathology
- Autosomal dominant, trinucleotide repeat disorder.
- A mutation of distal short arm of chromosome four leads to degeneration of neuronal cells in basal ganglia and caudate nucleus resulting in a progressive, terminal neurological disease.

Clinical features
a Physical
- Jerky, random, involuntary movements – 'chorea'.
- Lack of coordination.
- Unsteady gait.
- Difficulty with speech and swallowing.

b Cognitive
- Lack of concentration.
- Short-term memory loss.

c Psychological
- Anxiety.
- Depression.

- Aggressive behaviour.
- Compulsivity.

Treatment

a Medical

- Antidepressants for low mood.
- Antipsychotics for psychotic symptoms.

b Multidisciplinary

- Speech therapy for speech and swallowing problems.
- Social services and occupational therapy for home adaptations.

Prognosis

- Onset of HD is related to the number of CAG repeats in the gene.
- The higher the number of repeats, the sooner the onset.
- Onset usually occurs at 30–40 years of age. Life expectancy is 10–25 years after the onset of symptoms.
- Death usually occurs due to pneumonia or other infections. Other causes include falls and suicide.

Genetic screening

TABLE 2.5 Examples of autosomal dominant, autosomal recessive and X-linked recessive conditions

AUTOSOMAL DOMINANT	AUTOSOMAL RECESSIVE	X-LINKED RECESSIVE
HD	Sickle-cell anaemia	Duchenne muscular dystrophy
Charcot–Marie–Tooth disease	Cystic fibrosis	Becker's muscular dystrophy
Neurofibromatosis	Thalassaemia	Fragile X syndrome
Myotonic dystrophy		Haemophilia A and B
Osteogenesis imperfecta		
Haemochromatosis		
Polycystic kidney disease		

Further reading

- Huntington's Disease Association website. www.hda.org.uk (accessed 22 November 2010).
- Genetics Home Reference. *Genetic Conditions.* US National Library of Medicine; 2011. Available at: http://ghr.nlm.nih.gov/BrowseConditions (accessed 22 November 2010).
- Bradley-Smith G, Hope S, Firth HV, *et al. Oxford Handbook of Genetics.* Oxford: Oxford University Press; 2009.

Station 2.5

St Wonderful Hospital
St Wonderful Road
St Wonderful
ST1 WOND

Dear GP

Thank you for referring this gentleman who has a four-month history of worsening tremor.

He clearly has a diagnosis of PD and I have advised him to start on Sinemet 62.5 mg tds. I have given him a prescription today.

I would be grateful if you could continue prescribing this for him and I will review him again in three months to see how he is getting on.

Kind regards
Dr B Rain

Actor's notes
Background
- You are Jack Spade, a 70-year-old retired music teacher.

Opening statement
- 'Hello Doctor. I wanted your advice about these tablets.'

History
- You saw a specialist last week who told you that you have Parkinson's disease (PD). You have not heard of this condition before, and the specialist was too busy to explain it to you properly.
- He gave you a prescription for some tablets that 'act on the brain'. You collected the tablets from the hospital pharmacy, but have not started taking them as you are concerned about taking tablets that affect your brain.

Ideas, concerns and expectations
- You do not understand what PD is, or why it has happened.
- You want to know whether this condition can be passed on to your children, and if they need to have any tests now.
- You are worried about taking tablets that 'act on the brain' and the multiple side effects that you have read in the leaflet. You are unsure how the tablets would help your symptoms.

- You are worried that you have a brain tumour that the specialist has missed.
- You have come to the GP to find out more about PD, the medications and to ask whether you need a brain scan or second opinion from another specialist.

Further history candidate may elicit
- You noticed a mild tremor in your hands a few months ago, which is worse on the right side.
- It occurs at rest and disappears when you move your hand or arm. It is becoming progressively worse.
- Movements of your hands seem to be getting slower. This is particularly noticeable when you are playing the piano because you cannot seem to move your hands quickly enough. You find this very frustrating, so saw the GP for advice, who suggested you see a specialist.
- You saw the hospital doctor last week who examined you and said you had PD.
- You asked him about this and he told you it was a 'brain disorder'. He gave you some tablets that 'act on the brain'. He was rushed and you did not have an opportunity to ask him more.
- You collected the tablets from the hospital pharmacy and read the side effects on the leaflet, noting they included movement disorders. You did not take the tablets as you are worried they may make your symptoms worse, and wonder if the specialist gave you the correct medication.
- If asked, your legs seem stiff, and it is getting more difficult for you to stand up from a chair.
- If asked, your wife has mentioned you do not smile much these days, but you have not noticed any change in your mood. You have been drooling from the mouth recently.
- If asked, your handwriting seems less neat and is smaller than before.
- You are mainly concerned about the tremor and slowness of your hands. You have put these changes down to 'old age'.
- You have had no falls, constipation, urinary incontinence or difficulties with balance, speech, swallowing or memory. You have not had any headaches, syncope or visual problems.

Medical history
- PD.

Drug history
- Sinemet 62.5 mg tds.

Family history
- Nil relevant.

Social history
- You drink occasionally and do not smoke.
- You are a retired music teacher who still plays the piano daily.
- You live with your wife in a three-bedroom house.
- You have two sons and several grandchildren who live locally.

Approach to scenario
- You are mainly concerned about the slowness of your hand movements and the effect this has on playing the piano – you have played the piano with ease for 60 years and are distressed that you are struggling to play pieces of music that you have played for years.
- You are worried that the specialist suggested there is something wrong with your brain and ask the doctor 'Would Parkinson's disease cause a brain tumour? Is that the problem?'
- You want to know if you should have a 'brain scan' to show up any abnormality.
- You ask the doctor if PD is a condition you pass on to your children, and wonder if they need to be tested.
- Having read the multiple side effects, you are scared of starting the medications the specialist recommended. You wonder if the specialist has given you the wrong medication because the leaflet that came with the tablets suggested you could develop problems with movements of

your arms and legs – you are worried that if you take these tablets the tremor and slowness of your hands will get worse and you will not be able to play the piano.

- You want to know how the tremor and slowness in your hands can get better, and if you need a second opinion.
- If the doctor comes across well and is able to explain what PD is, how it can be treated and reassure you that you do not have a brain tumour, you agree to take the medication and see how you do.
- If the doctor does not come across well, is unable to effectively explain what PD is, or cannot provide reassurance about the medication, you refuse to take the medication and demand a second opinion, stating 'I think you have missed a brain tumour'.

Information gathering
Presenting complaint
a Tremor
- Ask when the tremor began.
- Check if it is unilateral or bilateral.
- Check if it affects the upper limbs, lower limbs or both.

b Rigidity
- Ask about muscle pain and stiffness.
- Ask about falls and poor balance.

c Poverty of movement
- Drooling of saliva.
- Slowness of movement (bradykinesia).
- Difficulty in writing (micrographia).
- Difficulty turning in bed.
- Change in voice (voice often softer in PD).
- Lack of facial expression.

d Other symptoms
- Constipation.
- Urinary incontinence.
- Memory loss.
- Changes in behaviour.
- Swallowing difficulties.

e Neurological history
- Fits.
- Syncope.
- Headache.
- Visual problems.

Medical history
- Encephalitis or brain injury.

Family history
- Parkinson's or other neurological disease.

Drug history
- Parkinson's medications.
- Use of neuroleptics (reserpine) and metoclopramide.

Social history
- Occupation.
- Smoking and alcohol.
- Home and financial circumstances.

Patient's agenda
- Explore his understanding of PD.
- Explore his concerns about his symptoms, medications and possible brain tumour.
- Clarify what help he would like from you.

Examination
- Offer to examine his upper limbs, cranial nerves and perform fundoscopy.
- 'If it's okay with you, I will check the nerves to your arms and face, and your eyes.'

Examination card

General examination	Mask-like facies
Neurological examination	Upper limbs = bradykinesia of hands
	Resting right-sided tremor
	Tremor resolves on action
	Tone = cog-wheel rigidity
	Power = normal
	Reflexes = normal
	Sensation = normal
	Coordination = normal
	Fundoscopy = normal

Clinical management
1 Discuss the diagnosis of Parkinson's disease
- Reassure him that his history and examination does not suggest a brain tumour, but does suggest PD. This condition is not associated with brain tumours.
- Explain that PD is a progressive degenerative neurological condition that occurs due to degeneration of dopamine neurones in the substantia nigra.
- This leads to low levels of dopamine, which results in impairment of movement. Outline that although the condition deteriorates with time, the speed of progression varies from person to person and cannot be predicted.
- Explain that PD is diagnosed on the basis of a clinical history (tremor, rigidity and poverty in movements) and a positive response to the drug dopamine.
- Explain that there is no 'diagnostic test' – brain imaging is not routinely required, and is only used to exclude other possible diagnoses.
- Explain that PD is not usually inherited, so his children and grandchildren are unlikely to be affected. There is no test available for screening.

2 Discuss the management of Parkinson's disease
- Explain that PD can be treated with medication that increases dopamine levels in the brain.
- Reassure the patient that the specialist **has** prescribed the correct medication – this increases the dopamine levels in the brain, so improving the symptoms of tremor, rigidity and bradykinesia.
- Discuss the side effects of levodopa, explaining that nausea is common but less likely if the initial dose is low and increased slowly.
- Explain that patients often have a very positive response to levodopa. However, it works less well over time, and so the dose may need to be increased.

- Explain that the involuntary movement side effects are associated with long-term use:
  — 'on-off' effects where the patient switches from being 'on' and mobile to 'off' and immobile
  — dyskinesias causing jerky and involuntary movements.
- Advise the patient that other drugs are available if levodopa is not beneficial.
- Outline that other therapies are available:
  — physiotherapy to help maintain posture and walking
  — occupational therapy to advise on home adaptations.

3 Offer follow-up
- Reassure the patient that he does not need brain imaging or a second opinion at present.
- Provide him with the details of the Parkinson's Disease Society (www.parkinsons.org.uk) so he can access information and support.
- Offer him leaflets on PD.
- Suggest he returns to see you in a few weeks to review his response to the levodopa.

Interpersonal skills
- During this case, the candidate would be expected to make a diagnosis of PD based on the clinical presentation. In addition, the candidate needs to address the concerns of the patient and manage the uncertainty of the disease progression.
- The candidate should explain the diagnosis to the patient without using complex medical terms.
  — 'Firstly, I want to reassure you that the symptoms you have described do not point to a brain tumour. However, your symptoms do point towards PD, which the specialist mentioned to you. Have you heard of this condition before, or discussed it with anyone since speaking to the specialist?'
  — 'People with Parkinson's disease have many of the symptoms that you have, such as a tremor of the hand or arm, slow movements of the arms or legs and muscle stiffness. There is no specific test, like a blood test or brain scan, that can diagnose Parkinson's disease.'
  — 'Parkinson's disease occurs because the brain cells in one part of the brain start to deteriorate. These brain cells control your muscles, and as they deteriorate your movements are affected more and more. We don't know why the cells are damaged in the first place, but the result is that the level of a special chemical called dopamine, falls.'
  — 'Dopamine is a special chemical that works in the brain and helps you move your muscles properly. The medication the specialist prescribed works by increasing the level of this chemical back to normal and helping the muscles work properly again.'
  — 'Many patients find this drug very useful, but with time it can become less effective. As you read in the leaflet, if you use this drug for a long time, you could start developing some involuntary movements that happen automatically, but obviously we would monitor you for side effects and may need to switch drugs if that happened.'
  — 'Many people have Parkinson's disease and lead a normal life for many years with this drug. It is an unpredictable condition and unfortunately I cannot say when it will get worse. However, I would encourage you to try the medication because it could help you keep playing the piano for some time to come.'

O⊶ **Key summary**
- Reassure the patient they do not have a brain tumour.
- Recognise the clinical features of PD.
- Be able to explain the diagnosis and management to the patient.
- Manage the uncertainty of a progressive disease.
- Address concerns about the need for further tests and the side effects of the medications.

Drugs used in Parkinson's disease
- Drugs are used to correct the imbalance of neurotransmitters, but do not correct the underlying destruction of dopamine neurones. Treatment for PD should be initiated by a consultant and patients should be reviewed every 6–12 months.

Dopaminergic drugs
a L-dopa
- Usually first-line treatment for people with early PD.
- This is a precursor of dopamine and increases dopamine levels in the substantia nigra.
- Helps with bradykinesia and rigidity but does not help tremor much.
- Comes in preparations combined with an inhibitor of peripheral dopa decarboxylase (co-beneldopa or co-careldopa) to prevent peripheral breakdown of L-dopa to dopamine and reduce side effects of nausea, vomiting and cardiovascular effects.
- Side effects include involuntary movements, 'on-off' fluctuations and 'end of dose' effect.

b Dopamine receptor (D2) agonists
- These drugs act directly on dopamine receptors.
- Can be an alternative first-line treatment in early PD because it:
  — can control motor symptoms (although less effective than L-dopa).
  — is associated with fewer motor complications than L-dopa.
- Can be used in conjunction with L-dopa in advanced disease to control fluctuations in response.
- Two types of preparations are available:
  — ergot-related, e.g. bromocriptine, cabergoline, lisuride and pergolide
  — non-ergot-related, e.g. ropinirole, pramipexole and rotigotine.
- Non-ergot-related drugs are preferred as ergot preparations are associated with fibrotic disease.
- Ergot-related preparations should be considered if CXR, spirometry, creatinine and ESR are normal. These drugs should be stopped if dyspnoea, persistent cough, cardiac failure or abdominal tenderness develops.

c Apomorphine
- This is a potent dopamine agonist that can be useful in advanced disease to decrease 'off' periods with L-dopa.
- It is administered via subcutaneous injection or subcutaneous infusion.

d Amantadine
- Weak dopamine agonist that improves mild bradykinesia, tremor, rigidity.
- May be useful for dyskinesias in more advanced disease.

e Monoamine oxidase type B (MAO-B) inhibitors
- Examples include rasagiline and selegiline.
- Selegiline can be used in early PD to postpone treatment with L-dopa.
- Both drugs can be used in advanced PD to reduce 'end of dose' effect with L-dopa.

f Catechol-O-methyltransferase (COMT) inhibitors
- Examples include entacapone and tolcapone.
- Act by inhibiting the COMT enzyme, thus preventing the peripheral breakdown of L-dopa, allowing more levodopa to reach the brain.
- Second-line treatment used as an adjunct to co-beneldopa or co-careldopa for patients who experience 'end of dose' deteriorations.

Anticholinergic drugs
- Examples include benzhexol, orphenadrine and procyclidine.
- Act by reducing the relative central cholinergic excess that results from dopamine deficiency.
- Can be useful in drug-induced parkinsonism but generally not used in idiopathic PD because they are less effective than dopaminergic drugs.
- Effective for tremor and rigidity, but little affect on bradykinesia.

Diagnosis of Parkinson's disease
- PD results from progressive degeneration of dopaminergic cells of the substantia nigra, resulting in disruption of the normal dopamine:acetylcholine ratio.
- PD is a clinical diagnosis based on the presence of bradykinesia plus ≥1 of:
  — muscular rigidity
  — rest tremor (4 to 6 Hz)
  — postural instability (unrelated to visual, cerebellar, vestibular or proprioceptive dysfunction).

Parkinsonism
- 'Parkinsonism' denotes a syndrome that appears to be clinically similar to idiopathic PD but has a different pathological or aetiological basis.

TABLE 2.6 Causes of a parkinsonian syndrome

CAUSE	EXAMPLE
Neurological disease	Multiple cerebral infarction
	Alzheimer's disease
	Progressive supranuclear palsy (Steele–Richardson–Olszewski syndrome)
	Multiple system atrophy (Shy–Drager syndrome)
Drugs (especially dopamine antagonists)	Phenothiazines
	Reserpine
	Haloperidol
Toxins	1-methyl-4-phenyl-1.2.3.6-tetrahydropyridine (MPTP)
Trauma	Repetitive head injury, e.g. boxing

Further reading
- Parkinson's Disease Society website. www.parkinsons.org.uk (accessed 22 November 2010).
- National Institute for Health and Clinical Excellence. Parkinson's Disease: NICE guideline 35. London: NIHCE; 2006. http://guidance.nice.org.uk/CG35 (accessed 22 November 2010).
- Manji H, Connolly S, Dorward N, *et al*. *Oxford Handbook of Neurology*. Oxford: Oxford University Press; 2006.

Station 2.6

Actor's notes

Background
- You are Judy Child, a 40-year-old lawyer.

Opening statement
- 'Doctor, I've come for my 36-week antenatal check-up.'

History
- This is your first pregnancy and you feel well.
- Your ankles and feet are very swollen but you know this is common in pregnancy.
- Your midwife reassured you 'everything's fine' when you saw her four weeks ago.

Ideas, concerns and expectations
- You are excited to be pregnant and looking forward to the birth of your baby.
- Your sister had pre-eclampsia and her baby was stillborn.
- You are worried about developing pre-eclampsia because you think your baby would be brain damaged or stillborn.

Further history candidate may elicit
- This is your first pregnancy. Unfortunately, you were unable to conceive naturally with your partner, so opted for IVF. The first cycle was unsuccessful and you were scared that you would never conceive.
- You and your partner were delighted to hear the second cycle was successful and you were pregnant. You and your family are very excited about the pregnancy.
- You know the baby is a boy. You and your partner have chosen the name 'Matthew'.
- Over the last two weeks, you have been working very hard at work so that you can complete as much as possible before you go on maternity leave. Your work colleagues are happy for you and have been very supportive.
- You have had some vague headaches over the last few days, which you think are a result of working long hours. You did not take any painkillers because you want to avoid medication in pregnancy. The headaches occur intermittently through the day. They are getting worse.
- You have felt nauseous over the last few days but have not vomited. The nausea can occur with or without the headaches. Your ankles are swollen. You think the nausea and ankle swelling are normal in pregnancy.
- You do not have any migrainous features, visual problems, epigastric pain or urinary symptoms.
- You have felt the baby move every day.

Medical history
- Nil.

Drug history
- Folic acid for the first trimester of pregnancy.

Social history
- You do not smoke and have not had any alcohol since becoming pregnant.
- You are a successful lawyer in a large law firm and are married to an IT consultant.
- Your husband is very supportive and you are very close to your family.

Family history
- You have one younger sister who developed pre-eclampsia in her first pregnancy.
- Unfortunately, this resulted in a stillbirth. She subsequently had two healthy children.
- Your mother had two pregnancies with no complications.

Approach to scenario
- At the start of the consultation, you are bright and cheerful. You come across excited about having your baby, but become anxious during the consultation when you are made aware that there may be problems.
- You mention the headaches and nausea only if the doctor asks. You do not seem to attribute much significance to these symptoms and comment 'I'm sure most women feel sick in pregnancy'.
- If asked about headaches, you begin by saying 'I have had some headaches for the last two weeks or so, probably because of the long hours I've been working. But I'm sure they will settle down'.
- If the GP explains that your baby is not growing normally, you become alarmed and ask 'Is my baby brain damaged?'
- If the doctor explains you may have pre-eclampsia or need further investigation, you become extremely concerned and tearful, asking 'Is my baby going to die like my sister's baby?'
- You want to know why this has happened, if it is your fault and related to the long hours at work.
- You want to know what the consequences are and what treatment is available.
- If the doctor mentions you may have to deliver the baby early, you become anxious and say 'It's too soon for my baby to be born. Isn't it safer to leave him inside? What will happen to him?'
- If the doctor comes across well and reassures you that there are special units to look after premature babies, you stop crying.
- If the doctor does not come across well, you continue crying and become more upset.

Information gathering
Presenting complaint
a Current pregnancy
- Confirm her expected date of delivery (EDD) and how many weeks pregnant she is.
- Confirm she has had regular antenatal appointments.
- Ask about:
  — foetal movements
  — problems in this pregnancy.

b IVF treatment
- Enquire about reasons for IVF and the number of cycles needed.

c *Previous pregnancies*
- Ask about previous pregnancies, complications and delivery.

d *Symptoms of pre-eclampsia*
- Enquire about:
  - headaches
  - blurred vision
  - epigastric pain
  - ankle, face or hand swelling.

e *Other symptoms*
- Enquire about:
  - per vaginam (PV) bleeding
  - PV discharge.

Medical history
- Any other medical condition, particularly:
  - hypertension
  - diabetes
  - autoimmune disease
  - cardiac or renal disease
  - thromboembolic disease.

Family history
- Pre-eclampsia affecting pregnancies of mother or sisters.

Drug history
- Current medications.

Social history
- Enquire about:
  - alcohol and smoking
  - current occupation
  - plans for maternity leave
  - marital status and support from partner.

Patient's agenda
- Explore her understanding of pre-eclampsia.
- Explore her concerns about losing her baby.

Examination
- Offer to examine her abdomen, ankles, perform fundoscopy, check her BP and dipstick her urine.
- 'If it's okay, I'll check your tummy and listen to the baby's heart. After that I'll check the back of your eyes, your blood pressure and urine.'

Examination card
General

| Urine dipstick | = protein ++ | BP | = 155/95 mmHg |
| | no blood or leucocytes | BP at booking clinic | = 111/77 mmHg |

Abdominal

| SFH | = 32 cm | Foetal movements | = felt |
| Foetal position | = cephalic | Foetal heartbeat | = 140/minute |

Other

| Fundoscopy | = normal | Ankles | = bilateral oedema |

Clinical management

1 Explain your findings of the antenatal check-up

- Explain that her BP is elevated and she has protein in her urine.
- Explain that the baby appears to be 'smaller than expected' but reassure her that the heartbeat is normal and you can feel the baby move.
- Advise her that in view of the examination findings, and taking into account her symptoms of headache and nausea, she is likely to have developed pre-eclampsia.

2 Discuss the aetiology and complications of pre-eclampsia

a Aetiology

- Reassure her that this condition is not her fault, and not related to working long hours.
- Explain that any woman can develop pre-eclampsia, but particular risk factors include:
  — maternal age <17 years or >40 years
  — first pregnancy or first pregnancy with a new partner
  — history of pre-eclampsia
  — family history of pre-eclampsia
  — pregnancy with twins or triplets
  — history of hypertension, diabetes, systemic lupus erythematosus (SLE) or renal disease prior to getting pregnant.
- Explain that the exact cause of pre-eclampsia is unknown but may be related to abnormal development of blood vessels in the placenta, which affects the transfer of oxygen and nutrients to the baby.
- Explain that pre-eclampsia is progressive and unpredictable. It is often treated with antihypertensives while being monitored on an antenatal ward. Delivery is the only definitive cure but this decision would be made by an obstetrician in hospital.

b Complications

- Discuss the maternal complications associated with pre-eclampsia:
  — stroke
  — seizures
  — pulmonary oedema
  — liver and renal failure
  — blood clotting disorders and severe bleeding from the placenta.
- Discuss the complications for the baby:
  — intrauterine growth restriction
  — stillbirth due to placental abruption.

3 Discuss urgent referral to hospital

- Advise her to attend hospital immediately.
- Explain you will refer her to the obstetric team who will monitor her and the baby to prevent any further complications. They will do some further tests:
  — 24-hour protein measurement

— monitoring of BP
— cardiotochography (CTG)
— ultrasound to assess foetal growth
— blood tests to check maternal hepatic and renal function.

4 Explain the management of pre-eclampsia

- Antihypertensive drugs to reduce BP.
- Magnesium sulphate used for eclampsia.
- Steroids may be given to promote foetal pulmonary maturity if gestation is <34 weeks.
- Delivery of the baby if the pre-eclampsia is severe or uncontrolled. This may be through inducing pregnancy or by caesarean section.
- Reassure her that specialist units are available to care for premature babies.

5 Other suggestions

- Offer to contact her husband to explain the situation and accompany/meet her at hospital.

Interpersonal skills

- During this station, the candidate should be able to diagnose pre-eclampsia and the need for urgent admission under the care of the obstetrics team, whilst delivering this news delicately to the expectant mother.
- The findings of the antenatal examination should be explained clearly and sensitively, recognising that the patient will be alarmed to hear that a complication has arisen.
  - 'I've finished the antenatal check-up and I want to explain what I've found. Unfortunately, your blood pressure is mildly raised at 145/90 mmHg. Ideally, it should be below 140/90 mmHg. In addition, I found some protein in your urine. Normally, this is not present.'
  - 'When I examined your tummy, I noticed your tummy is smaller than I'd expect it to be. This suggests that your baby isn't growing as normally as we'd expect.'
  - 'However, I would like to reassure you that currently the baby's heartbeat is normal and he is moving well.'
  - 'Your headaches and nausea are probably related to your high blood pressure and the protein in the urine. I think you may have developed a condition that only occurs in pregnancy called pre-eclampsia. This can affect the baby's growth. Have you heard about this?'
- It is important to provide an explanation of the condition in lay terms and reassure the patient that it is unrelated to her work pattern.
  - 'Pre-eclampsia does not happen because of working long hours. This is not your fault and there is nothing you did to make it happen.'
  - 'Pre-eclampsia is a condition that affects pregnant women. Although the exact cause is unknown, it is thought that the blood vessels in the placenta, which provide oxygen and nutrients to the baby, are abnormal. This can affect the growth of the baby.'
  - 'Although your baby seems smaller than expected, I can't say whether there has been any damage to the brain. We need to do some urgent tests on you and the baby to keep you both well.'
- The candidate would be expected to show empathy and understanding of her concern and distress about possibly losing her baby. Use of silence at appropriate times may aid the consultation.
  - 'I can understand how special this pregnancy is for you. Going through IVF could not have been easy.'
  - 'Seeing your sister lose her baby because of pre-eclampsia must have been extremely distressing for all of you.'
  - 'Of course you and your baby's health and well-being are of high priority to everyone who is involved in your care. By treating you as soon as possible, the risks to you and your baby are reduced.'

Pre-eclampsia

- Pre-eclampsia is a disease unique to pregnancy after 20 weeks' gestation.
- It is characterised by pregnancy-induced hypertension and proteinuria, which is often accompanied by oedema.
- The BHS criteria for the diagnosis of pre-eclampsia are:
  — BP rise of >15 mmHg diastolic or >30 mmHg systolic from early pregnancy **or**
  — dBP >90 mmHg on two occasions 4 hours apart **or**
  — dBP >110 mmHg on one occasion **and** proteinuria.

Pathogenesis

- Studies suggest that pre-eclampsia results from poor placental perfusion, which occurs due to:
  — a large placenta
  — abnormal trophoblast implantation and spiral artery atherosis
  — microvascular disease due to pre-existing hypertension or diabetes.
- Poor placental perfusion results in the release of substances that cause endothelial cell dysfunction, increased sensitivity to normal circulating pressor agents, increased intracellular coagulation and increased fluid loss from the intravascular compartment.

Risk factors
a Maternal factors
- Primiparity or first pregnancy with a new partner.
- Previous pre-eclampsia.
- Family history of pre-eclampsia.
- BMI >35.
- Age <20 or >40 years.
- Idiopathic hypertension, chronic renal disease, diabetes, SLE or thrombophilia.
- Multiple pregnancy.

b Foetal factors (associated with increased placental size)
- Multiple pregnancy.
- Hydrops.
- Hydatiform mole.

Clinical features
- Often asymptomatic and detected by routine screening alone.

TABLE 2.7 Clinical features of pre-eclampsia

SYMPTOMS	SIGNS
Headache	Hypertension
Epigastric pain	Proteinuria
Vomiting	Ascites
Oedema of face, hands or ankles	Hyper-reflexia
Visual disturbance with flashing lights	Excessive weight gain
	Foetus small for gestational age

Complications

Maternal

- Eclampsia.
- Disseminated intravascular coagulation (DIC).
- Cerebral haemorrhage.
- HELLP syndrome (see below on this page).
- Liver failure and hepatic rupture.
- Renal failure due to acute renal tubular and/or cortical rupture.
- Pulmonary oedema.
- Placental abruption.
- Maternal death (resulting from any of these complications).

Foetal

- Intrauterine growth retardation.
- Pre-term delivery and complications of prematurity.
- Stillbirth – often due to placental abruption or hypoxia.

HELLP syndrome

- H: haemolysis, EL: elevated liver enzymes, LP: low platelets.
- Due to clotting abnormalities and hepatic dysfunction.
- Can be life threatening with hepatic necrosis, rupture and exsanguination.

Treatment

- The only cure for pre-eclampsia is to deliver the baby and placenta, despite possible risk to the foetus. Delivery may be induced or performed via caesarean section. The decision to deliver involves considering maternal factors (what symptoms and signs are present in the mother, whether a pre-eclamptic crisis is imminent) and foetal factors (gestational age – if it would be safer in a neonatal unit or remaining inside the maternal environment).
- Antihypertensives may be used. Methyldopa is the drug of choice in pregnancy. Calcium antagonists, hydralazine and labetalol are also used.
- Magnesium sulphate is the treatment of choice for convulsions in eclampsia and reduces the risk of eclampsia for women with pre-eclampsia.
- Low-dose aspirin can be used in women at risk of pre-eclampsia.
- Calcium supplementation during pregnancy has been shown to reduce the risk of pre-eclampsia, particularly in women with low dietary calcium intake.

Further reading

- Preeclampsia Foundation website. www.preeclampsia.org (accessed 22 November 2010).
- Simon C, Everitt H, van Dorp F. *Oxford Handbook of General Practice.* 3rd ed. Oxford: Oxford University Press; 2010.
- Impey L, Child T. *Obstetrics and Gynaecology.* 3rd ed. Oxford: Wiley-Blackwell; 2008.
- Collier J, Longmore M, Turmezei T, *et al. Oxford Handbook of Clinical Specialties.* 8th ed. Oxford: Oxford University Press; 2009.

Station 2.7

Actor's notes

Background

- You are Ivy Milk, a 22-year-old economics student.

Opening statement

- 'Doctor, I'm a bit concerned I haven't had a period in 10 months.'

History

- You went to China eight months ago as part of your final-year university exchange programme.
- You missed a period before going to China – you were doing your exams at the time.
- You did not have a period when you were away.
- You came home a month ago and have still not had a period.
- You were worried that you might be pregnant because you have had some nipple discharge, but have had four negative pregnancy tests.

Ideas, concerns and expectations

- Initially, you thought you missed your period because of the stress of exams.
- When you did not get your period in China, you put this down to travelling to a foreign country.
- However, you expected your period to return when you came back to the UK.
- Last week, you were watching a 'chat show' with your mother where women with premature menopause described their experiences, including an abrupt stop in their periods.
- You told your mother that you had not had a period in some months, and she became concerned that you may be experiencing a premature menopause, and advised you to see the GP.
- You are concerned that you may be going through a premature menopause and will never be able to have children.
- You have lost interest in sex, and this is causing pressure on your relationship with your boyfriend.
- You have come to the GP to have some tests and to be referred to a specialist.

Further history candidate may elicit

- When in China, your boyfriend visited you for a few weeks, and you did have sex. He used a condom. You noticed an intermittent milky discharge from your breasts and became concerned that you may be pregnant, so you did a pregnancy test, which was negative.
- You repeated the test several times, and it was always negative.
- Your mother advised you repeat the pregnancy test in the UK last week – this was negative.

- If asked, you mention slight blurring at the edges of your vision. You have bumped into the edge of the doorway on occasion. You are short-sighted, and wear contact lenses or glasses.
- You think your prescription may have changed and so are going to see the optician next week.
- If asked, you admit you have had some vague headaches over the last few weeks. You have been working hard with your coursework that needs to be written up for university and assume the headaches are because of the long hours you are working. There are no migrainous features or vomiting associated with the headaches. You do not need painkillers and the headaches usually resolve within a few hours.
- If asked, you have lost interest in sex. This is causing a strain on your relationship because your boyfriend thinks you have 'gone off him' and cannot understand what is wrong.
- If asked, you deny any excess or increase in hair growth, acne, hot flushes, vaginal dryness, weight changes, symptoms of thyroid disease and have not noticed any breast lumps.
- If asked, you rarely exercise as you are busy studying. You do not drive.
- You have found the coursework and exams stressful but there are no other issues.

Obstetric and gynaecological history
- Prior to the 10 months of amenorrhoea, you had regular periods, every month.
- These lasted four to five days and were not heavy or painful.
- You have never taken the oral contraceptive pill and use condoms with your boyfriend.
- You have never been pregnant.

Medical history and drug history
- Nil.

Family history
- Your mother is 49 and still has regular periods. Your sister is 25 and has regular periods.

Social history
- You do not smoke or use recreational drugs. You drink on occasions when with your friends.
- You are a final-year economics student, who lives at home with your mother and sister.
- Your parents are divorced and you rarely see your father who now lives in the USA.

Approach to scenario
- You are concerned that you have not had a period in 10 months and are worried this is related to a premature menopause. You are worried that you may be unable to conceive.
- You want to have some tests, but are not sure which tests are needed. You would like the doctor to explain any tests they suggest.
- You are embarrassed to tell the doctor that you have lost interest in sex, and feel concerned at how this is impacting on your relationship with your boyfriend.
- If the doctor suggests you may have a brain tumour, you look shocked and ask 'Do I have cancer?'
- You are scared of brain surgery because of the potential brain damage that could occur, and do not want any scars. You are scared of taking medication to reduce the tumour because you know that people with tumours who have chemotherapy lose their hair and vomit a lot.
- You want to know if your periods will return, and if your fertility will be preserved. You want to know if the medication you may need to reduce the tumour will affect your fertility.
- If the doctor comes across well, and explains in a caring manner the cause for your symptoms and further management, you feel reassured.
- However, if the doctor does not come across well, you start to cry because you have a brain tumour and think this is going to spread around your body.

Information gathering
Presenting complaint
a Secondary amenorrhoea
- Enquire about her periods, including:
  — last menstrual period (LMP)
  — cycle length
  — painful periods
  — any new changes in periods.

b Consider underlying cause
i Pregnancy
- Ask about UPSI or if she could she be pregnant.
- Check if a pregnancy test has been performed and if so, when.

ii Emotional and physical stress
- Concerns about exams, relationships, finances, etc.
- Ask about exercise and rapid weight loss.

iii Prolactinoma
- Headaches.
- Galactorrhoea.
- Loss of libido.
- Vaginal dryness.
- Visual disturbances.

iv PCOS
- Acne.
- Hirsutism.
- Weight gain.

v Thyroid disorders
- Symptoms of hyper- and hypothyroidism:
  — weight gain or weight loss
  — constipation or diarrhoea
  — intolerance of cold or hot weather

vi Premature menopause
- Hot flushes.
- Vaginal dryness.

Menstrual history
- Age of menarche.
- Frequency of periods.
- Length of periods.
- Heaviness of periods.

Medical history
- Previous abdominal, pelvic or cranial radiotherapy.

Family history
- Premature menopause: ask about mother and sister(s).

Drug history
- Contraceptive pill and history of chemotherapy.

Social history
- Occupation, smoking and alcohol.
- Personal circumstances and relationships.

Patient's agenda
- Explore her understanding of premature menopause.
- Explore her concerns about amenorrhoea and future fertility.
- Explore the impact of loss of libido on her relationship.

Examination
- Offer a chaperone. Offer to check her BP, breasts, cranial nerves, perform fundoscopy and a pregnancy test.
- 'If it's okay with you, I will check your blood pressure and the nerves to your eyes, your breasts, and repeat a pregnancy test.'

Examination card	
General examination	Looks well, no acne or hirsutism
	BMI = 22 kg/m^2
	BP = 125/73 mmHg
	Pregnancy test = negative
Neurological examination	Visual fields = bitemporal hemianopia
	Fundoscopy = optic atrophy
Breast examination	Slight milky discharge from nipples bilaterally
	No breast lump or axillary lymphadenopathy

Clinical management
1 Discuss the cause of secondary amenorrhoea
- Agree with the patient that she needs to be investigated for secondary amenorrhoea.
- Explain there are several causes for secondary amenorrhoea, which can be determined through further tests.
- Reassure her that she does not have features of premature menopause, which include vaginal dryness, hot flushes and a family history.
- Explain that her symptoms of secondary amenorrhoea and galactorrhoea suggest she may have high levels of the hormone prolactin, which is made by the pituitary gland in the brain.
- Explain that this hormone is responsible for lactation and is usually raised in pregnancy and breastfeeding. However, it can be raised with certain medications, or due to a prolactinoma, which is a non-cancerous, benign tumour of the pituitary gland.
- Explain that in view of the headaches and peripheral vision impairment, you feel the likely diagnosis is a prolactinoma. Explain that this is likely to be causing the loss in libido.
- Reassure her that a prolactinoma is not a cancer, and will not spread to other parts of the body.
- Explain that the main problem with prolactinomas results from pressure on the optic chiasm, which can affect vision.
- Fertility is usually preserved once the prolactin levels become normal, and periods and libido return.

2 Discuss further investigations and management
- Advise the patient she will need a blood test to check her hormone levels, including prolactin.
- Explain you can check for other hormones, such as follicle stimulating hormone (FSH)

and luteinising hormone (LH) that are linked to ovulation and so determine if she has premature menopause.

- Explain that you will refer her to the hospital specialist who will arrange for an MRI of the brain to look at the pituitary gland in detail, and decide on further treatment.
- Explain that prolactinomas are usually successfully treated with medications that suppress the levels of prolactin. These medications do not affect fertility.
- Reassure the patient that surgery to remove the tumour is rarely needed. It is usually reserved for cases where treatment with the medication is not successful.

3 Offer follow-up
- Offer her a follow-up appointment to discuss the results of the blood test, or once she has seen the hospital specialist.
- Provide her with information leaflets about prolactinoma.

Interpersonal skills
- This is a difficult case where the patient is concerned that the underlying diagnosis is premature menopause and is worried about the effect this has on future fertility. She also presents with a loss of libido that has impacted on her relationship.
- The key to this case is to take a complete history, which suggests a diagnosis of prolactinoma, recognise and discuss her concerns, and explain the diagnosis to the patient.
  — 'I think the reason you have not had a period for 10 months is because one of the hormones in your body is higher than it should be, **not** because you are going through a premature menopause.'
  — 'This hormone is called prolactin and it is made in a special part of the brain called the pituitary gland. It is usually made in large amounts when women become pregnant, and it helps the breasts produce milk for the baby.'
  — 'However, you have had four negative pregnancy tests, and the test today is negative too, suggesting there is a different reason why your prolactin levels are high.'
  — 'I think your prolactin levels are higher than normal because the gland that produces it is bigger than normal. It is probably putting pressure on the nerves to the eyes, making your vision blurry at the sides.'
  — 'The condition is called a prolactinoma or pituitary gland tumour, but I can reassure you that even though it may be called 'tumour' it is **not** cancerous. Most cases are managed by tablets that reduce the size of the gland. Surgery is usually not needed.'

O⚷ Key summary
- Recognise the patient's concerns of amenorrhoea on future fertility.
- Assess the impact of her loss of libido on her relationship with her boyfriend.
- Be familiar with the causes of secondary amenorrhoea.
- Ask a detailed history to elicit the underlying diagnosis.
- Manage her concern about having a 'brain tumour'.

Secondary amenorrhoea
- Prolactinomas are the cause of secondary amenorrhoea in **30%** of cases.
- Prolactinomas can present with symptoms due to:
  — hyperprolactinaemia (*see* Table 2.9)
  — hypopituitarism (tumour reduces pituitary function): hypogonadism, depression, hair loss
  — local pressure effects: headache, bitemporal hemianopia or cranial nerve palsies.

TABLE 2.8 Causes of secondary amenorrhoea

ORIGIN	EXAMPLE
Outflow obstruction	Intrauterine adhesions (Asherman's syndrome)
Gonadal disorders	Pregnancy
	Anovulation
	Menopause
	Premature menopause
	PCOS
	Drug induced
Thyroid disorders	Hypothyroidism
	Hyperthyroidism
Pituitary disorders	Sheehan's syndrome
	Hyperprolactinaemia
	Haemochromatosis
Hypothalamic disorders	Stress
	Weight loss
	Excessive exercise
	Eating disorders (obesity, anorexia nervosa or bulimia)

Hyperprolactinaemia

- Women present with amenorrhoea, galactorrhoea, loss of libido, vaginal dryness and osteoporosis (due to reduced levels of oestrogen as a result of amenorrhoea).
- Men present with decreased libido, ED, and infertility. Men often present late, with other features of the underlying cause (headaches and visual field defects if due to prolactinoma) because they do not have a reliable indicator, such as menstruation, to signal a problem.
- Hyperprolactinaemia can lead to osteoporosis.

TABLE 2.9 Causes of hyperprolactinaemia

CAUSE	EXAMPLE
Physiological	Pregnancy
	Breastfeeding
Psychological	Stress
Pituitary disorders	Prolactinoma
	Acromegaly
	Cushing's disease
Ovarian disorders	PCOS
Thyroid disorders	Hypothyroidism
Drugs	Phenothiazines, e.g. haloperidol
	Metoclopramide
	Domperidone
Systemic disorders	Sarcoidosis
	Chronic renal failure

Further reading

- Simon C, Everitt H, van Dorp F. *Oxford Handbook of General Practice.* 3rd ed. Oxford: Oxford University Press; 2010.
- Longmore M, Wilkinson I, Davidson E, *et al. Oxford Handbook of Clinical Medicine.* 8th ed. Oxford: Oxford University Press; 2010.
- Impey L, Child T. *Obstetrics and Gynaecology.* 3rd ed. Oxford: Wiley-Blackwell; 2008.

Station 2.8

Actor's notes

Background
- You are Christina Taylor, a 29-year-old lady who owns a hair salon.

Opening statement
- 'I won't keep you, Doctor. I just need a prescription for some sleeping tablets, please.'

History
- For the past four weeks you have had trouble sleeping.
- This is becoming progressively worse and for the past week you have hardly slept.
- You are sleeping a maximum of 2–3 hours per night.
- You have not used sleeping tablets in the past.

Ideas, concerns and expectations
- You worry at night about financial problems and how to keep your business afloat.
- You are concerned because you cannot sleep and feel more tired in the day.
- You believe sleeping tablets will solve the problem and help you function better in the day.

Further history candidate may elicit
- You lie awake tossing and turning for most of the night.
- You have tried leaving the room, reading a book and watching television. These measures have made little difference.
- You fall asleep easily during the day. This is now disrupting your work and personal life.
- You have been running a hair salon for five years, and recently encountered financial difficulties.
- You are struggling to pay off business loans and the mortgage on the salon.
- Last month your accountant advised you that if the current circumstances continue, you may have to sell the business in the next six months.
- You would then have to seek alternative work, which is likely to be low paid since you have no qualifications.
- Your accountant advised you to reduce your staff to help delay, or avoid, the business collapsing.
- You work in a team of 10 people and are close to all of them, having worked together since the salon first opened.
- Until the past year, business was thriving. Since then, the recession has had a significant impact and despite a reduction in prices there is a lot less demand for your services.
- You feel terrible about having to cut staff. You are unsure how to do this and which staff to select.

- You recently took out your frustrations on staff at work by shouting at several people for making small mistakes.
- Your boyfriend has been very supportive but you find you are now also irritable around him.
- You are normally very friendly and get on with most people. You recognise that you are not your normal self.
- You may answer 'no' to any other questions posed about your psychological or physical well-being.

Medical and drug history
- Nil.

Social history
- You do not smoke or use recreational drugs. You drink two to three units of alcohol on special occasions.
- You live with your boyfriend and have no children.
- You used to play a lot of sport and go for walks. Nowadays you seem to be too busy and preoccupied to pursue these interests.
- You have been with your partner for three years. You have a very good relationship.

Family history
- Nil significant.

Approach to scenario
- You go into the consultation believing that sleeping tablets are the simple solution to the problem.
- You feel tired, and if asked other questions about work and personal circumstances, you initially become irritated because you feel that discussing these issues will not help your situation.
- You simply want to sleep properly and feel the only way to achieve this is with sleeping tablets.
- You become irritable with the doctor's questions and want to know why you cannot simply be given a prescription for sleeping tablets and then 'I'll be on my way'.
- If the questions lead into enquiries about your financial difficulties, you become upset, particularly at the prospect of having to make staff cuts and losing the business you care so much about.
- If the doctor adopts a sensitive approach and comes across as interested in your circumstances, you begin to open up and speak more freely about the situation.
- You will then recognise and accept that these factors are contributing towards your sleep problems.
- However, you still wish to get a few weeks' supply of sleeping tablets to get through this difficult time.
- You will be disappointed if the doctor does not agree to prescribe sleeping tablets or only agrees to issue a small supply.
- If the doctor addresses your concerns about not sleeping, and explains why they are only prescribing a short course of sleeping tablets, you will find this acceptable.
- If the doctor cannot offer you a reasonable explanation for not issuing a few weeks' supply, does not agree to issuing sleeping tablets at all or fails to come across sympathetically, you maintain your request for several weeks' supply.
- If this is declined you will take what is offered but leave unhappy. You will say 'I'm still going to be in the same pickle when this tiny supply runs out, aren't I?'

Information gathering
Presenting complaint
- Enquire about the reasons for requesting sleeping tablets.

a Sleep history
- Difficulties initiating sleep.
- Early morning wakening.
- Estimated time she is sleeping per night.
- Time course for current problems.
- Clarify when she last had a good night's sleep.
- Daytime sleeping/tiredness/napping.
- Exacerbating factors, e.g. noise, caffeine intake and frequent travel.
- Ask about any measures taken to help her sleep, e.g.
  — reading
  — hot bath
  — leaving the room
  — watching television.

b Anxiety and depression
- Screen for anxiety and depression.
- Ask about any worries that may stop her from sleeping:
  — family problems
  — work problems
  — financial problems
  — recent bereavement.

c Other conditions
- Consider other medical conditions, e.g.
  — hyperthyroidism
  — obstructive sleep apnoea.

Medical history
- Depression and anxiety.
- Past sleep problems.
- Previous requests for sleeping tablets.

Drug history
- Over-the-counter medication to help sleep, e.g. natural remedies.

Family history
- History of anxiety and depression.

Social history
- Smoking and alcohol.
- Recreational drug use.
- Marital status and dependents, e.g. children, sick relatives.
- Occupation.
- Financial circumstances.

Patient's agenda
- Enquire why she thinks she is not sleeping.
- Explore any underlying worries that lead to the sleep disturbances.
- Identify the patient's views of what she thinks could help her sleep.

Examination

- Offer to check her BP, pulse and perform a thyroid examination.
- 'If it's okay with you, I would like to check your blood pressure, pulse and check for any signs that your thyroid gland might be overactive.'

Examination card

General examination	BP =115/78 mmHg
	Pulse = 75/minute and regular
Thyroid examination	Patient is clinically euthyroid with no goitre

---

Clinical management

1 Provide an explanation
- Explain you think the main factors affecting sleep are related to the stressful situation surrounding her financial circumstances.

2 Discuss conservative measures
a *Sleep hygiene*
- Discuss sleep hygiene measures:
  — exercising later in the day
  — relaxation therapies
  — reduce alcohol and caffeine
  — ensure a quiet, relaxed sleeping environment
  — avoid heavy meals before going to bed
  — leave the bedroom if not successfully falling asleep within half an hour
  — arrange to read a book or watch television.

b *Stress management*
- Discuss stress management and methods that might help her relax:
  — yoga
  — meditation
  — aromatherapy
  — hobbies
  — exercise.

3 Offer support services
- Suggest psychological treatments such as counselling or CBT.
- Explore ways for her to seek help with her debts and finances, e.g. by contacting her bank and arranging to meet the bank manager to discuss mortgage payments.
- Inform her of support groups such as the Sleep Council (www.sleepcouncil.org.uk).

4 Consider medical treatments
- Explain that sleeping tablets are only a short-term solution (a few days up to two weeks), they do not address the root of the problem, and if used long term could lead to dependence.
- Discuss the side effects of sleeping tablets such as daytime tiredness and explain that patients can build up tolerance, which means higher doses are required.
- Offer a short course and follow-up soon after.

5 Consider time off work
- Discuss the possibility of taking annual leave to have a break, or taking sick leave.

6 Offer follow-up

- Offer a follow-up appointment to review her progress.
- Provide her with information leaflets about insomnia.

Interpersonal skills

- Be prepared to listen to the patient's reasons for requesting sleeping tablets through use of open questions.
  — 'Can you talk to me about your sleep patterns?'
- Be attentive to various non-verbal and verbal cues to help explore why the patient wishes to have sleeping tablets.
  — 'You mentioned that you feel you can't sleep because you think about things. What is it that you are thinking about?'
  — 'You seemed upset when we talked about work. How are things going at work at the moment?'
- Be prepared to revert to closed questions when the need arises.
  — 'Would you mind if I asked you some specific questions for a moment?'
  — 'How much sleep do you think you have been getting in the past few days?'
- Be sensitive when exploring personal issues.
  — 'Have you made any decisions about how you will stay afloat?'
  — 'It is obviously a very tough decision having to lay off staff. What thoughts have you had so far?'
- Remain polite and caring even if the patient shows her irritation.
  — 'I am really sorry to ask these questions. I do understand you want the sleeping tablets. It is important that we explore this a little further so that we can help you with the sleep problems. Would that be okay?'
- Explain to the patient what you think is wrong, being sure to check on patient understanding and to avoid medical jargon.
  — 'The sleep problems are very much connected with the financial difficulties you have been experiencing. What are your thoughts?'
  — 'I think if the problems with the business are sorted out, you will be able to sleep better. What do you think?'
- Offer shared management options, but do not be afraid to stand your ground whilst negotiating; relating this to the patient's ideas and concerns will aid patient satisfaction.
  — 'One option might be to offer a very short course of sleeping tablets for a week or so. I don't think providing a long-term course of sleeping tablets would be in your best interest.'
  — 'There can be problems with addiction and daytime drowsiness. And a long course is more likely to lead to these problems, which will affect you even more. How about we explore some of the other options that may help your sleep?'

⚏ Key summary

- Take a detailed sleep history.
- Elicit the underlying reasons for requesting sleeping tablets.
- Address any associated medical or psychosocial issues at play.
- Recognise the long-term effects of sleeping tablets such as zopiclone.
- Offer counselling and CBT.

Insomnia

Introduction

- One in five people have some form of sleep disturbance. Females are more frequently affected than males.
- Insomnia is more common with age. It is a common problem in older people.
- Insomnia can take various forms:
  - early morning wakening
  - problems falling asleep
  - waking up at regular intervals during the night and failing to return to sleep
  - feeling poorly refreshed following a night's sleep.
- Consider any underlying triggers for sleep disorders as well as any associated problems such as anxiety and depression.

Primary and secondary insomnia

- Primary insomnia occurs when there are no associated underlying conditions.
- Secondary insomnia is associated with underlying conditions:
  - psychological illness, e.g. bipolar disorder, depression and anxiety
  - physical illness, e.g. sleep apnoea, asthma, hyperthyroidism, heart failure
  - drug use, e.g. antidepressants, antiepileptics, β-blockers, oral theophyllines and steroids.

Management of short-term and long-term insomnia

- Insomnia can be divided into short-term (<4 weeks) and long-term insomnia (>4 weeks).

a Short-term insomnia management

- Discuss sleep hygiene measures (also useful to discuss for long-term insomnia management).
- Consider a short course of sleeping tablets:
  - Advise the patient that sleeping tablets cannot be repeatedly prescribed.
  - Start at a low dose and warn about side effects.
- If after two weeks the patient still has sleeping problems then consider CBT.

b Long-term insomnia management

- Offer psychological therapies (*see* Table 2.10).
- Avoid use of hypnotics for long-term insomnia except for acute relapses.
- There is not enough evidence to support the use of antidepressants, antihistamines and barbiturates for insomnia.
- However, consider patients individually when making these decisions – if anxiety or depression is the underlying cause, then antidepressants might be a worthwhile approach.

TABLE 2.10 Psychological therapies for treatment of insomnia

Relaxation classes	Audio material Meditation
CBT	Helps to re-train the patient's thoughts regarding sleep and falling asleep
Biofeedback	Trains the patient to control certain physiological processes, such as heart rate, breathing rate and BP
Sleep restriction therapies	Patients are advised to restrict their sleeping hours so that they eventually become tired again and establish new routines of falling asleep

Referral

- Consider referral to a sleep clinic in patients with:
  - — primary insomnia
  - — long-term insomnia not responding to treatment
  - — diagnostic uncertainty.

Further reading

- Semple D, Smyth R. *Oxford Handbook of Psychiatry*. 2nd ed. Oxford: Oxford University Press; 2009.
- National Institute for Health and Clinical Excellence. Insomnia: newer hypnotic drugs; NICE technology appraisal 77. London: NIHCE; 2004. www.nice.org.uk/TA77 (accessed 22 November 2010).
- Sleep Council website (provides an emphasis on beds and sleep). www.sleepcouncil.org.uk (accessed 22 November 2010).
- Patient UK. *Insomnia (Poor Sleep)*. Patient UK; 2009 (useful patient information leaflet). Available at: www.patient.co.uk/health/Insomnia-Poor-Sleep.htm (accessed 22 November 2010).

Station 2.9

Actor's notes

Background
- You are Melissa Calvin, a 30-year-old lady sales representative for a pharmaceutical company.

Opening statement
- 'Hello Doctor, my periods are really heavy and now I need to see a specialist urgently please.'

History
- You have had increasingly heavy menstrual periods for the last six months and are now fed up.

Ideas, concerns and expectations
- You find having heavy periods very inconvenient in your personal and professional life.
- You read about the possible causes of heavy periods on the internet and were alarmed to read that heavy periods can be a sign of cancer, such as endometrial cancer.
- You have come to see the GP to arrange to see a specialist this week and have taken a few days of annual leave for this reason.

Further history candidate may elicit
- Your periods occur regularly every 28 days. Previously they lasted four days but now last eight days.
- You use tampons during your period.
- On occasion your period has leaked through your underwear and clothes, which has been extremely embarrassing.
- Previously you changed tampons every 5–7 hours, but now need to change every 3–4 hours.
- You have noticed large blood clots in the past two cycles, which can be 3–4 cm in size.
- Your periods have always been painful at the onset, and settle as the period finishes – this has not changed. You usually take ibuprofen for the pain, which is only slightly beneficial.
- The heavy bleeding and pain are distressing. You have to take four to five days off work each month and find it difficult to travel to meet clients when you have your period.
- Work has become increasingly stressful with targets to meet. As a result of the days lost you are now falling behind with your work and concerned about how your colleagues perceive you.
- In terms of your personal life, you avoid exercising or going out when you have your period, since it is difficult to keep going to the toilet.
- Life is extremely busy and you have taken a few days of annual leave to see the GP for a referral to a specialist whom you expect to see this week.

- You do not believe in private healthcare and you believe it is your right to be referred urgently within the NHS since you are a taxpayer.
- If asked, you have not experienced any intermenstrual bleeding, postcoital bleeding nor any pain during sexual intercourse.
- You have not had any weight loss, change in appetite or fevers, but lately you have been feeling more tired than usual.
- If asked about any other symptoms you can say 'no'. You otherwise feel well in yourself.

Medical history
- Nil significant.

Drug history
- Ibuprofen 200 mg tds for period pains.

Obstetric and gynaecological history
- Your periods began when you were 12 years old.
- You have had no previous pregnancies.
- Your last cervical smear was four years ago and was negative.

Sexual history
- You have not been sexually active in the last six months.
- You have had two previous sexual partners.
- A routine sexual health screen performed two years ago was all clear.

Family history
- Nil significant.

Social history
- You drink alcohol in moderation, up to a maximum of 12 units per week. You do not smoke.
- You are single and live by yourself.
- Your parents and younger brother live locally.
- You travel once every fortnight for work to meet your clients who are based around Europe.

Approach to scenario
- You are very upset by these symptoms. You are a very busy person and you have had to go to great efforts to free up your schedule to attend the surgery today.
- You like to solve problems as soon as possible, especially when they are health related.
- You ask the doctor a lot of questions about what this could be and particularly want to know if you have cancer.
- If the doctor says it is unlikely to be cancer, you ask 'But how do you know for sure, Doctor?'
- You become upset if the doctor says you cannot be seen this week by a gynaecologist on the NHS. You cannot understand why patients cannot be referred urgently to a specialist on the NHS, particularly if a problem has lasted a long time.
- If the doctor continues to resist your request for urgent referral, you become upset and angry.
- If the doctor communicates well what the likely possibilities are, and offers a plan which makes you feel something is being done, as well as arranging early follow-up, you gradually come to accept postponing a referral for now.
- You will still be keen, however, to leave the option open to be referred when you next visit the doctor.
- If rapport with the doctor is poor, or you do not feel you have been offered a thorough plan of action, you continue to insist on an urgent referral.
- You would reluctantly accept a private referral in this instance, but be very upset about this.

Information gathering
Presenting complaint
a Menstrual bleeding
- Establish the extent of bleeding by asking about:
  — usage of pads or tampons
  — frequency of changing pads or tampons
  — whether pads or tampons are soaked
  — presence of flooding
  — presence of clots, including approximate size.

b Associated symptoms
- Ask about:
  — dysmenorrhoea
  — intermenstrual bleeding
  — postcoital bleeding
  — dyspareunia
  — pelvic pain and vaginal discharge.

c Systemic review
- Enquire about constitutional symptoms:
  — fevers
  — weight loss
  — loss of appetite
  — abdominal symptoms, e.g. bloating and altered bowel habit
  — symptoms of anaemia, e.g. light-headedness and tiredness.

Gynaecological history
- Endometriosis.
- Fibroids.
- Cervical smear history.

Obstetric history
- Parity and gravidity.

Medical history
- Thyroid disorders.
- Bleeding disorders.

Family history
- Gynaecological disorders or cancers.

Drug history
- Contraceptive pill.
- Copper coil.
- Anticoagulants.
- Antiplatelet drugs.

Social history
- Alcohol and smoking.
- Occupation.
- Marital status.

Patient's agenda
- Explore the impact of her symptoms on personal and work life.

- Explore her concerns and what she thinks is wrong.
- Identify her reasons for requesting an urgent referral.

Examination

- Offer to check her pulse, BP and look for any signs of anaemia.
- Offer to examine her abdomen and pelvis and perform a speculum examination to take a smear and swabs.
- Offer a chaperone in view of the examination involved.
- 'I would like to check your blood pressure and do a general examination. I would also like to examine your abdomen. Looking at your notes, I see you are also due a smear test. I suggest we do that and send off some swabs to make sure there is no infection. How do you feel about that?'
- 'Would you like a female staff member here?'

Examination card

General examination	No pallor of the conjunctiva
	Pulse = 66/minute and regular
	BP = 115/70 mmHg
Abdominal examination	Normal
Pelvic examination	Bimanual palpation reveals no masses
	The uterus is an appropriate size
Speculum examination	Normal looking cervix
	No masses, polyps and no signs of bleeding
	Smear performed and swabs taken

Clinical management

1 Provide an explanation for heavy periods

- Explain that there are several possible causes of heavy periods, e.g. endometriosis, fibroids.
- Reassure her that in view of her symptoms and normal examination, this is unlikely to be cancer.

2 Offer investigations

- Suggest initial investigations with blood tests and a USS of her pelvis.
- Explain that the blood tests will check for anaemia, iron deficiency, clotting abnormalities and thyroid gland disorders.
- Explain that a pelvic ultrasound would look at the uterus and ovaries in detail, looking for endometriosis, fibroids and would help to rule out cancer.

3 Offer medical treatment

- Discuss the various options available to treat menorrhagia.

a Tranexamic acid

- Explain that it can be taken as a 1 g tablet three times a day for days one to four of the menstrual period.
- It inhibits fibrinolysis, which means it interferes with the clotting mechanisms in the blood to decrease bleeding and reduce the heaviness of the period.

b Mefenamic acid

- Explain that this is taken at a dose of 500 mg three times a day for days one to four of the menstrual period.

- It reduces period pains and menorrhagia through its anti-inflammatory actions. This acts quite specifically on the uterine muscle.
- It can be taken along with tranexamic acid.

c Further analgesia for dysmenorrhoea
- Suggest other painkillers, such as codeine-based medication, to help alleviate the pain.

d Contraception
- Suggest the Mirena coil so she does not have to worry about taking tablets when travelling or have problems with different time zones.
- Explain she could also try the oral contraceptive pill.

4 Offer general support
- Discuss the option of a sick note or time off work, or a letter of support for her work, e.g. a letter stating that she is not currently fit for long business trips whilst the condition is being treated.

5 Discuss referral
- Reassure her that she is not acutely unwell and has no red-flag symptoms such as weight loss that would suggest she needed an urgent referral.
- Explain that an urgent referral to the gynaecologist may be difficult to arrange on the NHS.
- However, possible options that could be negotiated would include:
  — Making a request for the bloods and USS to be performed urgently and reviewing her when the results are back.
  — Agreeing to discuss the case with the gynaecology registrar over the telephone; this may help to reassure the patient.
  — Carrying out the blood tests and scan and making a routine referral to the gynaecologist anyway.
  — Offering the option of seeing someone privately.

6 Arrange follow-up
- Arrange early follow-up to review the results and advise her to come back at any stage if she needs to.

Interpersonal skills
- This is a challenging consultation. It is important not to react negatively to the immediate request for an urgent referral. The patient may have a valid reason for wanting to see a gynaecologist, so it is best to show you care, show that you are listening and take a history.
  — 'Things must be quite bad for you. Why don't we discuss this some more?'
  — 'Tell me about your symptoms.'
- Incorporate the patient's social issues into the consultation, i.e. the impact of her symptoms on her job and personal life. It is also important to see how this is affecting her emotionally and in terms of any stress there might be.
  — 'You mentioned that you have had bad periods while you've travelled abroad. How have you managed to work and attend meetings when it has been that bad?'
  — 'Have the symptoms been getting you down?'
- Pay attention to verbal and non-verbal cues as well as using silence and active listening.
  — 'You seem very upset by all of this . . . (silence) . . .'
- The patient's main concern is cancer. Addressing this concern is therefore very important.
  — 'I understand that you are worried. If you want, I can arrange some urgent tests. However, cancer in your particular case is unlikely.'
  — 'Having examined you, I can assure you that the cervix looks completely normal. When I examined you down below I was checking for any unusual lumps or masses, and I am pleased to say that I did not find anything untoward.'

— 'The fact that you are young without any family history of cancers also goes significantly in your favour.'

- Negotiation is an important part of the clinical management plan. The patient's agenda is a referral. The doctor's agenda should be to remain objective, adopt a shared management plan and outline the options. Demonstrating that you are on the patient's side will be the key to arriving at a mutually agreeable plan.
  — 'As I mentioned, we should start investigating these symptoms as soon as possible so that we can find out what is wrong and start treatment.'
  — 'I don't think I can arrange for a gynaecologist to see you straight away. However, I suggest I refer you for these blood tests and the scan straight away. If any of the tests show any suspicion of cancer, then of course the specialist would see you urgently.'
  — 'A specialist would also wish for you to have the tests I am suggesting, done first. If they are all normal then that would be very reassuring.'
- Showing you care by offering follow-up advice will also help gain the patient's trust.
  — 'I would like to see you once the results of the blood tests are back. How does that sound?'
  — 'If you suddenly feel very light-headed or dizzy after bleeding alot, then you should seek medical advice straight away.'

> **O━ Key summary**
> - Take a focussed history for menorrhagia.
> - Reassure the patient about cancer.
> - Be familiar with treatment options for menorrhagia.
> - Negotiate with the patient to avoid urgent referral to a specialist.

Menorrhagia
Definition
- This is menstrual loss that is considered to be excessive and interfering with a patient's life.
- It is usually a subjective symptom and difficult to quantify.
- However, studies have revealed that anything >80 mL/month is considered as menorrhagia.

Common causes

TABLE 2.11 Common causes of menorrhagia

SYSTEM	CAUSES
Gynaecological	Dysfunctional uterine bleeding (commonest cause)
	Fibroids
	Endometriosis
	Pelvic inflammatory disease
Neoplastic	Endometrial cancer
	Cervical cancer
Systemic	Hypothyroidism
	Bleeding disorders
	Drugs, e.g. anticoagulants

Investigations
- Blood tests: FBC, iron studies, thyroid function test (TFT), clotting screen.
- Ensure smears are up to date.
- Endocervical swabs to rule out infective cause.
- Pelvic USS +/− transvaginal scan.

When to refer to secondary care

- Age > 45 years
- Postcoital bleeding
- Intermenstrual bleeding
- Failure to respond to treatment

- This is a guide only and each case should be considered on its own merit.
- As this case highlights, always be prepared to negotiate.
- A good guide about when to refer is shown below.

Management

- Treatment is influenced by the underlying cause.
- Any associated iron deficiency should be treated with oral iron therapy.

NICE guidelines, 2007

(Reproduced with permission of National Institute of Health and Clinical Excellence.)

Drug treatments

TABLE 2.12 Drug treatments for menorrhagia

First line	• Mirena coil (highly effective)
Second line	• Tranexamic acid • NSAIDs, e.g. mefenamic acid • Combined oral contraceptive
Third line	• Oral progestogens, e.g. norethisterone 15 mg tds during days 5–26 of the menstrual cycle • Injectable progestogens

Other
a Medical options
- Gonadotrophin-releasing-hormone-analogue treatments are initiated by a specialist.

b Surgical options

TABLE 2.13 Surgical options for menorrhagia

Endometrial ablation	• Used when the patient does not wish to bear children • Patients must have a normal uterus or fibroids <3 cm in size • Technique is preferred over hysterectomy if uterus is <10/40 size
Uterine artery embolisation	• Used in women who wish to preserve their womb and not have a hysterectomy • Used in women with fibroids >3 cm in size
Myomectomy	• Used in women with fibroids >3 cm in size • Useful in women who wish to preserve their womb • Can be performed as an open procedure or hysteroscopically
Hysterectomy	• This option is used as a last resort

Further reading
- Impey L, Child T. *Obstetrics and Gynaecology*. 3rd ed. Oxford: Wiley-Blackwell; 2008.
- National Institute for Health and Clinical Excellence. Heavy Menstrual Bleeding: NICE guideline 44. London: NIHCE; 2007. www.nice.org.uk/CG44 (accessed 23 November 2010).
- Santer M. Heavy menstrual bleeding: delivering patient-centred care. *BJ Gen Pract.* 2008; **58**(548): 151–2. Available at: www.ncbi.nlm.nih.gov/pmc/articles/PMC2249789/pdf/bjgp58–151.pdf (accessed 12 December 2010).

Station 2.10

Actor's notes

Background
- You are Sarah Smith, a 15-year-old girl, attending the practice on your own.

Opening statement
- 'I need to get an abortion but my parents must not find out or I'll be in serious trouble.'

History
- You discovered you are pregnant two days ago.
- You performed a pregnancy test, which was positive.
- You do not want this baby and want to have an abortion.

Ideas, concerns and expectations
- You feel guilty about having had sexual intercourse before marriage and falling pregnant.
- You are terrified of your parents' reaction – your cousin fell pregnant when she was a teenager a few years ago and was disowned by the family.
- You are particularly concerned that the doctor may inform your parents and you want the consultation to be kept confidential.
- You want the doctor to make a referral to have an abortion so the whole thing is over with as soon as possible.

Further history candidate may elicit
- You missed your period last week. Over the last few days, you have noticed your breasts feeling tender and your nipples are sore.
- You spoke to your best friend who advised you to take a pregnancy test, which you purchased from the chemist and used at school.
- You followed the instructions on how to use the test and discovered it was positive. You burst into tears and told your best friend immediately. She advised you to see a doctor to arrange for an abortion.
- You started having sexual intercourse three months ago with your 16-year-old boyfriend.
- You know your boyfriend from school and the two of you have been together six months.
- He is your first and only sexual partner.
- You used condoms occasionally but sometimes your boyfriend forgot in the heat of the moment.
- You never pushed him to use a condom because you were scared this would upset him.
- You have not told him you are pregnant because you are scared of his reaction and worried he may tell others.
- Your parents are devout Catholics and do not believe in sex before marriage.

- They do not like you mixing with boys and would be extremely angry if they knew you had a boyfriend. Your father is particularly strict – you are very scared of him and think he would 'go mad' if he discovered you had a boyfriend. You are terrified of him finding out that you are sexually active and pregnant.
- You feel very guilty and feel you have let everyone down, including God.

Medical and drug history
- Nil.

Social history
- You do not smoke, drink alcohol or use recreational drugs.
- You attend a local private school and are a high achiever. You feel pressurised by your parents to constantly do well and are unsure about what you want to do after completing school.
- You live with your parents and seven-year-old sister in a large house. Your father works long hours as a city lawyer and your mother is a teacher in another school. As a family, you attend church every Sunday.
- Your boyfriend is in the year ahead at a local school. You have been meeting at his house after school when his family have not been at home.

Obstetric and gynaecological history
- Your periods started when you were about 12 years old. They occur regularly, every 28 days.
- They last four to five days and are not heavy.
- You have never had any abnormal vaginal discharge or symptoms of STDs.
- You have never been tested for STDs.
- You have never been pregnant before. You use condoms only, for contraception.
- You have had the human papillomavirus (HPV) vaccination at school.

Family history
- Nil significant.

Approach to scenario
- Going into the consultation you are very worried and nervous.
- Your main concern is ensuring that your parents do not find out what has happened.
- At the start of the consultation, you repeatedly seek reassurance that the information is kept confidential.
- Initially you will be guarded and confine your answers to brief replies.
- You are mature for your age and can understand the doctor's advice, you ask questions when unsure about anything and are able to justify your reasons for wishing to have the abortion.
- If the doctor is caring and reassures you that the information is kept confidential, you begin to open up and trust the doctor.
- You will then discuss options of keeping the child, or adoption, as well as future contraception methods. However, at the end of the discussion you still wish to go ahead with an abortion.
- You will not agree to tell your parents or boyfriend under any circumstances, because you are too scared of what might happen.
- If the doctor maintains a sympathetic approach, emphasises that this is a big decision, and asks you if there are any close adults you would be willing to tell, you reveal that you have an aunt who is 10 years older.
- You trust her to keep the pregnancy quiet and are prepared to bring her with you to see the doctor.
- If the doctor cannot reassure you about confidentiality, then you say 'I can't afford for my mum and dad to find out. I'll go to a family planning clinic where they don't know my parents.'

- If the doctor fails to communicate effectively, or does not explore your underlying concerns, then you will not raise the issue of your aunt, but simply say 'I have made my mind up. I'd like to go ahead and be referred, please.'

Information gathering
Presenting complaint
- Explore her reasons for requesting a termination of pregnancy (TOP).

a Pregnancy
- Clarify how she came to know she was pregnant.
- Ensure she correctly performed the pregnancy test.
- Enquire about LMP and regularity of periods.
- Ask about other symptoms:
  — nausea and vomiting
  — abdominal pain
  — vaginal bleeding
  — breast tenderness and sore nipples.

b Partner
- Age.
- Casual or regular partner.
- Check if he is in a position of power, e.g. priest or teacher.
- Ask if he is aware of the pregnancy.
- Clarify that sex was consensual and rule out any form of abuse.

Sexual history
- Confirm when she first became sexually active.
- Ask about the number and age of previous sexual partners.
- Check if she and her partner have had a sexual health screen.

Obstetric history
- Previous pregnancies.

Gynaecological history
- Ask about age of menarche.
- Previous abortions or miscarriages.
- Check she has had the HPV vaccine.

Medical history
- Previous significant medical history.

Drug history and allergies
- Contraceptive use, including emergency contraception.

Family history
- Any significant illnesses.

Social history
- Religious beliefs.
- Details of schooling:
  — bullying
  — relationships with teachers.
- Educational achievements and career aspirations.

- Family dynamics, e.g. relationship with parents and siblings.
- Support networks, e.g. family, relatives and friends she can trust.
- Occupation of parents and financial circumstances.

Patient's agenda
- Explore her concerns about being pregnant.
- Clarify her understanding about an abortion.
- Explore her understanding of the options available to her.

Examination
- Offer to check her BP and calculate the gestational age using a gestational wheel.
- 'I would like to check your blood pressure if that's okay.'

Examination card
General examination	BP = 105/62 mmHg
Gestational age calculation	Four weeks and six days

Clinical management
1 Discuss confidentiality and TOP
- Reassure her that the information will be kept confidential and you will not inform her parents.
- Inform her that patients often experience symptoms of guilt and regret following a TOP.
- Inform her she is about five weeks pregnant and there are different methods to end this pregnancy.

a Medical abortion
- Explain that this is the most likely method that she would pursue.
- Medical terminations are possible until nine weeks of pregnancy; they are performed in a special clinic.
- At the first appointment, she would need to swallow a tablet (mifepristone), which blocks the hormone that supports the pregnancy.
- At a second appointment, another tablet (misoprostol) is placed in the vagina; it acts in a few hours, causing the womb to cramp and the lining to break down. Bleeding can last 7–14 days.
- Explain that the pregnancy is lost in the bleeding that follows, as happens with a miscarriage.
- After this, she would go to the clinic after one to two weeks to repeat the pregnancy test and make sure the treatment has worked.
- Reassure her that the treatment is safe, and she can take someone with her to the clinic.
- If asked, reassure her that the most common side effects are diarrhoea and vomiting.

b Surgical abortion
- Explain that in this procedure, she would receive a local anaesthetic.
- The uterus is then emptied using a gentle manual or electric vacuum.
- This is generally performed between 7 and 10 weeks' gestation.

2 Discuss alternative options
- Discuss the options of keeping the child or adoption.
- Go through the implications of each of these options, e.g. having to tell her family, the idea of bringing up a child, or allowing another couple to bring up a child if adopting.
- Suggest speaking to a priest for spiritual advice, given she is from a religious background.

3 Assess if she is Fraser competent

- (*See* Gillick competence and the Fraser guidelines, page 167).
- Assess how **not** having the TOP may affect her physically or mentally.
- Assess her state of mind and level of maturity to make the decision to have a TOP.
- Assess her understanding of your advice and encourage her as much as possible to tell her family and the father. If she is adamant against informing her parents but is competent, try to negotiate that she speaks to an adult she trusts, e.g. another family member.
- If you deem the patient to be Fraser competent, and believe it to be in her best interests, then agree to refer her for TOP. Suggest she take someone with her for moral support.
- If you are uncertain, explain that you need to take advice yourself from your practice colleagues (but assure her that confidentiality will be maintained) and offer early follow-up.

4 Discuss general sexual health issues

- Briefly discuss the option of different contraceptive methods, such as the contraceptive pill, and LARC – explain she can consider having a coil inserted following a TOP.
- Briefly discuss the risk of STIs from unprotected sex, emphasising the importance of condoms.
- Suggest she and her partner have a sexual health screen at the surgery or family planning clinic.

5 Arrange follow-up

- Offer an early follow-up appointment (e.g. in the next few days) to further explore the issues about abortion, sexual health and contraception. Suggest she brings an adult with her.
- Offer leaflets on abortion, sexual health and contraception, or suggest websites if she does not want leaflets in case her family see them.

Interpersonal skills

- Use all available verbal and non-verbal cues to ensure the patient is at ease.
  — 'Don't worry, you are in a safe place. Take your time and talk me through things.'
- Maintain a caring, non-judgemental approach.
  — 'Becoming pregnant must have come as a complete shock to you. Talk me through your reasons for not wishing to tell your parents.'
- Keep the language plain and simple, avoiding any jargon.
  — 'I have a diary here. Can you tell me the last time you had a period?'
  — 'What was the first day of that period?'
- Try and gain the patient's trust by offering her reassurance and addressing her concerns.
  — 'I would like to reassure you that what you tell me will not leave this room. I know you are worried that your parents will find out, but if you say you do not want them to find out then I won't tell them, even if I see them again soon.'
  — 'Tell me more about your cousin who fell pregnant.'
- Put forward the counter-arguments to the patient, but do so in a way that helps the patient think through the issues in a constructive way.
  — 'Might there be any advantages to telling your parents about the pregnancy?'
  — 'I know it seems a terrible thought explaining this to your parents. Would you like my help in doing that?'
- Use open questions as much as possible, especially when assessing Fraser competence.
  — 'What do you understand about the abortion procedures we have just discussed?'
- Be honest and open with the patient, do not be afraid to communicate your own uncertainty.
  — 'I can see you have arrived at this decision quite rationally. Obviously, this is a big decision to make. Perhaps it might be a good idea to digest what has been discussed.'
  — 'I would like to make sure we are managing this in the best possible way and so I will take advice myself – don't worry, I won't mention your name at all. How about I make you an appointment to come and see me tomorrow?'

Key summary

- Reassure the patient about confidentiality.
- Ensure there are no child-protection issues.
- Be aware of the Fraser guidelines.
- Consider any sexual health and contraceptive issues.
- Referral for TOP would be justified if she is Fraser competent, but aim to persuade her to share this information with a close relative.

Gillick competence and the Fraser guidelines

For a minor to be classed as Fraser competent, the following guidelines should all apply:

- The person understands the doctor's advice.
- The doctor is unable to persuade the patient to tell their parents.
- The patient is likely to continue having sexual intercourse regardless of whether contraception is prescribed.
- Declining the requested treatment is likely to have an adverse physical or mental impact on them.
- It is in the patient's best interests to have the treatment with or without parental consent.

FIGURE 2.2 Fraser competence

- It is very important to assess if the patient is Fraser competent. Even if she is deemed to meet the criteria, it is still very important to encourage her to let her parents know.
- If you deem the child to be Fraser competent, then they have the right to withhold all medical records from their parents. However, it is good practice to encourage parental involvement.
- The terms 'Gillick competence' and 'Fraser guidelines' are often used interchangeably by doctors.
- The Fraser guidelines technically apply to a child consenting to contraceptive treatment, whereas Gillick competence applies to medical treatments in general.
- Although the Fraser guidelines refer to contraceptive treatments, the principles can be applied to other forms of treatment, such as a request for abortion (as in this case).
- If a patient is considered not competent to make this decision, aim to act in their best interests. This involves making a judgement of the likely consequences of her telling her parents, compared with the likely impact of her concealing the proposed treatment.
- If you conclude that her parents do need to be informed, explain to the patient that this is in her best interest, and unless she tells her parents, then you would have to do so yourself.
- Aim to keep her on side as much as possible to maintain trust and reassure her about confidentiality.
- If there is any suggestion of abuse, e.g. rape, sexual relations with someone older or child abuse, you will need to involve social services.

Further reading

- Impey L, Child T. *Obstetrics and Gynaecology*. 3rd ed. Oxford: Wiley-Blackwell; 2008.
- Department of Children, Schools and Families and Department of Health. *Teenage Pregnancy Strategy: beyond 2010*. London: Department of Children, Schools and Families and Department of Health; 2010. Available at: www.education.gov.uk/consultations/downloadableDocs/4287_Teenage%20pregnancy%20strategy_aw8.pdf (accessed 15 January 2011).
- Wheeler R. Gillick or Fraser? A plea for consistency over competence in children: Gillick and

Fraser are not interchangeable. *BMJ*. 2006; **332**(7545): 807. Available at: www.ncbi.nlm.nih.gov/pmc/articles/PMC1432156/ (accessed 12 December 2010).

- Marie Stopes website (provides information on abortion, contraceptive methods as well as sexual health advice) www.mariestopes.org.uk (accessed 23 November 2010).

Station 2.11

Actor's notes

Background
- You are Stephen Brown, a 59-year-old headmaster at a secondary school.

Opening statement
- 'Hello Doctor, I received a note to say I needed a blood pressure check, but I also wanted to see you about another problem?'

History
- You have had some trouble maintaining erections during intercourse in the past three months.
- You usually have morning erections. You have not had any problems with erections in the past.

Ideas, concerns and expectations
- You are upset that you cannot maintain an erection during intercourse and feel 'old'.
- You have been avoiding having sex with your partner because you feel embarrassed about the situation.
- Your partner believes this is because you no longer find her attractive and have lost interest in her.
- You are worried this will affect your relationship and she may leave you if you cannot 'perform'.
- A friend mentioned he had a similar problem and Viagra® has helped improve his sex life.
- You have come to see the GP today to ask for Viagra® but feel very embarrassed.

Further history candidate may elicit
- Your late wife of 30 years passed away 18 months ago following a road traffic accident.
- For the first month you were in a state of shock. You then immersed yourself in your work.
- Your friends encouraged you to go out and you met your partner at a friend's 60th birthday party.
- You began a relationship with her six months ago and started to have sexual intercourse after a few months. This is the first relationship you have had since your wife passed away.
- You are very happy with your new partner and share many common interests.
- You cannot remember an instance when you had problems maintaining an erection with your wife.

- Since beginning this relationship, however, you have never been able to maintain an erection normally.
- When you are intimate with your new partner you develop an erection initially, but soon after intercourse the problem starts.
- You have avoided discussing the issue with your partner. When you become impotent, you tend to make an excuse that you feel tired and then stop having sex.
- You are careful to always use a condom as your partner is still having periods and neither of you want to have children.
- You feel guilty about being so happy in a new relationship and often wonder if you are betraying your late wife.
- You do not consider yourself to be depressed. If asked any further specific questions about your mood you answer 'no'.
- You have not attended the practice for a while because you have been busy with work.

Medical history
- Hypertension diagnosed three years ago.

Drug history
- Amlodipine 5 mg od.

Social history
- You share a bottle of wine one to two nights a week with your partner.
- You are an ex-smoker of 20 cigarettes per day but stopped when you were diagnosed with hypertension.
- You have two children in their early 30s who are both married. You see them every few weeks.
- You enjoy your work as a headmaster.
- You stay active, swimming and walking regularly.

Family history
- Nil relevant.

Approach to scenario
- You are very embarrassed to discuss this problem, and your main agenda coming into the consultation is to obtain a prescription for Viagra®.
- Initially, you try to focus on the reasons for not attending the practice, saying 'I have been really busy with work and kept meaning to come', and ask the doctor to check your BP.
- If the doctor makes you feel at ease and takes an interest in your 'other problem', then you answer their questions but keep your answers short because you feel awkward.
- If the doctor enquires about your current relationship, you speak fondly of your new partner and this helps you feel relaxed. You are then be able to speak more freely about the impotence.
- If the subject of your late wife comes up, you become very upset and say 'I came here for Viagra®, not to talk about my wife'.
- If the doctor is sensitive to this and gently suggests you may not have fully grieved the loss of your wife, then you accept this and be prepared to take up offers of help.
- If you develop a particularly good rapport, you would also be willing to come back and see the doctor with your partner.
- If the doctor fails to explore your problems in a sympathetic fashion, or does not make you feel relaxed, then you close the subject of your late wife.
- If advised that the prescription will be a private one, then you become upset and question this.
- At first you insist on a standard NHS prescription because you do not see why you should have to pay extra.

- If the doctor explains the reasons in a friendly and sympathetic manner, as well as providing good reasons, you accept this.
- If the doctor is unsympathetic about the private prescription, or does not provide plausible reasons for it, then you show you are angry with this decision.
- If it does not go your way, then you say 'In that case, I'll purchase it on the internet, it's a lot cheaper there'.

Information gathering
Presenting complaint
- Enquire about the 'other problem'.

a Erectile dysfunction
- Ask about erections:
  — Check when problem arose.
  — Ask how intercourse is affected.
  — Ask about the presence of normal morning erections.
  — Check if he has had normal erections with any previous partners.

b Hypopituitarism
- Loss of libido.
- Premature ejaculation.
- Depression and anxiety.
- Hair loss.
- Anorexia.

c Sexual history
- Ask about sexual partners:
  — length of time he has known his current partner
  — when they first became sexually involved
  — use of contraception and condoms.

d Hypertension
- Ask about:
  — associated symptoms, e.g. headaches
  — concordance with antihypertensive medication
  — side effects of medications, e.g. ankle swelling.

Medical history
- Significant medical conditions.
- STIs.

Drug history
- Past use of drugs for impotence.

Social history
- Smoking and alcohol.
- Occupational history.
- Marital status.
- Financial issues.

Patient's agenda
- Explore his understanding of ED.
- Explore how this is affecting his relationship.
- Explore his expectations of the consultation.

Examination
- Offer to examine his genitalia, check his BP and dipstick his urine.
- 'I would like to check your blood pressure and examine your testicles, because certain hormonal disorders can lead to impotence and a reduction in their size. I would also like to check the urine for any glucose if that's okay.'

Examination card

General examination	BP = 151/85 mmHg
	BMI = 26.2 kg/m^2
Urine dipstick	All negative, including glucose
Testicular examination	Normal size and no lumps palpable

Clinical management

1 Discuss 'the problem'
- Explain to the patient that he has ED.
- Reassure him that this is a common problem.
- Explain it is likely to be caused by a combination of anxiety and a history of hypertension, because this affects the blood supply to the penis.

2 Explore any underlying issues
- Address the underlying psychosocial issues arising, in this case the loss of his wife 18 months ago.
- Offer general lifestyle advice, explaining that addressing areas such as reducing alcohol intake, losing weight (through diet and exercise), will help with his BP control and reduce his cholesterol, both of which are associated with ED.

3 Offer support
- Encourage him to discuss the problem with his partner, and offer to see them together.
- Offer psychosexual and relationship counselling.
- Offer to refer for bereavement counselling.
- Raise the issue of family planning methods and offer sexual health screening.

4 Discuss the hypertension
- Explain his BP should be maintained at <140/80 mmHg and is raised today.
- Underline the importance of good BP control, which may help his erectile problems.
- Advise him that if his BP remains elevated, he may need to increase the amlodipine to 10 mg.

5 Discuss medical treatments
- Offer an explanation about sildenafil.
  - Its action – smooth-muscle relaxation and vasodilatation resulting in increased arterial flow. This leads to an erection.
  - It should be taken about an hour before intercourse. Starting dose in adults is usually 50 mg and this can be increased to 100 mg according to response.
- Discuss common side effects, e.g. headache, flushing and indigestion.
- Outline the more serious side effects, e.g. it can precipitate subclinical heart disease, liver dysfunction and visual impairment.
- Alert him to the fact that there are alternatives, e.g. vardenafil and tadalafil, which he could try if sildenafil is not effective.
- Explain that all three drugs are similarly efficacious. Most patients tend to prefer tadalafil. The frequent reason cited is because of the ability to have an erection long after administering the medication.

- Inform the patient of the requirement to issue the medication as a private prescription.

6 Arrange blood tests
- Arrange blood tests as part of an annual hypertension review.
- Also arrange blood tests to investigate his ED, including testosterone levels.

7 Offer follow-up
- Suggest he makes a follow-up appointment to monitor his BP, review the blood tests and discuss if sildenafil has helped.
- Offer written information such as leaflets.

Interpersonal skills
- If the patient is embarrassed, then set the patient at ease from the outset.
  — 'So what was the other issue you would like to discuss with me today?'
  — 'Don't worry, this is a very common. Talk to me about your partner and your relationship.'
- Sensitively confirm that the patient has ED.
  — 'So tell me your reason for requesting Viagra® at this stage.'
  — 'What do you mean when you say you are having trouble in bed?'
- Explore his ideas and health beliefs.
  — 'Have you any thoughts about why this has started happening?'
  — 'Did you have any thoughts about when you might raise this issue with your partner?'
- If the patient is reluctant to open up, be prepared to move to closed questions.
  — 'How often do you experience these episodes?'
- Be sensitive when exploring underlying factors that may be affecting the patient's current problems, through use of open questions and by picking up on cues.
  — 'You mentioned that thoughts run through your mind when you are intimate with your partner. Tell me about those thoughts?'
  — 'I'm sorry to hear about your late wife. What happened?'
- If the patient becomes upset or angry, then be prepared to apologise and show you care.
  — 'I am sorry that I upset you. We can leave the subject if you would prefer.'
- Avoid being confrontational when exploring the reasons why the patient has not attended his health checks.
  — 'I notice we haven't seen you here at the surgery for a while.'
  — 'A lot has happened over the past few months. Do you feel you might have neglected your general health?'
- Offer a simple explanation about the problem, keeping language in simple terms and paying attention to verbal and non-verbal cues.
  — 'An erection occurs when blood flows to the penis. There are various factors that can disturb this blood flow and so cause impotence. Does that make sense so far?'
  — 'You seem confused, shall I try and explain that again?'
- Adopt a patient-centred approach to the management of the problem, ensuring that relevant options are discussed.
  — 'Taking Viagra® for erectile dysfunction is one option that we can pursue. There are special kinds of counselling which could also be of help. Would that be something you'd like to explore?'
  — 'Would it help to arrange an appointment to come back and see me with your partner?'
- Remain calm and provide a carefully laid out explanation when discussing private prescribing.
  — 'I am afraid that this particular medicine is not prescribable on the NHS except for certain medical conditions that I mentioned earlier. But I can prescribe this privately for you.'

— 'I do understand that the tablets are more expensive on a private prescription. I agree, it is difficult to understand the full reasoning behind these guidelines.'
— 'It is better that I prescribe it than you buy it off the internet, since you can't be sure of the quality of medicine from the internet.'

O⟶ Key summary
- Take a focussed history for ED.
- Perform a BP review.
- Be aware of the causes of ED (physical and psychological).
- Recognise the options for treating ED (conservative and medical treatments).
- Be aware of the investigations for ED.

Erectile dysfunction
Investigations
- Be guided by the clinical circumstances as to how far to investigate.
- Standard investigations would be to look at cardiac risk factors (fasting glucose/lipids) and checking serum testosterone (taken between 8 and 11 a.m.).
- If the serum testosterone level is borderline or low then repeat the sample along with LH, FSH and prolactin levels. Offer referral if any of these tests are abnormal.
- Consider more specialised investigations:
  — in younger patients
  — in those with a history of trauma
  — when a problem is found in the testes or penis
  — in patients who are difficult to treat in primary care.

Treatment (as recommended by the British Society for Sexual Medicine)
a First line
i Phosphodiesterase inhibitors
- Sildenafil and vardenafil should be taken an hour before sexual activity, whilst tadalafil can be taken at least half an hour before.
- Sildenafil and vardenafil tend to last for about 4 hours.
- Tadalafil is longer acting. Some patients report it lasting for longer than 24 hours.

Efficacy
- These drugs have a 75% satisfaction rate.
- There is no significant difference in efficacy among the three drugs but patients often prefer tadalafil because of the ability to have an erection for much longer after taking it.

Drug interactions
- Absolute contraindication with nitrates due to hypotension.
- Caution with alpha blockers.
- Use with caution in:
  — structural problems with the penis, e.g. Peyronie's disease
  — cardiac disease (*see* Figures 2.3 and 2.4)
  — those with tendencies to priapism, e.g. sickle-cell disease.

Non-responders
- Before deciding that a patient does not respond to phosphodiesterase inhibitors, they should have tried the maximum tolerated dose of at least two drugs, at least four times.

ii Vacuum erection devices
- The penis is inserted into a tube which has a pump connected to it. A vacuum effect is created by pumping air out of the tube. This results in increased penile blood flow and an erection. A ring is attached to the base of the penis to maintain the erection.
- These devices have a very mixed satisfaction rate.
- Patients who get on well with them tend to continue using them longer term.
- The main side effects tend to be confined locally to the penis, e.g. pain, problems with ejaculation and bruising.
- The device should not be used by those at risk of bleeding.

b Second line
i Intracavernous injection therapies
- Alprostadil is a prostaglandin analogue that works by stimulating penile blood flow. If used alone, efficacy rates can be as high as 80%.
- Alprostadil can also be used as part of combination therapy, e.g. with papaverine or phentolamine.
- An alternative intracavernous treatment is aviptadil and phentolamine combination therapy. There is evidence suggesting it has a similar efficacy as alprostadil.

ii Intraurethral alprostadil
- A pellet containing alprostadil is inserted into the urethra after urination. The pellet is applied via an applicator. The penis is then massaged to allow the drug to be absorbed into the corpus cavernosum.
- It has an efficacy rate of 30–60%.

c Third line
i Penile prosthesis
- This can be malleable or inflatable.
- Patients do not require medication.
- Very good satisfaction rates.

Management and grading of risk for patients with erectile dysfunction

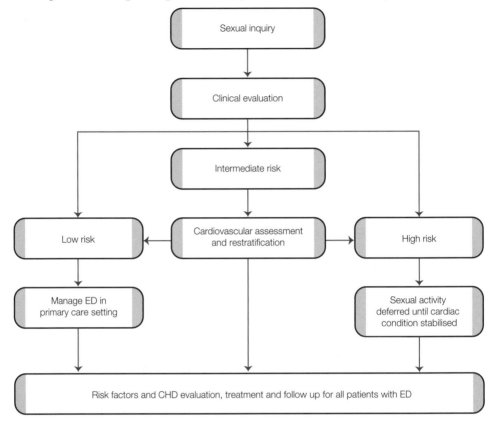

FIGURE 2.3 Algorithm according to graded risk for ED

(Reproduced with permission of the British Society of Sexual Medicine.)

British Society for Sexual Medicine. *British Society for Sexual Medicine Guidelines on the Management of Erectile Dysfunction.* Fisherwick: British Society for Sexual Medicine; 2007. Available at: www.bssm.org.uk/downloads/BSSM_ED_Management_Guidelines_2007.pdf (accessed 12 December 2010).

Prescribing drugs for erectile dysfunction on the NHS

- This is restricted to the following circumstances:
  — diabetes
  — polio
  — kidney patients on dialysis or following renal transplant
  — neurological disorders, e.g. spina bifida, spinal cord injury, multiple sclerosis (MS) and PD
  — pelvic conditions, e.g. following severe trauma and radical surgery
  — prostatic conditions, e.g. cancer and surgery, including transurethral resection of prostate (TURP) and prostatectomy
  — patients with severe distress as a result of the condition (needs to be reviewed by a specialist)
  — patients who were already receiving the drug on 14 September 1998.

Grading of risk	Cardiovascular status upon presentation	ED management recommendations for the primary care physician
Low risk	• Controlled hypertension • Asymptomatic ≤ 3 risk factors for CAD excluding age and gender • Mild valvular disease • Minimal/mild stable angina • Post successful revascularisation • CHF (I)	• Manage within the primary care setting • Review treatment options with patient and his partner (where possible)
Intermediate risk	• Recent MI or CVA (i.e. within last 6 weeks) • Asymptomatic but > risk factors for CAD — excluding age and gender • LVD/CHF (II) • Murmur of unknown cause • Moderate stable angina • Heart transplant • Recurrent TIAs	• Specialised evaluation recommended (e.g. exercise test for angina, echo for murmur) • Patient to be placed in high or low risk category, depending upon outcome of testing
High risk	• Severe or unstable or refractory angina • Uncontrolled hypertension (SBP > 180 mmHg) • CHF (III, IV) • Recent MI or CVA (i.e. within last 14 days) • High risk arrhythmias • Hypertrophic cardiomyopathy • Moderate/severe valve disease	• Refer for specialised cardiac evaluation and management • Treatment for ED to be deferred until cardiac condition established and/or specialist evaluation completed

FIGURE 2.4 Grading of risk and management considerations for patients with ED
(Reproduced with permission of the British Society of Sexual Medicine.)

British Society for Sexual Medicine. *British Society for Sexual Medicine Guidelines on the Management of Erectile Dysfunction.* Fisherwick: British Society for Sexual Medicine; 2007. Available at: www.bssm.org.uk/downloads/BSSM_ED_Management_Guidelines_2007.pdf (accessed 12 December 2010).

Further reading

- British National Formulary (BNF). Drugs for erectile dysfunction. Look at the most up-to-date edition for the latest information. Available at: www.bnf.org (accessed 23 November 2010).
- British Society for Sexual Medicine. *British Society for Sexual Medicine Guidelines on the Management of Erectile Dysfunction.* Fisherwick: British Society for Sexual Medicine; 2007. Available at: www.bssm.org.uk/downloads/BSSM_ED_Management_Guidelines_2007.pdf (accessed 12 December 2010).
- Reynard J, Brewster S, Biers S. *Oxford Handbook of Urology.* 2nd ed. Oxford: Oxford University Press; 2009.

Station 2.12

Actor's notes
Background
- You are Rio Terry, a 23-year-old gentleman who works in a car dealership.

Opening statement
- 'Hi Doctor, could you check my knee please, it's been causing me some gyp.'

History
- You have had right knee pain for almost a month, which is gradually getting worse.
- Ibuprofen helped initially but has been ineffective in the past week.

Ideas, concerns and expectations
- You do not think there is anything seriously wrong.
- You expect the doctor to examine you and prescribe some stronger painkillers.
- You have attended today because some of your colleagues insisted you see a doctor.
- You want to ensure the pain in your knee settles so you can continue to play football.

Further history candidate may elicit
- The pain began during a football game a month ago. You were passed the ball, but as you made contact with it you changed direction and in doing so twisted your knee.
- You recall the knee being painful but played through the pain as there was only 20 minutes of the match left. You remember limping and had to rest for the remainder of the day.
- The pain is located mainly on the inner side of the right knee and is worse when playing football.
- The knee swells intermittently. This is happening more frequently, and exacerbated by any form of exercise.
- The knee often locks. You find that you can unlock the knee by giving it a nudge.
- It does not 'give way'. You manage stairs without any pain and have no other symptoms.
- In the past week you have played two games but have been struggling. The pain is quite bad in the second half of the match, and you cannot run fast but have continued to play.
- You play football regularly as part of a Sunday amateur team who are progressing through a national league tournament. If successful, your team could play at Wembley stadium in the final.
- You are the team's main striker and do not want to miss playing. The next game is in two days.
- Your colleagues, particularly the team manager, insisted you see the doctor today because your performance has declined in the last few games. Prior to your injury, you scored at least one goal in every match. Now that hardly ever happens.
- Playing football has given you a new lease of life. You started playing for this local team after

a friend got you involved at the start of the season, and are excited that your team is playing well.

- Prior to joining the football team, you felt life did not have much to offer. The recession hit hard at work and although you managed to keep your job, you lost a lot of good work colleagues. You also had to take a significant pay cut, which meant you had to give up living in a rented flat with your friends.
- You have had to move back home with your parents and lost much of your independence.
- The pain has not affected your performance at work. Your knee sometimes feels a little sore, but you tend to get on with things and forget about it.

Medical history
- Nil significant.

Drug history
- Ibuprofen 400 mg tds for one week.

Social history
- You are a non-smoker.
- You drink four to five pints of beer on a Friday night and sometimes more if it is a big night out.
- You have worked full-time for the same company since leaving school at age 16.
- You are single and live with your parents.

Family history
- There are no significant illnesses in the family.
- Your parents are both alive and well in their early 50s.
- You have a younger brother aged 15 and sister aged 17. They are both still at school.

Approach to scenario
- You appear rushed in the consultation because you are keen to get it over with and have the doctor give you the all clear so you can tell your colleagues/football manager that everything is okay.
- You confine yourself to brief answers and appear cagey when mentioning how the injury occurred.
- If the doctor appears empathic, you begin to open up more about your passion for football and reasons for not wanting to take a break.
- If the doctor advises that the pain is linked to playing football, you become defensive, and explain that you have to be able to play in the remaining football games.
- You will not agree under any circumstances to miss the next football game.
- However, if the doctor perseveres and comes across as being on your side, you agree to be investigated and managed by a specialist or physiotherapist. In these circumstances, if the doctor asks, you would also agree to visit the doctor again and consider not playing in future games if the symptoms worsen.
- If the doctor does not provide a good explanation about what is wrong, or fails to take into account your concerns about playing football, you decline any offers of further management and brush aside their suggestions, saying 'I'll be fine Doctor. I'll make sure I take the painkillers.'
- If the doctor is concerned about this, you may agree to come back for a follow-up appointment.

Information gathering
Presenting complaint
- Enquire about the knee pain:
  - — nature
  - — location and radiation
  - — exacerbating and alleviating factors
  - — locking, giving way and clicking
  - — swelling – immediate or gradual onset
  - — history of trauma and the mechanism of injury, e.g. twisting or direct blow
  - — treatments used, e.g. resting, ice packs, exercises and compression bandages.
- Ask about pain in other joints, e.g. back pain.
- Ask about inflammatory features:
  - — improvement when mobilising
  - — pain worse in the morning or when resting.
- Screen for depression.

Medical history
- Knee problems.

Drug history
- Enquire about analgesia taken, e.g. NSAIDs.

Family history
- Joint and knee problems.

Social history
- Smoking and alcohol.
- Occupational history.
- Friends and family.
- Financial circumstances.

Patient agenda
- Explore how the knee pain is impacting on his work, recreational activities and personal life.
- Explore his understanding about what might be wrong.
- Explore his expectations of the consultation, e.g. referral, painkillers.

Examination
- Offer a full examination of both knees.
- 'I would like to examine your knees if that's okay.'

Examination card	
Right knee examination	No scars
	Mild effusion with a positive patellar tap
	Straight-leg raising intact
	Significant medial joint line tenderness
	No ligamentous laxity
	McMurray's test positive
Gait examination	Normal

Clinical management
1 Explain your provisional diagnosis
- Explain that this is likely to be a meniscal injury.
- Provide an explanation about what the menisci are and their function. Explain that they are in the shape of a half moon, sitting on top of the shin bone. They act as shock absorbers for the knee, preventing the joint cartilage from becoming easily damaged.
- Explain the complications of a meniscal tear:
  — bucket handle tear
  — associated anterior cruciate ligament (ACL) rupture
  — secondary osteoarthritis.
- Offer information in the form of fact sheets and answer any questions he may have.

2 Suggest simple measures
- Discuss conservative measures such as rest, elevation and using ice packs for flare ups of pain and swelling.
- Advise that any potential triggers, e.g. strenuous activities, should be avoided at least for the short term.
- Offer support with his job if this is applicable, e.g. sick note, letter suggesting lighter duties.

3 Explore medications
- Consider optimising the dose of ibuprofen or changing to a stronger anti-inflammatory, e.g. diclofenac.
- Enquire about any contraindications to NSAIDs, e.g. GI symptoms, asthma. If so, then consider alternative analgesia, e.g. paracetamol, co-codamol.

4 Discuss further management
- Offer referral to an orthopaedic department. Given that he is an active person, offer to request an urgent assessment.
- Discuss physiotherapy as the most likely course of action and explain that surgery is not commonly undertaken.
- Explain that the preferred investigation for a meniscal tear is MRI scanning. This would be organised by a specialist.
- If the patient wishes to seek further information, mention that if there is a torn cartilage, this can often be dealt with by keyhole surgery, and that sometimes patients have a keyhole procedure to make the diagnosis and treat at the same time.

5 Offer follow-up
- Offer to review the patient again. If he decides to play in the next football game, offer an appointment afterwards to assess his progress and allow him a chance to consider the discussions.

Interpersonal skills
- Maintain a good rapport with the patient. Showing an interest in what is important to the patient, by picking up on cues, is a good way to help move the discussion forward.
  — 'You mentioned you get the pain when playing football. How often do you play?'
- Explore the patient's concerns through open questions and maintaining positive, non-verbal communication.
  — 'You mentioned being given a new lease of life since the start of the season. Tell me more about that.'
  — 'In what way do you feel life has not been so good in the last year?'
  — 'I'm sorry to hear that many of your friends were laid off at work. How did you feel at that time?'

- Provide an explanation about what is wrong. Use simple, easy-to-follow language, clarifying what is meant if you have to use medical jargon.
  — 'There is a piece of rubbery tissue that sits in this part of the knee here (*point to the medial compartment*). It is called a meniscus. There is also one on the opposite side. When you twisted your knee, it is quite likely that this structure was torn.'
- Arrive at a mutually agreed management plan by being prepared to negotiate.
  — 'Do you think taking a break from playing might be good for the knee and help you start scoring goals again?'
  — 'I understand you will definitely be playing this Sunday. Just so we know that your knee holds up okay with all the playing, how about we have the problem looked into by a specialist? How does that sound?'
- If there is a lot of negotiating, and consequently a lot of detail discussed, summarise the management plan so both the doctor and patient feel they understand each other's advice.
  — 'Okay, just to summarise what we have agreed on. You wish to continue playing football for now. I shall try and get you to see one of our local orthopaedic doctors as soon as possible and I shall prescribe you a stronger anti-inflammatory.'
- If you feel the knee problem is not being managed appropriately despite your best efforts, be prepared to offer early follow-up as a compromise.
  — 'How about we have another appointment in a week's time so that I can re-examine your knee and see how you are after your next game?'

○━ **Key summary**
- Take a detailed history of the knee pain.
- Recognise the features of a meniscal injury.
- Be willing to negotiate and offer best help even if the patient disregards your main advice.

Meniscal injuries

- These commonly occur from sporting injuries, e.g. football and rugby, by a 'twisting' mechanism.
- Another possible mechanism is degeneration, which is usually seen in older patients.
- They can be associated with an ACL rupture.
- Examination findings to look out for include tenderness over the joint line and a positive McMurray's test (*see* page 183).
- Management can be conservative or surgical. Surgical options usually involve arthroscopy, during which the torn fragment can be excised.

ACL and PCL injuries

- Common mechanism for an ACL injury is following a blow to the back of the knee, with or without twisting of the knee.
- The main examination findings include a knee effusion and a positive anterior draw test.
- PCL injuries commonly occur with a direct blow to the front of the knee, e.g. in a road traffic accident.
- Management for ACL and PCL injuries is usually conservative with a cast and physiotherapy.
- A minority of cases will go on to require operative intervention. Refer to orthopaedics if you suspect an ACL or PCL injury.

Medial and lateral collateral ligament injuries

- These injuries commonly occur from direct impact, often in sports people.
- There is often tenderness over the affected area +/– effusion. Stress testing of the affected

ligament is usually normal but >5 degrees of deviation implies ligament rupture (in which case the patient should be referred to orthopaedics with a view to surgery).
- Management is usually conservative as for a soft tissue injury.

McMurray's test
- This test helps to elicit a torn meniscus. It should be performed with the patient in a supine position.
- Placing the fingers of one hand along the medial joint line, use your other hand to flex the knee to 90 degrees by holding the sole of the foot.
- Apply valgus stress to the knee, then extend the knee and externally rotate the leg.
- If a click or pop with pain is elicited then this indicates a medial meniscal tear.
- To examine the lateral meniscus, place the fingers from one hand along the lateral joint line of the knee. Hold the sole of the foot with the other hand and flex the knee to 90 degrees.
- Apply varus stress to the knee, then internally rotate the leg and extend the knee.
- As above, if there is a click or pop with pain then this indicates a lateral meniscus tear.
- To complete the examination both knees should be examined.

Further reading
- Collier J, Longmore M, Turmezei T, *et al*. *Oxford Handbook of Clinical Specialties*. 8th ed. Oxford: Oxford University Press; 2009.
- Duckworth AD, Porter DE, Ralston SH. *Orthopaedics, Trauma and Rheumatology*. Oxford: Churchill Livingstone Elsevier; 2009.
- Wheeless CR, editor. *Wheeless' Textbook of Orthopaedics*. Durham, NC: Duke University Medical Center Division of Orthopedic Surgery and Data Trace Internet Publishing; n.d. Available at: www.wheelessonline.com (accessed 23 November 2010).

Station 2.13

Fax
Dr O'Ncology
Local Hospital NHS Trust
Local Lane
Locality

Dr AN Other
Treewood Medical Centre
Treewood Lane
Treehamshire

URGENT ATTENTION OF DR AN OTHER

Re: Mrs Margaret Smith, date of birth 1/1/1965

Dear Dr Other

We have made several unsuccessful attempts to contact this patient over the past 12 days. She presented to this department two weeks ago having been referred with a recent history of a breast lump. An USS, fine needle aspirate and biopsy were performed. Histology confirms an infiltrating ductal carcinoma.

We had intended to inform the patient of the result within two days of the biopsy, but Mrs Smith has failed to respond to telephone calls and letters. We would be most grateful if you could also try and get the patient to contact this department and we will arrange to see her.

Yours sincerely
Dr O'Ncology

Actor's notes

Background
- You are Margaret Smith, a 45-year-old lady who works part time in a supermarket.

Opening statement
- 'I was asked to come in urgently, the receptionist mentioned that the results of the biopsy were back. She wouldn't tell me the result. Is everything okay?'

History
- You noticed a lump in your right breast for about one month before you visited the doctor.
- It was getting bigger and becoming painful.
- You eventually visited the GP three weeks ago.
- The GP referred you to a specialist to be seen within two weeks.
- You saw the breast specialist at the local hospital and then had some investigations.

Ideas, concerns and expectations
- You are terrified, and believe that you have breast cancer, like your mother.
- You feel guilty about the emotional and financial effects this would have on your family.
- Finances have been very tight lately and you are worried how mortgage payments will be met if you have to stop working.
- Your husband convinced you to see the GP today for the results.

Further history candidate may elicit
- The specialist explained that you needed to have further tests to determine the nature of the lump and if it is cancerous. He was running late and failed to answer most of your questions.
- You ignored the letters and phone calls from the hospital because you are scared of the results.
- Since leaving the last outpatient appointment, you convinced yourself that the lump is cancerous.
- Your mother was diagnosed with breast cancer when she was 40 and died a year after diagnosis.
- Memories of your mother's illness and the difficulties your family faced when your mother's condition deteriorated have been at the forefront of your mind over the last few days.
- You recall her being in significant pain, losing her hair and making frequent visits to the hospital.
- She became particularly unwell whilst undergoing chemotherapy, with recurrent infections.
- You were 15 years old at the time and your whole life was turned upside down.
- Your father was extremely supportive, but being an only child, you felt quite lonely for a long time. Your schoolwork suffered and you had to see a counsellor at the time.
- You are scared that you will suffer the same fate, and worry about your own mortality.
- You have come to see the GP today because your husband insisted you come for this appointment.
- He is also worried but has been very supportive. You have a very good relationship.
- You have not told your children that you have a breast lump.
- Finances have been tight at home because your eldest child has gone to university and needed some financial support, which you are determined to give since you did not have the opportunity to go to university yourself.

Medical and drug history
- Nil.

Social history
- You smoke five cigarettes per day and drink socially.
- You are married and your husband works at the local butcher.
- You have two children, aged 18 and 16, and live in a rented flat. You are a close-knit family.

Family history
- Your mother died of breast cancer aged 40.

Approach to scenario
- Coming into the consultation, part of you is expecting the worst.
- You avoided the calls and letters from the hospital because you dreaded the idea of being diagnosed with breast cancer. Were it not for your husband's insistence, you probably wouldn't have attended today.
- You keep thinking about your mother's suffering and the impact it had on your father and yourself.
- When told you have breast cancer you feel shocked and very upset. You feel numb and remain speechless initially, for up to a minute.
- After this, you find it hard to engage in the conversation and sometimes repeat your question because you did not listen to the answer properly the first time.
- If the doctor is sensitive, you let them console you.
- After the initial silence is over you ask the doctor questions, including what this means, how long you have to live and whether there is a cure.
- You are particularly concerned about the implications for your family in terms of having to look after you, how they will cope financially and how they will come to terms with the situation.
- You refuse to go back to the hospital because you feel chemotherapy is a humiliating experience that is pointless if you are going to die anyway.
- After being tearful and upset, you become angry towards the doctor if they suggest you see the specialist again.
- If the doctor explores your worries, reassures you about the advances in cancer medicine over the past years, and helps you feel that you should not give up, you agree to see the hospital specialist.
- If the doctor does not address your concerns effectively, particularly about the benefits of cancer treatment, or take the time to sympathetically explore the experiences with your mother, then you will be reluctant to engage with secondary care any further.
- You may agree to come back and see the GP with your husband. If you do not have good rapport with the doctor then you say 'I'm not up to this at the moment. I'll get in touch when I've got my head around the situation.'

Information gathering
Presenting complaint
- Check the patient's current understanding of her condition.
- Ask about her reasons for not responding to the hospital:
  — holiday
  — difficulty getting time off work
  — difficulty coming to terms with potential diagnosis.

Medical history
- Previous breast lumps.

Drug history
- Contraceptive pill or hormone replacement therapy (HRT).

Family history
- Breast, ovarian, cervical or endometrial cancer.

Social history
- Marital status and dependents, e.g. children.
- Social support, e.g. family and friends.
- Occupation.
- Financial circumstances.

Patient's agenda
- Explore her understanding of breast cancer.
- Explore how she feels about further tests and treatment.
- Explore her understanding of available treatments.

Clinical management
1 Breaking the bad news
- Explain that her investigations have shown she has breast cancer.

2 General discussion
- Emphasise that breast cancer carries a much better prognosis now, compared to when her mother had breast cancer. If treated, the overall five-year survival for breast cancer is 80%.
- Encourage her to inform her family about the diagnosis.
- Offer to help with this if she would like you to speak to her husband.
- Try and persuade her to engage with hospital services.
- Offer to call the specialist to answer any further questions, and slot her back into the system.

3 Further management
- Explain that further treatment depends how advanced the tumour is.
- Explain that the hospital will need to do some further investigations to 'stage' the tumour, to find out how far it has spread, and look at the 'grade' to see how aggressive it is.
- Emphasise the importance of engaging with the specialist as soon as possible to reduce the chances of the cancer spreading and thereby influencing her prognosis.
- Suggest that further tests may include lymph node biopsy, and special scans of her liver and chest.
- Explain that treatment options include radiotherapy, surgery and chemotherapy.
- Explain that treatment is individualised according to the patient as well as the stage and grade of the cancer.
- Explain the principles of treatment.
  — Most breast tumours are treated with surgery, either by lumpectomy or mastectomy (with breast reconstruction).
  — Surgery is sometimes supplemented with chemotherapy or hormonal treatments that can be given before or after surgery.
  — Radiotherapy may be used after surgery to destroy any residual breast tumour cells.
  — Other treatments are available if there is a recurrence, e.g. Herceptin.

4 Offer support
- Offer to put her in touch with a patient who has successfully come through the treatment for breast cancer (subject to obtaining consent).
- Reassure her there is a full team of trained professionals to help guide her through this difficult time, such as the McMillan Nurses, oncologists, the GP, practice nurse and counsellors.

5 Closing the consultation
- Offer an early appointment and suggest she brings her husband.
- Offer written information; provide fact sheets and leaflets.
- Provide information about support groups, e.g. Breast Cancer Care (www.breastcancercare.org.uk) and Macmillan Cancer Support (www.macmillan.org.uk).

Interpersonal skills

- Set the scene and avoid having a table between the patient and yourself. Keep tissues handy, ask reception staff not to disturb you unless urgent.
- Maintain a caring and empathic approach. Be aware of her concerns, picking up on cues and using open questions to identify her reasons for not wishing to engage with hospital services.
  — 'Tell me about your reasons for not replying to the hospital's letters and phone calls.'
  — 'I am sorry to hear about what happened to your mother. That must have been a very difficult time for you.'
- Maintaining effective use of verbal and non-verbal communication skills is important when breaking bad news. Avoid using medical jargon. Use lay terminology. For example, instead of saying 'fine needle aspiration and biopsy' you could instead say:
  — 'A fine needle is inserted into the lump and a sample sent to the lab.'
- Be attentive to the patient's verbal and non-verbal cues and check for understanding when offering explanations. It may become obvious that she is not listening when she hears the news, in which case it would be appropriate to allow for silences.
- Deliver the news in stages. Be supportive if she starts crying. When delivering the news, explain the background first.
  — 'As you know, we found a lump that was suspicious, therefore you were referred urgently to the breast specialist. They carried out tests in the form of a scan and by removing a small sample of tissue.'
  — 'The sample is sent to the laboratory where the cells are examined closely for any signs of cancerous change.'
- Fire a 'warning shot':
  — 'As you know, we received a fax earlier from the specialist. The result of the biopsy has come back and I am sorry to tell you that it is not good news.'
- This can then be followed by the bad news.
  — 'I am very sorry to have to tell you that the results confirm that you have breast cancer.'
- Allow the patient to respond to the news in her own way, e.g. crying, shock and anger. Be comfortable with prolonged silence and maintain a sensitive, calm demeanour at all times.
- Be guided by the patient in terms of how much information she may want about diagnosis, management and follow-up. There is a chance she will not remember much of the information, which is why written information, as well as early follow-up, should be offered.
- Emphasise that prognosis depends on a few factors, including the type of cancer and the 'staging'.
  — 'How things go from here depends on whether there is any spread of the tumour beyond the breast tissue; the cancer can spread through tissue, through the gland system or through the blood. This information helps to determine if you just need to have the lump removed, or if other measures are required, like removing the breast, chemotherapy or radiotherapy.'
- Answer questions honestly, and be prepared to say if there is something you do not know. Make a note of it and offer to find out and let her know at a follow-up appointment.
- Gently try and persuade the patient to engage with secondary care by being positive, whilst at the same time not giving false hope.
  — 'Breast cancer is much more treatable nowadays. Many women are completely cured from this cancer, but it depends on how much it has spread. The earlier this is looked into, the more likely we are able to prevent things getting worse and ultimately improve your chances of recovery, possibly even providing a complete cure.'
  — 'How about you think about what we have discussed and I arrange to see you with your husband tomorrow?'

- Closing the consultation requires careful attention. It is important to avoid the patient leaving the building or driving home if she is distraught. Offer her the chance to spend time with someone, e.g. a receptionist, or to sit in another room whilst you see other patients.
- Offer to telephone her husband/a family member to collect her.

O⎯ᴍ   Key summary
- Recognise how to break the bad news.
- Explore underlying worries and understand how they relate to the patient avoiding contact with the hospital.
- Discuss the treatments for breast cancer, the effectiveness of treatments and support available.
- Use good interpersonal skills to try and persuade her to engage with secondary care.

Breast cancer
Epidemiology
- Commonest cancer affecting women in the UK. Affects one in nine women in their lifetime.
- Breast cancer is usually an adenocarcinoma.

Risk factors
- Increased risk with age.
- Being born in North America or Northern Europe.
- Family history – particularly having a mother or sister affected.
- Early menarche, late menopause.
- Nulliparity.
- Age >30 years at first pregnancy.
- Oestrogen-containing medication, i.e. oral contraceptives and HRT.
- Higher socio-economic group.
- *BRCA1/BRCA2* and *TP53* genes.

Treatment options
- Options include surgery, radiotherapy, hormonal treatments (e.g. tamoxifen), chemotherapy and biological agents (e.g. Herceptin).
- The choice of treatment depends on several factors including stage, grade, onset of menopause and receptor types of the cancer cells.
- Where possible, the specialist will also take account of patient factors, e.g. a patient determined to preserve the breast, when deciding on the best treatment options.
- Surgery is commonly carried out. This can take the form of lumpectomy (often with radiotherapy) or mastectomy (with breast reconstruction).
- Those cancers that are high grade are likely to require chemotherapy. Chemotherapy can be offered as neo-adjuvant (before surgery) or adjuvant (after surgery).

Staging of breast cancer

TABLE 2.14 Breast cancer staging and five-year survival figures in the UK

STAGE	DESCRIPTION	FIVE-YEAR SURVIVAL RATE
0	Carcinoma-in-situ	>99%
I	Tumour size >2 cm diameter Without lymph node involvement or metastases	80%
II	Tumour size 2–5 cm diameter **and/or** Spread to the ipsilateral axillary lymph nodes, not fixed	68%
III	Tumour size >5 cm diameter **or** Lymph nodes are fixed	40%
IV	Spread past the breast, internal mammary nodes and axilla	10%

Overall five-year survival = 80%.

Further reading

- National Institute for Health and Clinical Excellence. Breast Cancer (early and locally advanced): NICE guideline 80. London: NIHCE; 2009. www.nice.org.uk/CG80 (accessed 23 November 2010).
- National Institute for Health and Clinical Excellence. Breast Cancer (advanced): NICE guideline 81. London: NIHCE; 2009. www.nice.org.uk/CG81 (accessed 23 November 2010).
- Cassidy J, Bissett D, Spence RAJ, *et al. Oxford Handbook of Oncology.* 3rd ed. Oxford: Oxford University Press: 2010.
- Patient support: www.breastcancercare.org.uk (accessed 23 November 2010) and www.macmillan.org.uk (accessed 23 November 2010).
- Patient UK. *Breaking Bad News.* Patient UK; 2010. Available at: www.patient.co.uk/doctor/Breaking-Bad-News.htm (accessed 23 November 2010).
- Fujimori M, Uchitomi Y. Preferences of cancer patients regarding communication of bad news: a systematic literature review. *Jpn J Clin Oncol.* 2009; **39**(4): 201–16.

Circuit 3

Station 3.1

Actor's notes

Background
- You are Holly Nicholas, a 33-year-old Caucasian secretary.

Opening statement
- 'Doctor, I changed my child's nappy and I noticed a bruise on her bottom.'

History
- Your daughter, Emma, stayed with her father over the weekend.
- She is dry in the day (potty trained) but still wears nappies at night.
- She was brought back home by her father last night.
- You changed her nappy this morning and noticed a bruise on her bottom.
- The bruise looks very straight, and measures about 5 cm by 2 cm.
- Emma is at the toddler's group. You have come alone today, to speak to the doctor.

Ideas, concerns and expectations
- You think the bruise has occurred because your ex-husband or his girlfriend has hit your daughter.
- You are currently separated from your husband and going through a messy divorce. You feel he is unfit to be a father, and do not want him to have access to your children any more.
- You have come to see the GP to see what to do next – your children's safety is paramount.

Further history candidate may elicit
- You separated from your husband about six months ago, and are going through a messy divorce.
- You have a three-year-old daughter, Emma, and a five-year-old son, Frank, who were fathered by him. Both children live with you.
- Emma is quieter than normal but is otherwise well and is drinking and eating.
- Frank is behaving normally.
- You were married and lived together for seven years. Problems in the marriage started about four years ago when you became pregnant with your second child.
- Arguments happened daily, and some nights he would punch you after drinking heavily. You never went to hospital and have never disclosed the violence to anyone before.
- He has never hit the children in front of you, but has shouted at them before. Although you agreed that he could look after the children on the weekends, he often cancels and actually only sees them once or twice a month. He has forgotten their birthdays in the past.
- You have agreed to his access to the children on an informal basis.
- He moved into a separate flat and his new girlfriend moved in with him two months ago.
- He does not offer any financial support. You pay the mortgage, bills and childcare yourself.

- You are claiming child benefits and just about manage financially, although finances are tight.
- You work full-time and do not have any support from your family because they live far away.
- You do feel low occasionally and sometimes feel overwhelmed. However, you are not depressed and do not have any thoughts of suicide or self-harm.
- Your children are your main concern and will do anything to protect them from any harm.

Medical history
- Nil relevant.

Drugs and vaccination history
- Emma does not take any medications.
- She is up to date with her vaccinations.

Birth and development history
- Emma was born by normal vaginal delivery at term.
- She has had no significant problems since birth and seems to be developing well.

Social history
- Emma lives with you and Frank in a two-bedroom private flat.
- You are separated from your husband, and he lives with his girlfriend.
- You work full-time and pay for childcare. Frank is in school.
- You do not smoke and rarely drink. You do not use recreational drugs.
- You ex-husband smokes and drinks. He has been a heavy drinker in the past but cut down more recently. He does not use recreational drugs.
- There are no other family members that live close by.

Family history
- Nil relevant.

Approach to scenario
- You are angry that your ex-husband or his girlfriend hurt your child.
- You are worried that this may have happened before or may happen again.
- You feel guilty that you let him see the children – he has hit you in the past and you 'should have known better than to leave your children with him'.
- You want to ensure that your ex-husband does not have access to your children again.
- You feel a lot less anxious about the situation if the doctor takes your side and accepts your point of view and then you can take the appropriate steps to ensure that your children no longer see their father and his girlfriend.
- If the GP communicates well and explains to you that they cannot take sides, but will report the case urgently, then you accept this.
- If, however, the doctor does not communicate well, or does not satisfactorily take account of your concerns about your children, then you become more anxious and upset, saying 'You don't really understand, do you, Doctor?'

Information gathering
Presenting complaint
a The bruise
- Check when the bruise was first noticed.
- Ask where it is and what it looks like.
- Enquire about other marks on the rest of the body.
- Check if the mother noticed any bruises or marks before.
- Ask if Emma bruises easily.
- Determine the last time the mother noted the bottom was normal, with no bruise.
- Enquire further about who has been looking after the child since the time the bottom was last normal.

b The incident
- Ask what the mother thinks has happened.
- Enquire if she has asked Emma what happened.
- Check if Emma had been involved in any accidents recently.
- Ask if Emma is walking normally.
- Ask if Emma's behaviour has changed.

c Other information
- Enquire who lives at home.
- Ask who looks after Emma.
- Check if any new people have been in contact with Emma, and if so, who.
- Check that Emma is growing well.

d Mother
- Check how is she coping.
- Screen for depression.

e The abuser
- Ask who the mother suspects as being the abuser.
- Check if they still have access to the child.
- Ask how often they have been left alone with the child.
- Ask if they use alcohol or drugs.
- Check if they have a history of mental health problems.

Medical history
- Ask if Emma is up to date with her immunisations.
- Ask if Emma was premature.
- Check if Emma has any disability.
- Check if Emma has any other physical injuries.
- Enquire about any hospital admissions.

Family history
- Check for a family history of mental illness.
- Ask about other children in the family.
- Check if any of these children could be at risk.

Drug history
- Current medications.

Social history
- Occupation of parents.
- Support from relatives, e.g. grandparents, social worker.

- Financial support from social benefits.
- Parental use of alcohol, smoking and recreational drugs.
- Living circumstances (house/flat, council/private owned).
- Childcare arrangements.

Patient's agenda
- Explore the mother's concerns.
- Explore how she feels about taking further action.

Clinical management
1 Safety of the child
- Explain to the mother that because concerns have been raised, further investigation is needed.
- Do not suggest you agree that the father or his new partner are responsible for the bruise. You must recognise that currently, you only have allegations from the mother, and that the child is not present for examination.
- Explain that you would need to contact social services, and will do so by speaking to them and faxing a referral letter.
- Explain that social services will contact her to speak to her and conduct an assessment. An examination of the child by a paediatrician may be necessary.

Note:
- In this case, referral to social services is the next most appropriate step forward. However, a candidate who suggests contacting the paediatric department for advice, would not be penalised.

2 Supporting the mother
- Explore social support mechanisms (family and friends).
- Advise her to make an appointment with you in the future if she feels low or is struggling.
- Suggest the health visitor could also help and support her.

3 Follow-up
- Offer her a follow-up appointment to further discuss how she is coping.
- Suggest a follow-up appointment with Emma to review the situation in the next week or so.

Interpersonal skills
- During this consultation, it is important to remain non-judgemental and recognise that the mother may feel guilty and responsible since she has let her children stay with the father and his partner, whom she blames for the abuse.
- However, it is also important to remain impartial – the only information available to you is from the mother. Her allegations need to be verified – she, or her own partner, may be responsible.
- Share your concerns with the mother and emphasise to her that you share her main priorities.
  — 'This story sounds very worrying. I am also concerned by what I have heard.'
  — 'Obviously, we don't wish to accuse anyone falsely and jump to conclusions. I'll get in touch with social services right away to arrange an investigation. How does that sound?'
- Explore the mother's concerns through open questions, while allowing her to lead the discussion.
  — 'So, what in particular concerns you about your ex-husband?'

— 'You mentioned problems in your marriage. Tell me some more about them.'

— 'Tell me some more about the children's relationship with their father's girlfriend.'

- Demonstrate empathy and show that you care.
  — 'It must be very difficult being a single mother.'
  — 'How do you manage looking after the children and working full-time?'
- Take a detailed history of the bruise. Avoid making her feel it is an interrogation. Remain friendly and calm.
  — 'I think we ought to concentrate some more on the bruise if that's okay. When exactly did you first notice the bruise?'
- Develop a feel for the social set up and identify any other adults involved in the children's lives.
  — 'So, apart from her father and his girlfriend, tell me who else she comes into contact with on a daily basis?'
  — 'What about her schooling? Briefly talk to me about that?'
  — 'Has Emma attended any nurseries or visited any friend's houses?'
- Offer support for the mother if you feel it is necessary.
  — 'I'm sure all of this must be taking its toll on you.'
  — 'Would it help to book yourself an appointment to come and see me?'
- After a difficult consultation, it sometimes helps to summarise at the end.
  — 'So, just to clarify then. We have agreed that I will contact social services. As soon as I have spoken to them, I'll call you with an update. I'll request that they attend to this matter as soon as possible. In the meantime, you have agreed to bring Emma in for me to assess, and you will make the appointment yourself. Was there anything else?'

⊶ Key summary
- Child abuse can manifest in many ways and should be considered in any child who presents with an injury. Other presentations are discussed on this page and overleaf on page 198.
- Perform a risk assessment to determine if the child is in immediate danger. If you feel they are at immediate risk, they must be taken to a place of safety such as a hospital.
- Referral to social services and follow-up are crucial.

Child abuse and child protection
- Every year, 2% of children are abused. In retrospective studies, 10% of men and 20% of women report abuse in their childhood.
- Abuse can be physical, emotional, sexual or neglect. They often overlap in the same child.

The role of the doctor
- A doctor's primary responsibility is the well-being of the child or children concerned.
- Where a child is at risk of serious harm, the interests of the child override those of parents or carers. Never delay taking emergency action.
- All doctors working with children, as well as parents and other adults in contact with children, should be able to recognise, and know how to act upon, signs that a child may be at risk of abuse or neglect, both in a home environment and in residential and other institutions.
- Efforts should be made to include children and young people in decisions that closely affect them. The views and wishes of children should therefore be listened to and respected according to their competence and the level of their understanding.
- When concerns about deliberate harm to children or young people have been raised, doctors must keep clear, accurate, comprehensive and contemporaneous notes.

Types of abuse
a Physical abuse
- Physical abuse comprises any action causing physical harm to a child.
- Physical harm may also be caused when a parent or carer feigns the symptoms of, or deliberately causes, ill health in a child whom they are looking after (Munchausen syndrome by proxy).
- Features of a history that may suggest child abuse include:
  — inconsistent history from carers
  — delay between the injury and the presentation
  — injury out of proportion to the alleged accident.
- The following investigations are mandatory in any case of suspected physical abuse:
  — full skeletal survey to look for old or undiagnosed fractures
  — blood tests including FBC for platelets, clotting, bone biochemistry
  — medical photography to document evidence of injuries.

b Emotional abuse
- Emotional abuse is the persistent emotional ill-treatment or neglect of a child that causes severe and persistent adverse effects on the child's emotional development.
- It may involve conveying to children that they are worthless or unloved, inadequate or valued only in so far as they meet the needs of another person.
- It may involve serious bullying (causing children to frequently feel frightened or in danger) or the exploitation or corruption of children.

c Sexual abuse
- Sexual abuse involves forcing or enticing a child or young person to take part in sexual activities, including prostitution, whether or not the child is aware of what is happening.
- The activities may involve physical contact, including penetrative or non-penetrative acts.
- They may include non-contact activities, such as involving children in looking at, or in the production of, pornographic material or watching sexual activities, or encouraging children to behave in sexually inappropriate ways.
- Child sexual abuse may present in a variety of ways in primary care, including:
  — anogenital bruising or injury
  — recurrent UTI
  — vaginal discharge
  — sexually precocious behaviour or language
  — behavioural problems – including enuresis, anorexia, sexualised behaviour or self-harm.

d Neglect
- Neglect is the persistent failure to meet a child's basic physical or psychological needs, which is likely to result in the serious impairment of the child's health or development.
- There are five types:
  1 **medical care neglect:** refusal of medical treatment by parents of child
  2 **gross safety neglect:** injury secondary to lack of supervision or hazardous environment
  3 **emotional deprivation:** failure to provide psychological caret
  4 **educational neglect:** persistent non-attendance at school >25 days/year without adequate reasons
  5 **physical neglect:** inadequate food, clothing or shelter that results in harm to normal development and which is not attended to by parents.

Risk factors
a Child factors
- Prematurity.
- Age <2 years.

- Demanding child.
- Physical or learning disability.

b Parental factors
- History of abuse.
- Substance abuse.
- Psychiatric problems.
- Chronic medical problems.
- Maternal age <30 years.
- Unwanted pregnancy.

c Environmental factors
- Family stresses.
- Social deprivation.
- Inadequate support.

O━ Key summary
- Take a history from the accompanying adult and, if possible, from the child.
- Fully examine the child, asking for an explanation of any injury.
- Further management depends on whether the child is at immediate risk:
  — Hospital admission for the child at immediate risk, for protection and more detailed assessment.
  — Liaise with social services child-protection team if the child is not at immediate risk.
- Keep detailed records of the consultation, with practice notes to state if the child is on the 'at risk' register, and also keep notes on siblings up to date.

Further reading
- NSPCC. *What is Child Abuse?* NSPCC; n.d. Available at: www.nspcc.org.uk/helpandadvice/whatchildabuse/whatischildabuse_wda36500.html (accessed 20 November 2010).
- Meadow R, Mok J, Rosenberg D. *ABC of Child Protection.* 4th ed. Oxford: Wiley-Blackwell; 2007.

Station 3.2

Actor's notes

Background

- You are Jane Jones, a 29-year-old sales assistant.

Opening statement

- 'Doctor, I've come to see you today for my results.'

History

- Three weeks ago, you noticed a change in your vaginal discharge.
- You came to see the nurse who suggested you have some swabs and a smear taken.
- You telephoned the practice for the results but the receptionist asked you to see the doctor.

Ideas, concerns and expectations

- You are very embarrassed about the vaginal discharge.
- You are worried you may have an infection because the discharge has not settled.
- You have never had a smear before and did not understand why the nurse performed it.
- You have come to see the GP for some treatment that will ensure the discharge resolves.

Further history candidate may elicit

- You broke up with your long-term partner one year ago. Since then, you have had several episodes of UPSI. The last occasion was one month ago with someone you met at a party. You have not met him again.
- You have been on the contraceptive pill for several years. You have not experienced any problems with it and take it regularly.
- You just started your period, since this is your pill-free week.
- You normally have some slight colourless vaginal discharge. However, three weeks ago, you developed a thick yellow vaginal discharge.
- It is not offensive and you have not experienced any itching.

- You mentioned it to your best friend who suggested you may have thrush. You tried using a cream you bought over the counter, for a few days, but this did not help.
- You spoke to your friend again, who advised you to have some tests.
- You became worried and saw the nurse, who suggested some vaginal swabs. The nurse also suggested you have a smear because you had not had one before.
- You felt so embarrassed about having the swabs that you did not ask the nurse what a smear was or why it was needed.
- Your best friend went on holiday, so you have not spoken to her about the smear.
- You only joined this practice one year ago, and have never received a letter to ask you to attend for a smear.
- Prior to that, you were registered with a GP in Manchester, but have been living in London for seven years.

Medical history and drug history
- Nil relevant.
- No previous smear.

Social history
- You do not smoke. You drink four to five units when you are at a party.
- You work as a sales assistant in a local clothes shop five days a week.
- You are currently single.
- You live with your best friend in a two-bedroom flat in London.
- You were born and brought up in Manchester, and moved to London seven years ago.
- Your parents and older brother still live in Manchester.

Family history
- Nil relevant.

Approach to scenario
- You are worried about coming to the doctor for the results and are embarrassed about the vaginal discharge. You want to discuss the results of the swabs first, and discuss the smear after.
- If the doctor explains you have chlamydia, you become alarmed and want to know if this has any long-lasting effects, especially on your fertility.
- You also want to know how to prevent getting further infections.
- If the doctor suggests you have an HIV test and use condoms in future, you agree.
- After you have discussed the vaginal discharge, you are ready to discuss the smear result, but want to know why you had it, and what it tests for.
- If the doctor explains the result is abnormal, you become concerned.
- If the doctor explains the abnormality can lead to cancer, you become particularly worried and want to know how you developed this abnormality, and how it can be treated.
- If the doctor suggests referring you to a specialist clinic for further treatment, you look frightened and ask 'Will I still be able to have a baby? Will this procedure stop me from having a baby?'
- If the doctor comes across well, you feel reassured that you do not have cancer and thank the doctor before you leave.
- If the doctor does not come across well, you become visibly upset.

Information gathering
Presenting complaint
a Vaginal discharge
- Ask about any changes in the vaginal discharge:
  — when it started
  — colour, e.g. green or yellow
  — consistency, e.g. thick
  — smell
  — frequency
  — relationship with menstrual cycle.

b Associated symptoms
- Ask about associated symptoms:
  — dyspareunia
  — urinary symptoms
  — vaginal itching
  — vaginal sores.

Sexual history
- Ask about use of condoms and UPSI.
- Ask about number of partners.

Medical history
- Smears.
- STIs.
- Sexual health check-ups including HIV tests.

Family history
- Ask about breast or gynaecological cancer in the family.

Drug history
- Check about current or past use of contraception.

Social history
- Occupation.
- Alcohol, smoking and use of recreational drugs.
- Relationship status.

Patient's agenda
- Explore her understanding of chlamydia.
- Discuss her understanding of STIs and what her thoughts are about the use of condoms.
- Explore her understanding of cervical cancer and HPV.
- Explore her concerns of developing cervical cancer and having further treatment.

Clinical management
1 Discuss the results of the swabs and treatment of chlamydia
- Explain the swab tests revealed she has chlamydia, which is an STI that can cause vaginal discharge.
- Underline the importance of treating chlamydia to prevent future complications such as pelvic inflammatory disease and infertility.
- Reassure her that treatment will prevent complications from developing.
- Advise her that there are several different antibiotics that can be taken, but the simplest one is a single dose of azithromycin.

- Outline the common side effects of the antibiotic – diarrhoea and vomiting.
- Reassure her that the potential side effects will be minimal since this is a single dose.

2 Discuss STIs in general
- Advise her to abstain from sex for seven days after treatment.
- Underline the importance of condom use for two weeks as the antibiotic can interact with the oral contraceptive pill and reduce its effectiveness.
- Emphasise the importance of contact tracing – she should notify any partners she has had sex with in the past six months. If she is not comfortable doing this herself, the practice nurse or GUM clinic can do so on her behalf.
- Underline the importance of condom use to prevent transmission of STDs and HIV in the future.
- Suggest she considers having an HIV test.

3 Discuss the smear results
- Explain that smears are used as a routine screening tool to look for any abnormalities of the cervix and involve taking a sample of cells from the cervix or 'neck of the womb'.
- Explain that her smear results revealed some moderately abnormal cells.
- Emphasise that although the cells are abnormal, she does not have cancer.
- Explain that these cells *can* return to normal, but could also become more abnormal and even cancerous in time, so are best treated now.
- Explain that the most common cause of abnormal cervical cells and cervical cancer is HPV.
- Explain HPV is transmitted during sex (and so is an STD) so she will have picked it up from a previous sexual partner.

4 Further treatment
- Advise her that you need to refer her to a specialist for further treatment to get a closer look at the abnormal cells.
- Discuss what this appointment would involve:
    - A closer examination of the cervix using a magnifying device.
    - Taking a biopsy or small sample of tissue to be viewed in the laboratory.
    - Removal of the abnormal cells, using local anaesthetic to numb the area.
    - Explain that the process is usually not painful but may be uncomfortable because of the position she will have to lie in.
- Explain briefly that the abnormal cells are usually removed using diathermy or a 'hot wire'.
- The purpose of this treatment is to remove the abnormal cells to help prevent cancer in the future.

5 Complications of treatment
- Reassure her that treatment for cervical dyskaryosis will not affect fertility or future pregnancies.
- Explain there is a small risk of developing an infection after treatment.

6 Follow-up
- Explain and emphasise the need for follow-up smears more frequently in the future, and that the schedule would be explained when treatment was completed.
- Offer her leaflets and a follow-up appointment in the next few weeks to discuss any further issues.

Interpersonal skills

- During the consultation, the candidate has to treat the patient for a STD, but also discuss the abnormal smear. One approach is to work through the problems systematically.
- When informing her she has chlamydia, ensure that she has the chance to take in the news. Some patients may not have heard of this infection, so seek feedback verbally and non-verbally to check for understanding. Take the time provide explanation according to her response.
  — 'The swabs show you have an infection called chlamydia (silence). Have you heard of this?'
  — 'Chlamydia is an infection passed through sexual contact. Condoms help to limit its spread.'
- Address any concerns at this stage about chlamydia, answering any questions in the process.
  — 'If we treat this now with antibiotics, then we have a very good chance of clearing the infection and preventing any complications.'
  — 'Chlamydia can cause fertility problems, especially when it is not treated. It is good that we did a swab and identified it.'
  — 'As I mentioned, wearing condoms helps prevent spread of all sexually transmitted disease, not just chlamydia. I will give you some information sheets about this so you can find out more. What are your thoughts so far?'
  — 'We mentioned infections being passed on by sexual contact. We have checked for most of the important ones and I am please to say the results showed you don't have them. However, we didn't check for HIV.'
- It is important to reassure the patient that she does not have cervical cancer, yet explain the importance for further treatment and long-term follow-up.
  — 'I would like to reassure you that the abnormal cells in your cervix are not cancer . . . (silence) . . . but the abnormal cells could in the future go on to become cancer, and that is why we have done the test. This way we can 'get in' early and destroy the bad cells, which will make it unlikely you will get cervical cancer.'
  — 'Obviously we need to perform smears regularly, just to check that the abnormal cells don't come back, but this is quite straightforward.'
- Allow the patient time to ask questions and explore her fears about future treatment.
  — 'You seem apprehensive about all of this. Is there anything worrying you?'
  — 'The colposcopy test we spoke about is a very common procedure carried out by doctors who do it on a very regular basis. The overwhelming majority of women with your conditions, chlamydia and abnormal cells, go on to have completely normal fertility.'
- Explaining that cervical cell dyskaryosis and cervical cancer are linked to HPV, an STD, can be difficult for the patient and needs to be handled sensitively.
  — 'There is a virus that is passed through sexual contact. It is called human papillomavirus or HPV. HPV can cause the abnormal cells that we spoke about earlier. As I mentioned, these abnormal cells can go on to become cancer in the future. This is how HPV and cervical cancer are linked . . . (silence) . . . Feel free to ask any questions.'
  — 'Going back to our earlier discussion about condoms. These will also help prevent spread of HPV and so this is another good reason to use them.'

O⌐ Key summary
- Be aware of the treatment and complications of STDs.
- Be able to counsel patients on sexual health, the importance of condoms and contact tracing.
- Explain the results to the patient, reassuring her that she does not have cervical cancer.
- Outline the relationship of HPV to cervical dyskaryosis and cervical cancer.
- Formulate a management plan with appropriate referral and follow-up.

The cervix

- The epithelium of the cervix is varied. The ectocervix, which is the distal part of cervix and continuous with the vagina, is lined with squamous epithelium. The endocervix, which is the proximal part of the cervix that opens into the uterine cavity, is lined with columnar epithelium.
- The transformational zone describes the border of squamous epithelium that undergoes metaplasia to columnar epithelium. Metaplasia normally occurs during puberty and pregnancy.
- Cells undergoing metaplasia are vulnerable to neoplastic change if exposed to certain agents, and cervical carcinoma usually originates from the cells in the transformational area.

Cervical intraepithelial neoplasia (CIN)

- CIN is the preinvasive stage to cervical cancer.
- It describes the presence of atypical, dyskaryotic cells in the squamous epithelium.
- If untreated, 30–40% of patients will develop invasive cervical cancer over 3–10 years.
- There are three stages – CIN I (mild) to CIN III (severe). CIN III is also known as carcinoma-in-situ.
- CIN I can progress to CIN III but more commonly regresses spontaneously.
- Risk factors include HPV (types 16, 18, 31 and 33), smoking and immunocompromised states (e.g. HIV and long-term steroid therapy).

Cervical screening

- By identifying women with CIN through the cervical screening programme and offering early treatment, the incidence of cervical cancer can be reduced.
- Currently, the cervical screening programme is available to women aged 25–64 years. Women aged 25–49 should be screened every three years and women aged 50–64 are screened every five years.
- Smears identify cellular abnormalities (dyskaryosis), rather than histological abnormalities.
- The degree of dyskaryosis is graded mild, moderate and severe.
- Dyskaryosis suggests the presence of CIN. The **grade** of dyskaryosis reflects the severity of CIN.
- The presence of mild dyskaryosis would suggest CIN I, whilst moderate dyskaryosis suggests CIN II and severe dyskaryosis suggests CIN III. However, a biopsy is needed to confirm the diagnosis and severity of CIN.

Management of abnormal smears

TABLE 3.1 Management of abnormal smears

SMEAR ABNORMALITY	FURTHER MANAGEMENT
Normal	Repeat every 3 or 5 years
Inflammatory	Take swabs Repeat in 6 months If persistent, proceed to colposcopy
Mild dyskaryosis	Repeat in 6 months If persistent, proceed to colposcopy
Moderate dyskaryosis	Refer for colposcopy
Severe dyskaryosis	Refer urgently for colposcopy

Colposcopy

- Colposcopy is performed if a cervical smear shows moderate or severe dyskaryosis, or if mild abnormalities persist. The cervix is examined using a magnifying device and biopsies are taken to determine the severity of CIN.

- If CIN II or III are confirmed, several procedures are available to remove the abnormal cells.
- Most commonly, large loop excision of the transformation zone (LLETZ) is used. This procedure involves excision of the transformation zone with diathermy, under local anaesthetic. The advantage of this procedure is that abnormal tissue is removed but not destroyed, so a histological diagnosis can be made at the same time as treatment. Subsequent pregnancies are unaffected.
- Other procedures, outlined in Table 3.2, destroy the area of abnormality, hence a histological diagnosis is not possible.

TABLE 3.2 Methods of treating abnormal cervical cells

LLETZ	Abnormal tissue is removed by diathermy The tissue is preserved for histological examination
Laser therapy	Abnormal cells are destroyed by laser ablation
Heat coagulation	Abnormal cells are destroyed by a hot probe
Cryotherapy	Abnormal cells are destroyed by a cold probe

Cervical cancer
- Risk factors include HPV infection, smoking and immunocompromised states such as HIV.
- Clinical features include postcoital, intermenstrual or postmenopausal bleeding. Offensive vaginal discharge and dyspareunia can also occur.
- Examination may reveal a palpable or visible cervical mass or ulcer.
- Microinvasive disease can be treated with a cone biopsy only. Complications of this procedure include postoperative haemorrhage, cervical stenosis and cervical incompetence.
- A caesarean section may needed if cervical stenosis occurs, and a cervical stitch may be needed to prevent premature delivery. In older women, simple hysterectomy is preferred.
- Stage 1 and 2a disease can be managed by radical abdominal hysterectomy (Wertheim's hysterectomy) which involves pelvic lymph node clearance, hysterectomy and removal of the parametrium and upper third of the vagina. The ovaries are left only in young women.
- Radiotherapy is then used after surgery if histological examination shows lymph node involvement.
- Radiotherapy can be used without surgery – survival rates are equivalent but complications are greater. This option is usually reserved for elderly women who are medically unfit for surgery.
- In later stages, the cancer has spread too widely and surgery is not an option. Patients are treated with radiotherapy.

Further reading
- CancerHelp UK. *Cervical Cancer*. London: Cancer Research UK; 2009. Available at: www.cancerhelp.org.uk/type/cervical-cancer/index.htm (accessed 23 November 2010).
- Impey L, Child T. *Obstetrics and Gynaecology*. 3rd ed. Oxford: Wiley-Blackwell; 2008.
- Collier J, Longmore M, Turmezei T, *et al. Oxford Handbook of Clinical Specialties*. 8th ed. Oxford: Oxford University Press; 2009.

Station 3.3

```
Candidate's notes
Name                    Tom Green
Age                     55
Medical history         Diabetes
Medication              Aspirin 75 mg od
                        Ramipril 5 mg od
                        Simvastatin 40 mg od
                        Metformin 500 mg qds
                        Gliclazide 160 mg bd
Allergies               Nil
Last consultation       Seen by diabetic nurse two months ago
                        Advised Hb A₁c raised at 8.5%
                        Neurovascular examination of lower limbs normal
                        BP = 125/77 mmHg
                        BMI = 30 kg/m²
                        Suggest repeat bloods in two months
                        Explained may need insulin if not controlled
                        Repeat blood test from last week shows Hb A₁c 9.8%
                        Serum lipids and renal function normal
                        Urinary ACR normal
                        Asked to see GP for review
```

Actor's notes

Background
- You are Tom Green, a 59-year-old financial executive.

Opening statement
- 'Doctor, the nurse told me to come to see you.'

History
- You saw the diabetic nurse two months ago who explained that your diabetes is poorly controlled.
- She explained that you may need insulin if there is no improvement in the overall control.
- She advised you to have your blood test repeated in two months and see the GP for a discussion about your diabetes since you may need to start on insulin.
- You repeated the blood test last week and have come today to find out the results.

Ideas, concerns and expectations
- You have many negative views about insulin because your father needed daily insulin for diabetes and he found it very problematic.
- You do not want to use insulin because you think using insulin is very complicated, do not like the thought of using needles to inject yourself and want to avoid the problems your father experienced.
- You are concerned that your diabetic control is not improving and are willing to take any advice or tablets the doctor has to offer, but you refuse to take insulin.

Further history candidate may elicit

- You were diagnosed with diabetes 18 months ago when you had a routine blood test.
- Your Hb A_{1c} has been poorly controlled ever since diagnosis despite you increasing the number of tablets to control your diabetes. You are always concordant with your medication, but do not measure your blood glucose routinely.
- You know you are overweight and rarely do any exercise. You eat a lot of fried food, junk food and red meat. You often snack on biscuits or chocolates.
- You do not have any symptoms of polydipsia, polyuria, weight loss or recurrent infections.
- Your vision is normal and you attend your annual eye screening.
- You have not noticed any loss of sensation in your feet.
- Your father had diabetes in his old age. He needed insulin daily, which he found very inconvenient, especially if he was eating at a restaurant or in front of guests. On several occasions his blood sugars would drop too low and he would have to go to hospital. He passed away a few years ago from colon cancer.
- You are aware of the complications of diabetes, but know you may well die from a condition unrelated to diabetes, like your father, who despite having excellent control of his diabetes fell ill for other reasons.
- You think using insulin is very complicated since it needs to be taken at specific times, which would be difficult since you travel a lot with work.
- You do not like the thought of using needles. You are not needle phobic, but because of your diabetes, have had many blood tests that have been painful.

Medical history

- Diabetes, diagnosed 18 months ago.
- Hypertension, diagnosed one year ago.

Drug history

- Aspirin 75 mg od.
- Ramipril 5 mg od.
- Simvastatin 40 mg od.
- Metformin 500 mg qds.
- Gliclazide 160 mg bd.

Family history

- Your father had type 2 diabetes and needed insulin. He died from colon cancer five years ago.
- Your mother died from a stroke three years ago.
- You have two younger brothers who have high BP but no diabetes.
- You are a financial executive and often have to travel around the UK or abroad for work.

Social history

- You do not smoke. You drink one or two pints on most days.
- You live with your wife. Your two children are in university.

Approach to scenario

- You are very disappointed to hear your Hb A_{1c} has risen and your diabetic control has worsened.
- You ask the doctor 'What do I have to do to make sure my diabetes improves?'
- You refuse insulin, even if the doctor is helpful and explains the complications of diabetes.
- However, you are willing to discuss other ways to improve your diabetic control, such as weight loss, dietary change and exercise.
- You are willing to try orlistat for weight loss and accept a referral to the local gym +/– dietician if the doctor suggests it.
- You will accept adding in another tablet for your diabetes, but not insulin.

- If the doctor communicates well and provides you with a range of options, you engage in conversation and inform the doctor 'This is a wake-up call for me – I'll work hard at my diet and do my best to lose weight.'
- If the doctor only considers insulin treatment, you become unhappy and repeatedly state 'I will not take insulin.'

Information gathering
Presenting complaint
a Diabetes
- Ask about polydipsia, polyuria and recurrent infections.
- Ask about vision and sensory disturbance of lower limbs.
- Ask about concordance with medication.
- Check if the patient measures blood sugar at home.

b Risk factors
- Smoking.
- Hypertension.
- Hypercholesterolaemia.
- Family history of heart disease or stroke.

c Weight control
- Ask about diet (portion size, junk food, snacks, drinks).
- Ask about exercise (walking, swimming or other activities).

Medical history
- Hypertension.
- Other autoimmune disease.

Family history
- Diabetes.
- Other autoimmune disease.

Drug history
- Confirm medications.
- Ask about side effects.
- Check concordance with medications.

Social history
- Occupation, e.g. driver.
- Smoking and alcohol.
- Home circumstances.

Patient's agenda
- Explore his understanding of diabetes.
- Explore his concerns about insulin treatment.
- Explore which options he would consider to improve control.

Clinical management

1 Explain the blood results
- Explain that the blood test, with an Hb A_{1c} of 9.8%, shows his diabetes is not under control.
- Discuss the complications of diabetes, emphasising the importance of diabetic control in reducing the risk of complications:
  - microvascular – diabetic retinopathy, nephropathy and neuropathy
  - macrovascular – ischaemic heart disease, MI and stroke.

2 Discuss treatment options

a *Insulin*
- Explain that diabetes results from a lack of insulin in the body, or insulin resistance.
- Insulin therapy therefore improves diabetic control and reduces the risk of diabetic complications.
- This would involve self-administered daily injections and checking blood glucose levels with finger-prick monitoring.
- Offer strategies to address his concerns.
  - Suggest trying insulin for one month and then review – stop if not suitable.
  - Explain that he may only need to add in a dose of insulin overnight, whilst continuing his tablets, which would be manageable even when travelling.
  - Explain that hypoglycaemic events are minimised by optimal control.
  - Reassure him that insulin needles are not like blood tests and are much less painful.

b *Oral hypoglycaemics*
- Explain importance of concordance.
- Explain that he is already on the maximum dose of metformin and gliclazide.
- Offer an alternative oral hypoglycaemic agent.
  - Gliptins would be the best choice for this patient as they are not associated with weight gain.
  - Glitazones can also be offered, but can cause weight gain.

3 Weight loss
- Explain that type 2 diabetes results from insulin resistance, which can be improved by weight loss.
- Outline lifestyle measures that can help weight loss.
  - Offer dietary advice, e.g. healthier eating and smaller portions.
  - Offer a referral to a dietician to provide further information.
  - Offer advice on exercise, e.g. start gently and build up over time.
  - Offer exercise referral to the local gym.
- Offer orlistat to augment weight loss.
  - Outline the action of orlistat in preventing absorption of fat.
  - Explain this needs to be taken three times a day.
  - Discuss common GI side effects.
  - Explain that this would not be a long-term option but to help kick-start his weight loss.

4 Follow-up
- Suggest looking at Diabetes UK website (www.diabetes.org.uk) and attending local diabetic groups to speak with others about the use of insulin.
- Offer follow-up appointment.
- Advise he needs to have his Hb A_{1c} rechecked in two months.
- Provide him with information leaflets about diabetes.

Note:
- Ideally, this patient should be managed in primary care, but if the candidate suggested a referral to the diabetic clinic, this would be acceptable.

Interpersonal skills

- Key aspects of this case include:
  - knowledge of NICE guidelines for the management of diabetes
  - understanding the concerns of the patient about insulin treatment
  - respecting his autonomy and decision to refuse treatment with insulin
  - working with him to formulate a shared management plan.
- The candidate would be expected to outline the benefits of insulin and appreciate the patient's concerns about insulin therapy.
  - 'The advantage of insulin is that it will control your blood sugar better, and so reduce the risk of you having a heart attack or stroke, or developing kidney, nerve and vision problems.'
  - 'Are there any reasons why you aren't so keen on taking insulin?'
  - 'I can understand why you want to hold off insulin. How about we discuss some of your concerns? . . . (silence) . . . Insulin injections are not as painful as blood tests. This is because they make the needles a lot smaller nowadays. Also, you may only need to take insulin at night, and be able to continue taking your tablets in the day. This means you wouldn't need regular insulin throughout the day. How do you feel about having a trial for one month to see how you get on?'
  - 'There have been many developments in diabetes treatment since your father used insulin. A lot of the newer insulins can be well tailored to meet your own individual lifestyle requirements.'
  - 'The alternative to insulin at this stage is to look at your overall health and add in another tablet. Losing weight would help improve your diabetes. Have you considered that before?'
  - 'Tell me about your diet. How do you think you could improve your diet?'
  - 'Exercise would help improve your diabetes control. Is there any type of exercise you enjoy?'
  - 'If you are not happy to try insulin, would you consider another tablet for your diabetes?'
- Summarise at the end and give the patient the opportunity to come back and see you.
  - 'I realise that there has been a lot to take in today. We have discussed the option of insulin, which I know you aren't keen on. We also discussed some of the lifestyle measures, such as weight reduction, for which you will also start orlistat. We will also be starting one of the newer diabetic medicines. And we will review things after the next blood test. Are there any questions you would like to ask?'

⌐ Key summary
- Be familiar with NICE guidelines on diabetes.
- Outline the complications of poor glycaemic control.
- Address the patient's concerns about insulin therapy.
- Discuss alternative hypoglycaemic drugs.
- Address management of other risk factors such as weight control.

Management of type 2 diabetes: lifestyle and other drugs
Diet
- Smaller portion size and fewer snacks – opt for healthier options.
- Limit intake of fried food.
- Reduce alcohol intake.
- Increase water intake and avoid artificial drinks.

Exercise
- Aim for 30 minutes a day.
- Consider 'exercise referral' to local gym.

Orlistat
a Mechanism of action
- Lipase inhibitor that reduces the absorption of dietary fat.

b Indications
- BMI of >30 **or** BMI >28 in the presence of other risk factors such as diabetes, hypertension or hypercholesterolaemia.
- Used in conjunction with other lifestyle measures, and may be continued for up to 12 months.

c Side effects and contraindications
- GI effects, e.g. flatulence, liquid/oily stools, abdominal distension and pain – minimised by reduced fat intake. Other side effects include headache, anxiety and fatigue.
- Contraindicated in malabsorption states.

d Dosage
- 120 mg up to three times a day.
- Continue treatment beyond 12 weeks only if >5% weight loss.

Antiplatelets
- Aspirin 75 mg daily if >50 years **and** BP <145/90 mmHg.
- Aspirin 75 mg daily if <50 years **and** significant cardiovascular risk factors.
- Clopidogrel should be used instead of aspirin **only** in those with clear aspirin intolerance.

BP
- Measure BP annually in patients with normal BP and no end-organ damage.
- Measure BP every six months if on antihypertensives.
- If end-organ damage (CVD, diabetic nephropathy or retinopathy), aim BP <130/80 mmHg.
- If no end-organ damage, aim BP <140/80 mmHg.
- Offer lifestyle advice regarding diet (including low salt), exercise and weight control.
- First-line antihypertensive is ACE inhibitor or ARB, second-line is calcium channel blocker.

Lipids
- Offer diet and lifestyle advice.
- Aim for total cholesterol <4.0 and LDL <2.0.
- Offer simvastatin 40 mg if >40 years **or** <40 years if CVD risk factors present, e.g. microalbuminuria or strong family history of premature cardiovascular disease.
- If target cholesterol not achieved, increase simvastatin to 80 mg or add ezetimibe.
- Offer a fibrate if triglycerides raised and not controlled with lifestyle or statin.

Management of type 2 diabetes: hypoglycaemic agents

- The choice of treatment should be made in conjunction with the patient.
- With all treatments, Hb A_{1c} should be checked every two to six months until diabetic control is stable.
- Once blood glucose and treatment are stable, Hb A_{1c} should be monitored every six months.

Biguanides, e.g. metformin
a Mechanism of action
- Decreases gluconeogenesis and increases peripheral utilisation of glucose.

b Important side effects
- Lactic acidosis.
- Diarrhoea and abdominal pain.

c Contraindications
- Impaired renal function – creatinine >150 or GFR <30.
- MI.
- Hepatic impairment.

d Monitoring – renal function
- Measure renal function before initiating metformin therapy and regularly throughout treatment.
- Check renal function annually in people with normal renal function, and twice a year in older persons.
- Review dose if creatinine >130 or GFR <30. Stop metformin if creatinine >150 or GFR <30.

e Indications
- First-line treatment for people who are overweight (BMI >25).
- Consider as first-line treatment or combination therapy for people who are not overweight.

Insulin secretagogues: sulfonylureas and meglitinides
a Mechanism of action
- Insulin secretagogues include the sulfonylureas (gliclazide, glimepiride and glipizide) and the rapid-acting insulin secretagogues (nateglinide and repaglinide).
- Sulfonylureas act by increasing insulin secretion.
- The rapid-acting insulin secretagogues (meglitinides), also stimulate insulin release. These drugs have a rapid onset of action and a short duration of activity.
- Patients should be educated about the risk of hypoglycaemia.

b Side effects
- Weight gain of 1–5 kg.
- Hypoglycaemia, e.g. frail, older, renal or hepatic impairment and those with irregular meal times.

c Contraindications
- Avoid using in people at increased risk of hypoglycaemia and in people with occupations where hypoglycaemia may present a problem (e.g. HGV drivers).

d Indications
- A sulfonylurea is first choice when an insulin secretagogue is indicated.
- Sulfonylureas should be considered first-line glucose-lowering therapy:
  — for people who are not overweight
  — if metformin is contraindicated or poorly tolerated
  — if a rapid response to therapy is required because of hyperglycaemic symptoms.

- Should be added as second treatment if blood glucose control is inadequate with metformin.

e Comments
- A rapid-acting insulin secretagogue may be preferred for people with erratic lifestyles leading to irregular meal times.

Glitazones or thiazolidinediones: pioglitazone and rosiglitazone
a Mechanism of action
- Peroxisome proliferator-activated receptor (PPAR)-gamma agonists.

b Important side effects
- Weight gain.
- Water retention and leg oedema.
- Hypoglycaemia (only when used in combination with a sulfonylurea).

c Contraindications
- Hepatic impairment.
- Heart failure or history of heart failure because they cause fluid retention.
- Avoid in women at risk of fractures as they double fracture risk in women (but not men).

d Monitoring
i Liver function
- Assess liver function prior to initiating therapy. Check every two months for the first year of treatment.
- If ALT levels increase >3× the upper limit of normal during treatment, recheck.
- If they remain >3× the upper limit of normal, treatment should be discontinued.

ii Fluid retention and cardiac failure
- Monitor for signs and symptoms of fluid retention (including weight gain or oedema).
- Stop glitazone if any deterioration is seen in cardiac function.

iii Blood glucose control
- Only continue glitazone therapy if the Hb A_{1c} falls by 0.5% in six months.

e Indications
i Dual therapy with metformin
- Consider adding a glitazone, instead of a sulfonylurea, to metformin **if**:
  — significant risk from hypoglycaemia or its consequences, e.g. older, social circumstances (living alone) and certain jobs (working at heights or with heavy machinery)
  — sulfonylurea not tolerated or is contraindicated.

ii Dual therapy with sulfonylurea
- **If** metformin is not tolerated or contraindicated.

iii Triple therapy with metformin and sulfonylurea
- **If** insulin is unacceptable or inappropriate (e.g. employment, social or recreational issues, injection anxieties or obesity).

iv Pioglitazone with insulin therapy
- **If**:
  — patient has previously had a marked glucose-lowering response to glitazone **or**
  — on high-dose insulin therapy and blood glucose is inadequately controlled.

Note:
- Glitazones may be preferable to dipeptidyl-peptidase 4 (DPP4) inhibitors **if:**
  — the person has marked insulin insensitivity
  — a DPP4 inhibitor is contraindicated
  — patient had previous poor response to, or did not tolerate, a DPP4 inhibitor.

DPP4 inhibitors: sitagliptin and vildagliptin
a Mechanism of action
- Inhibit the enzyme DPP4.
- The gliptins do not cause weight gain – an advantage to the glitazones.

b Contraindications
- Avoid either drug in renal impairment.
- Contraindicated in pregnancy and breastfeeding.
- Vildagliptin should be avoided in hepatic impairment.

c Monitoring
i Liver function (for vildagliptin, not sitagliptin)
- LFTs should be checked before initiating treatment with vildagliptin, every three months during the first year of treatment, and periodically thereafter.
- Stop the drug if ALT or AST increases >3× the upper limit of normal.

ii Blood glucose control
- Only continue gliptin therapy if the Hb A_{1c} has fallen 0.5% in six months.

d Indications
i Second-line therapy with metformin
- **If:**
  — significant risk of hypoglycaemia or its consequences
  — sulfonylurea not tolerated or a sulfonylurea is contraindicated.

ii 2nd-line therapy with sulphonylurea
- **If** metformin not tolerated or contraindicated.

iii 3rd-line therapy
- When insulin is inappropriate or unacceptable, e.g. in the above case.

e Further comments
- DPP4 inhibitors may be preferable to a thiazolidinedione **if:**
  — the patient has a high BMI **or**
  — thiazolidinediones are contraindicated **or**
  — the patient has had a poor response to, or did not tolerate, a thiazolidinedione.

Glucagon-like peptide-1 (GLP-1) mimetics: exenatide and liraglutide
a Administration
- Both drugs are administered by subcutaneous injection.
- Exenatide is administered twice daily and liraglutide once daily.
- Can be used to improve glycaemic control and induce weight loss.

b Important side effects
- GI side effects, e.g. nausea, vomiting and diarrhoea.
- Exenatide has been found to cause pancreatitis.

c Contraindications

- Severe GI disease, e.g. IBD, because of GI side effects.
- Renal impairment.
- Pregnancy and breastfeeding.
- Acute or history of pancreatitis.

d Monitoring

- Only continue exenatide therapy if the Hb A_{1c} has fallen >1% **and** patient has lost at least 3% of initial body weight in six months.
- NICE did not issue guidance on the continuation of liraglutide because it was not available at the time the guidance was published.

e Indications

i Triple therapy

- Consider adding exenatide to metformin and a sulfonylurea **if:**
  — BMI ≥35 in those of European descent (adjust for other ethnic groups) and specific psychological or medical problems associated with high body weight **or**
  — a BMI <35.0 kg/m^2, and therapy with insulin would have significant occupational implications or weight loss would benefit other significant obesity-related comorbidities.

Insulin

a Indications

- If patient agrees, start insulin therapy when blood glucose control remains or becomes inadequate (Hb A_{1c} ≥ 7.5%) with other measures.
- Consider insulin therapy **in preference** to adding other drugs in patients already on dual therapy unless the insulin is inappropriate or unacceptable.

b Issues to consider

- Patients should be aware of the need for self-monitoring and the management of hypoglycaemia.
- Drivers with diabetes who require insulin therapy have to inform the DVLA.

Further reading

- Diabetes UK website. www.diabetes.org.uk/ (accessed 24 November 2010).
- National Institute for Health and Clinical Excellence. Type 2 Diabetes: newer agents; NICE guideline 87. London: NIHCE; 2009. www.nice.org.uk/nicemedia/live/12165/44318/44318. pdf (accessed 24 November 2010).
- Simon C, Everitt H, van Dorp F. *Oxford Handbook of General Practice*. 3rd ed. Oxford: Oxford University Press; 2010.
- Longmore M, Wilkinson I, Davidson E, *et al*. *Oxford Handbook of Clinical Medicine*. 8th ed. Oxford: Oxford University Press; 2010.

Station 3.4

Vision Opticians
1 Eye Street
Eysleworth
EYE 1OP

Dear GP

This gentleman attended for an eye test today.
His visual acuity is 6/12 in both eyes and I have recommended he wears glasses.
On examination, he had mild cupping of both optic discs.

Intraocular pressure: right eye 20 mmHg,
                          left eye 21 mmHg.

Visual field examination was normal.
Kindly refer him to an ophthalmologist **routinely**, in view of the disc cupping.

Yours sincerely
I Sight
(Optician)

Actor's notes
Background
- You are Ican See, a 37-year-old Afro-Caribbean paramedic.

Opening statement
- 'Doctor, I've come to talk about my eyes.'

History
- You saw the optician last week for an eye test and were told you needed glasses. He also said that the nerve supplying your eyes looked abnormal and that the pressures were 'a bit high'.
- He suggested you may have glaucoma, and needed to see your GP so you could be referred to an eye specialist.

Ideas, concerns and expectations
- You are concerned you have glaucoma.
- You were alarmed to read on the internet that glaucoma can lead to deterioration in vision or blindness, and are extremely worried about going blind.

- You are about to start up a part-time business as a photographer and are scared that if your vision starts to fail, so will your business.
- You want an urgent referral to see a specialist so that you can start treatment immediately.

Further history candidate may elicit

- Over the last two or three months, you noticed that distant objects were slightly blurry and unfocussed. Nearby objects appear normal.
- Your wife noticed you were having difficulty reading street signs when driving so recommended you go to the optician.
- You saw the optician last week who checked your eyes and did some tests. He explained that you were slightly short-sighted and recommended glasses. He also explained that the nerve supplying both eyes looked abnormal, which could suggest the start of glaucoma. He advised you to see the GP for a referral to a specialist.
- You had not heard of glaucoma before and subsequently researched it on the internet and found that this condition can lead to blindness. You also read that patients with glaucoma may need treatment with laser therapy or surgery if the glaucoma is not treated quickly.
- You have come to the GP for an urgent referral to see the eye specialist this week so that you can start treatment quickly and avoid laser or surgery treatment, and preserve your eyesight.
- You do not have private medical insurance but have worked as a paramedic for the NHS for several years, and you believe that frontline NHS workers should get a degree of priority to healthcare. You enjoy your role as a paramedic but find the hours and shifts you work are affecting your home life.
- You have not had any headaches, haloes, pain or redness of the eyes.
- You are passionate about photography, which you started as a hobby two years ago.
- You are hoping to start up a part-time photography business in the next few months and ideally would like to become a full-time photographer in the next few years.
- You ordered a pair of glasses but are thinking about getting contact lenses, which would let you use your camera more easily.

Medical history

- Nil.

Drug history

- Nil.

Family history

- Your father died 11 years ago from lung cancer.
- You remember he used eye drops but cannot remember why.
- Your two older sisters and brother are all well.

Social history

- You drink two to three pints of beer on the weekends.
- You are an ex-smoker. From the age of 14 to 25 you smoked about ten cigarettes a day.
- You live with your wife, who is a school teacher, and two children in a three-bedroom house.
- Your parents are both Afro-Caribbean and emigrated from Jamaica before you were born. You have lived in the UK all your life.
- You spend your leisure time with your family or improving your photography skills.

Approach to scenario
* You are worried about being diagnosed with glaucoma and going blind.
* You have come to the GP today expecting an urgent referral to an eye specialist.
* You believe you should be seen urgently by the specialist because you may have a condition that can cause blindness, and because you have worked for the NHS for a number of years.
* You are frustrated to hear that you have to wait several weeks to see a specialist, and express your concern that a delay in potential treatment may affect your vision.
* You express your anger at working for the NHS for several years, yet not receiving support at your time of need.
* You cannot afford to see a specialist privately.
* You want to know if you definitely have glaucoma and how this condition develops.
* If the GP explains that glaucoma is treatable and does not always lead to blindness, you feel somewhat reassured.
* However, if the doctor does not communicate this in a confident manner, you will still be reluctant to accept the advice given.
* If the doctor comes across well, and reasonably explains that there are long waiting times to see a specialist, you agree to an NHS referral, provided the GP agrees to state that you are a paramedic and asks for you to be seen quickly.
* If the doctor does not seem caring or empathic, or fails to explain why they cannot have you seen urgently, you beat your fist on the table and say 'I want to see the specialist next week!'

Information gathering
Presenting complaint
* Clarify why the patient visited the optician (routine appointment or due to visual problems).
* Ask how long ago he noticed distance vision was problematic.
* Ask about symptoms of glaucoma:
  — eye pain
  — headaches
  — visual haloes
  — redness of the eyes.
* Ask about other visual symptoms:
  — floaters
  — colour vision
  — flashing lights.
* Explore what the optician has explained.
* Explore whether he has decided to use contact lenses or glasses.

Medical history
* Any other medical condition.

Family history
* Ask specifically about diabetes and glaucoma.

Drug history
* Current medication.

Social history
* Alcohol and smoking.
* Current occupation.
* Social activities.
* Home circumstances (marital status, dependents).

Patient's agenda
- Explore his understanding about glaucoma.
- Explore his concerns about blindness and the impact on his personal and professional life.
- Discuss his expectations regarding specialist referral and treatment options.

Clinical management
1 Explain the results of the eye test
- Explain the optician found he was short-sighted and noted bilateral optic disc cupping, along with raised intraocular pressures.
- Explain short-sightedness is:
  — very common
  — easily managed with glasses and contact lenses.
- Explain optic disc cupping with raised intraocular pressures:
  — can be, but is not always, related to glaucoma
  — needs to be assessed by an ophthalmologist to make the diagnosis.

2 Explain about glaucoma and how it is management
- Explain glaucoma usually results from increased intraocular pressure due to poor drainage of aqueous humour, which leads to damage of the optic nerve.
- Inform him risk factors include myopia, diabetes, a family history of glaucoma and Afro-Caribbean ethnicity.
- Emphasise the progression of glaucoma is generally very slow, requires monitoring over a long period and it is important that treatment is introduced at the appropriate time.
- Explain that treatment of glaucoma ranges from eye drops to laser treatment and surgery.
- Reassure him that most cases are managed with eye drops only.
- Reassure him that although glaucoma can lead to blindness, this is rare as early treatment prevents deterioration in vision, and patients can generally expect to have good eyesight indefinitely.

3 Negotiate a shared care management plan for specialist referral
- Explain that optic disc cupping is considered a non-urgent referral. Therefore, he is likely to wait four to six weeks before being seen by the specialist.
- Explain you recognise his years of hard work for the NHS, but this is unlikely to speed up the referral process.
- Suggest, however, you will emphasise this in your letter, together with the fact that he is concerned about developing glaucoma and his interest in photography.
- Explore whether he would consider seeing the specialist privately.

4 Follow-up
- Offer him leaflets about glaucoma.
- Advise him to return for further discussion if needed.

Interpersonal skills
- The focus of this station is to understand the patient's concerns about blindness and seeing a specialist quickly.
- An explanation of glaucoma must be delivered in lay terms, if possible with a simple diagram to clearly illustrate the pathology.
  — 'Our eyes need a certain amount of pressure to maintain the shape of the eyeball and let it function properly. A fluid known as the aqueous humour helps provide this pressure. It also provides nutrients to the eye. The aqueous humour is continually produced inside the eye and then drains out through special ducts.'

- 'However, sometimes the eye produces excessive amounts of aqueous humour, or it does not clear away effectively. As a result, the pressure in the eye builds up and can damage the optic nerve. The optic nerve is important because it carries information to the brain about what the eye sees. Does that make sense?'

- It is important to explain that he has not been diagnosed with glaucoma yet, but does have some risk factors, such as his ethnicity, short-sightedness and a possible family history.
  - 'The optician noticed the pressures were raised and saw some changes in the optic nerve that may suggest glaucoma. Glaucoma is more common in people who are over 40 years of age, have a family history, are short-sighted, are of Afro-Caribbean descent or have diabetes.'
  - 'You have some, but not all of the risk factors. In addition, many people can have the same changes in the optic discs that you have, but still have normal vision. At this stage, we cannot say you have glaucoma, but we do need to refer you to a specialist to arrange for some further tests.'
  - 'Glaucoma is common, but blindness associated with glaucoma is rare. These days, we have excellent treatments available to prevent eyesight from deteriorating or blindness from developing.'
- When discussing with the patient about getting a referral arranged quickly, it is important to take on board the patient's concerns, but stress that his condition does not require an urgent appointment.
  - 'I can understand your concern over your vision. I can also understand how frustrating it must be for you that you have to wait several weeks to see a specialist despite working for the NHS for many years.'
  - 'However, I want to reassure you that you do not have an urgent eye condition that needs to be dealt with immediately. If you are diagnosed with glaucoma, starting treatment in a few weeks will not be detrimental to your eyesight.'
  - 'Even though you are a paramedic, I cannot fast track your referral. However, I am more than happy to outline your concerns about your vision and explain you are a paramedic when I write to the specialist. Would that be acceptable?

Key summary

- Empathise with the patient regarding his concerns about blindness.
- Explain in simple terms how glaucoma develops, if possible illustrating with diagrams.
- Reassure the patient that blindness is a rare complication of glaucoma these days because of the effective treatments now available.
- Negotiate the outpatient referral to the specialist, whilst recognising the patient's frustration.

Glaucoma

Introduction

- Glaucoma is a major cause of blindness worldwide.
- Risk factors include age >40 years, family history, diabetes, short-sight and African or Afro-Caribbean origin (more likely to develop primary open-angle glaucoma).
- Early detection and treatment is very important to prevent deterioration of vision and blindness.
- People >40 years of age who have a first-degree relative (mother, father, sister or brother) with glaucoma are entitled to a free NHS eye test.

How the eye works

- The eyeball contains aqueous humour, which creates pressure in the eye to give it shape.
- Normally, this fluid constantly flows in and out of the eye to nourish it. It drains back into the bloodstream at the same rate that it is produced to maintain the correct pressure.
- Glaucoma occurs when the drainage tubes (trabecular meshwork) within the eye become

slightly blocked, preventing the aqueous humour from draining properly. The cause of blockage is unknown.

- It can also occur if the trabecular meshwork is obstructed by such things as blood or blood vessels, which prevent fluid from draining properly.
- When the fluid cannot drain properly, intraocular pressure rises, which can cause damage to the optic nerves and the nerve fibres from the retina.

Types of glaucoma
- Chronic primary open-angle glaucoma.
- Acute primary closed-angle glaucoma.
- Secondary glaucoma (chronic or acute).
- Congenital glaucoma.

a Chronic primary open-angle glaucoma
- This is the most common type of glaucoma and it develops slowly with a chronic rise in intraocular pressure (IOP).
- Usually asymptomatic and detected on routine eye test by noting cupping of the optic disc and peripheral visual field loss.
- Occurs when the trabecular meshwork becomes partially blocked, preventing the drainage of aqueous humour. This leads to an increase in IOP which leads to optic nerve damage.
- Insidious damage occurs to the retina and optic nerve fibres leading to loss of peripheral vision with central vision unaffected tunnel vision until late in the disease.

TABLE 3.3 NICE guidelines for chronic primary open-angle glaucoma (2009)

- Treatment with a prostaglandin analogue should be the initial therapy
- If this does not reduce the IOP sufficiently, check the person's adherence to their treatment and eye drop instillation technique
- If adherence and instillation technique are satisfactory then offer **one** of the following:
  — alternative pharmacological treatment with a prostaglandin analogue, beta blocker, carbonic anhydrase inhibitor or sympathomimetic
  — add a second agent to achieve target IOP
  — laser trabeculoplasty
  — surgery with pharmacological augmentation: mitomycin C (MMC), or 5-fluorouracil (5-FU)
- If IOP is still not controlled after trying two alternative pharmacological treatments, consider offering laser trabeculoplasty or surgery with pharmacological augmentation (MMC or 5-FU) as indicated

Treatment options
Topical medical treatment
(1) Prostaglandin analogues (e.g. latanoprost)
- First-line drugs. Only need to be administered once a day.
- Enhance outflow of aqueous humour through pathways other than the trabecular meshwork (uveoscleral drainage).
- Lower IOP effectively and have fewer side effects than other drugs.

(2) Beta blockers (e.g. timolol)
- Second-line drugs. Need to be administered twice a day.
- Reduce the amount of fluid produced inside the eye.
- Contraindicated in asthma (bronchospasm) and heart disease.

(3) Cholinergic agonists (e.g. pilocarpine)
- Third-line drugs. Need to be administered three or four times a day.
- Enhance outflow of aqueous humour through the trabecular meshwork.
- Side effects include headaches, eye ache and dark or blurred vision.

(4) Alpha agonists
- Administered two or three times a day.
- Help to reduce the amount of fluid that is produced in the eye, and help to improve the flow of fluid out of the eye.
- Side effects include a dry mouth.

(5) Carbonic anhydrase inhibitors (e.g. dorzolamide)
- Administered two or three times a day.
- Reduce the amount of fluid produced in the eye.
- Can be given systemically (acetazolamide), but often poorly tolerated due to side effects, such as GI upset, renal calculi, malaise and paraesthesiae.

⚷ Key summary
- Topical enhancement of aqueous flow:
  — prostaglandin analogues (uveoscleral route)
  — cholinergic agonists (trabecular meshwork).
- Topical aqueous humour suppression:
  — beta blockers
  — alpha agonists
  — carbonic anhydrase inhibitors.

Surgical treatment
(1) Laser treatment (argon laser trabeculoplasty)
- Argon laser induces changes in the trabecular meshwork that lower the IOP.
- The procedure is usually quick and painless, but the effect is not permanent. Repeat treatment is not effective.

(2) Surgery
- Trabeculectomy is the most common form of surgery for glaucoma. This removes part of the trabecular meshwork to allow increased drainage of the aqueous humour.
- Other surgical procedures include viscocanalostomy and deep sclerotomy.

b Acute primary closed-angle glaucoma
- In some individuals, the anatomy of the eye predisposes to blockage of aqueous humour flow through the pupil ('pupil block').
- This causes narrowing of the angle between the iris and sclera and reduced outflow through the trabecular meshwork, hence the name 'angle-closure' glaucoma.
- The narrowing often happens quickly, causing a sudden and painful rise in IOP. If not treated, visual loss is severe and often permanent. There may be a history of previous subacute attacks.

Symptoms	**Signs**
Intense pain in the eye	Cloudy cornea
Nausea and vomiting	Loss of red reflex
Headache	Oval, non-reactive pupil
Loss of vision	
Redness of the eye	
Halos around lights	

FIGURE 3.1 Symptoms and signs of acute primary closed-angle glaucoma

Management

- The elevated IOP must be treated **urgently** with topical and systemic (acetazolamide) aqueous suppressants. Acetazolamide may need to be administered intravenously as the patient may be nauseous or vomiting and so not tolerate oral administration.
- Patients may need systemic analgesics and antiemetics.
- Once the acute attack has resolved, treatment must be undertaken to prevent recurrence and prevent involvement of the contralateral eye.
- Creating a small hole in the iris, surgically or by laser iridotomy, allows aqueous humour to pass from the posterior to anterior chamber, bypassing the blocked pupil.
- Lifelong medical treatment is often required as the IOP can remain moderately elevated if the narrow angle does not reopen completely.

c *Secondary glaucoma*

- Secondary glaucoma can occur with an open angle or a closed angle. Therefore, it may present acutely, like angle-closure glaucoma, or insidiously, like primary open-angle glaucoma.
- Treatment involves managing the underlying condition and use of standard glaucoma treatment.

Causes

- Lens abnormalities (acute or chronic presentation).
- Steroid treatment, usually topical (chronic).
- Uveitis can cause glaucoma, either directly or secondary to prolonged steroid therapy (chronic).
- Iris neovascularisation (rubeosis), due to ocular ischaemia (from diabetic retinopathy or retinal vein occlusion), results in blockage of the trabecular meshwork (can present acutely or chronically).

d *Congenital glaucoma*

- Presents at birth or shortly after birth due to abnormal development of the anterior chamber angle.
- Clinical features include:
  - squint
  - sensitivity to light
  - cloudy appearance to eyes
  - buphthalmos – enlargement of the eye due to pressure causing the eye to expand.
- Treatment is usually surgical but prognosis is usually poor.

Further reading

- National Institute for Health and Clinical Excellence. Glaucoma: NICE guideline 85. London: NIHCE; 2009. www.nice.org.uk/guidance/CG85 (accessed 24 November 2010).
- RNIB (Royal National Institute of Blind People) website. www.rnib.org.uk/Pages/Home.aspx (accessed 24 November 2010).

Station 3.5

Actor's notes

Background
- You are Albert Freeman, a 57-year-old Afro-Caribbean trader in an investment bank.

Opening statement
- 'I don't have much time since you've kept me waiting for 35 minutes. My wife sent me here because she thinks my eyes have gone yellow.'

History
- Your wife spent hours making you a collage of photos for your twentieth wedding anniversary.
- She compared your photos from your holiday two weeks ago to photos earlier in the year, and noticed your eyes in recent photographs looked yellow.
- She spoke to you and suggested you see the doctor, even though you feel fine.

Ideas, concerns and expectations
- You wife is worried that your eyes look different and is concerned that 'something is wrong'.
- You are not very concerned about your health because you had a private medical performed two months ago that declared you fit.
- You are more interested in an explanation from the doctor as to why you have been kept waiting for 35 minutes.

Further history candidate may elicit
- Every year, your company arranges for you to have a private medical. Your last annual private medical was performed wo months ago. This involved a blood test, ECG, eye test, hearing test and 1-hour consultation with a doctor. Stool samples were sent off to screen for bowel cancer, and these were all negative.
- The doctor advised you that you were in excellent health since all your tests were normal. He suggested you lose some weight, since you had put on 5 kg in the last year.
- You were seen on time and found the service very professional.
- Following the medical, you spoke to your wife who suggested trying a 'detox' diet to lose weight.
- Over the last few weeks, you started to lose some weight. You attribute this to the detox diet.
- If asked, over the last week, your stool has gone a strange grey colour and your urine is darker than normal.
- You suspect this is a consequence of the 'detox' diet your wife has started you on.
- If asked, you do not have any bruises, are not scratching more than normal, do not have abdominal distension, gynaecomastia or ED. You have never used intravenous drugs, do not have tattoos and never had a blood transfusion or sex with a prostitute.

- You have to attend an important meeting at work and will be late because the doctor has not seen you on time.
- You asked the receptionist if you could see another doctor so you did not have to wait, but the receptionist explained that every doctor was running late.
- You do not come to the surgery often, but every time you do, you have to wait over half an hour to be seen. You cannot understand how it is acceptable that every doctor in the practice runs late daily and the appointment system has not been changed.
- You know that delays like this in the private sector would cost people their jobs.

Medical history
- Nil.

Drug history
- Nil.

Family history
- You have three younger brothers who are well.
- Your parents are both still alive and live separately. They are generally well.

Social history
- You do not smoke. You drink five to ten units a week.
- You are married and live with your wife in a large five-bedroom house.
- You are financially very secure, and enjoy a luxurious lifestyle.
- Your wife does not work but is head of several local charities.
- You do not have any children. Unfortunately your wife had a difficult pregnancy many years ago which resulted in an emergency hysterectomy. The baby was premature and did not survive.
- You are still deeply in love with your wife whom you consider your 'best friend'.
- You are still both very close and your recent 20th wedding anniversary was very special.

Approach to scenario
- You enter the consultation quite angry because the doctor you are seeing is running 35 minutes late. You are not verbally abusive or physically violent.
- After your opening statement, you ask the doctor 'Can you explain to me why all the doctors here are always running late?'
- You wait for the doctor to reply and ask 'Surely the practice should look at the appointment system. Do you really think it is acceptable that you have children, elderly and the working population waiting day in, day out to see a doctor?'
- You believe in customer satisfaction and want to know that something will be done to rectify the appointment system, stating 'Frankly, if any of you worked in the private sector you wouldn't last 2 minutes!'
- You will calm down if the doctor apologises and seems to mean it. However, if the apology sounds artificial, you comment 'You clearly don't really care, do you?'
- If the doctor suggests you write a letter of complaint, you agree.
- If the doctor reassures you that something will be done, you are happy to move on.
- If the doctor suggests that you could have cancer, you are left speechless.
- Eventually you ask 'Am I going to die?' and 'How long have I got?'
- You are looking forward to spending your retirement years with your wife.
- You grow concerned as to how she will cope, living alone with no children.
- You do not know how to explain the doctor's words to her tonight, saying 'What do I tell my wife, Doctor? I don't know how to tell her.'

Information gathering
Presenting complaint
a Jaundice
- Ask when the patient or wife first noticed the jaundice.
- Ask if they noticed a change in the sclera, skin or both.

b Other features
- Ask about other symptoms:
  — abdominal pain
  — abdominal distension
  — pruritus
  — discoloured stools or urine
  — haematemesis
  — fatigue and malaise
  — fever
  — weight loss
  — loss of appetite
  — peripheral oedema.

c Risk factors for hepatitis
- Blood transfusions.
- Tattoos or intravenous drug use.
- Sex with a prostitute.

Medical history
- Any previous episodes of jaundice.
- Liver or gallstone disorders.
- History of autoimmune disease.

Family history
- Liver disease.

Drug history
- Current medications.
- Use of painkillers such as paracetamol.
- Previous hepatitis A and B vaccination.

Social history
- Enquire about alcohol and smoking.
- Occupation.
- Marital status.

Patient's agenda
- Explore his understanding of jaundice.
- Explore his and his wife's concerns about his health.
- Explore his concerns about the appointment system.

Examination
- Offer to examine his abdomen.
- 'Is it okay if I feel your stomach?'

Examination card
General examination   Jaundice of the sclera
Abdominal examination   Hepatomegaly with liver edge 3 cm below right costal margin
                                 Liver edge is hard and knobbly

---

Clinical management
1 Apologise for the delay in his appointment
- Apologise sincerely for keeping him waiting, explaining that unpredictable things happened that slowed you down.
- Explain you understand his frustration and will speak to the other doctors and practice manager to review the appointment system.
- Advise him to write a letter to the practice manager to formalise the complaint if he wants to.

2 Discuss the likely cause of his jaundice
- Explain that you agree with his wife that his eyes appear 'yellow' or 'jaundiced'.
- Explain that jaundice occurs when there is an abnormal build up of waste products from the liver.
- Explain that there are many reasons why jaundice occurs.
- In view of the pale stool, dark urine and weight loss, explain that you are concerned he may have a pancreatic or biliary tract problem, such as a stone or polyp, or possibly even a tumour.
- Explain that he will need further tests to determine if he has cancer, and if so, the extent.
- Advise him that prognosis is dependent on the underlying cause.
- Advise him that it is not possible to comment further on prognosis or treatment until the cause is known.

3 Discuss the further management plan
- Explain that you need to refer him under the two-week rule to the gastroenterology department for further investigation, such as a computed tomography (CT) scan of his abdomen.
- Suggest an urgent blood test to check his liver function today.
- Discuss referring him through the NHS or privately if he has private medical insurance.

4 Discuss any other concerns
- Explain that his change in diet would not have affected the colour of his stools.
- Explain that the investigations he had as part of his private medical two months ago may have been normal at the time but do not prevent problems arising in the future.

5 Offer follow-up
- Offer a follow-up appointment in a few days to discuss the blood results and see how he is.
- Reassure him that you will not keep him waiting – offer him a double appointment or one at the end of the surgery.
- Explain that he can bring his wife to this appointment too, and offer to speak to his wife on his behalf.

Interpersonal skills

- This case involves managing an angry patient and determining the likely cause of his jaundice.
- Dealing with angry patients in the consultation can be extremely difficult. Remember to ensure your safety first, and if you feel threatened, terminate the consultation or press the panic alarm.
- In this case, try to defuse his anger by:
  - staying calm and remembering his anger is not directed at you personally
  - giving him space and time to ventilate
  - expressing empathy, concern and support: 'I can see how upset you are.'
  - acknowledging the cause of his anger: 'I understand this must be frustrating for you, especially as you have to go to work.'
  - apologising for running late: 'I'm really sorry you have had to wait for me.'
  - listening and exploring what has upset him and contributed to his anger
  - discuss how you can help:
     (i) 'Running late is a problem for many GPs. Its frustrating for patient and doctor.'
     (ii) I will definitely bring this up with the other doctors and the practice manager.'
     (iii) 'Would you like to write the practice to make your concerns formal? And we will respond to you, explaining what we will do in future.'
  - coming to a shared agreed plan: 'Does this sound reasonable to you? Is there anything else you suggest?'
  - checking his understanding of what you have agreed
  - ensuring you deliver your side of the deal
  - addressing your emotional 'housekeeping'
- When asking personal questions to assess risk factors for hepatitis B (such as asking about sex with prostitutes), first warn the patient that you will be asking some personal questions, and explain their relevance.
  - 'I do need to ask you some personal questions about your lifestyle as they can impact on your health. Is that okay?'
- Sensitively explain you will refer under the two-week rule to rule out cancer.
  - 'Your symptoms could indicate a problem in a small tube that comes from your gall bladder. This organ sits under your liver. There are a number of possible causes for this, some potentially serious, so I'll arrange an urgent referral to a specialist so that you are seen within two weeks. Is there anything else you would like me to clarify?'
- Offer the patient shared management options, but be prepared to state your overall opinion if you feel something is important.
  - 'Whilst we wait for your appointment to see the specialist, it might be a good idea to arrange some blood tests. The other option would be to do all the tests when you attend the hospital, but that might lead to delays. I personally would suggest we avoid any delays and we get a blood test organised for you today or tomorrow. What are your thoughts?'
- Let patients express their fear and shock about a potential diagnosis, especially if it is a serious one. It is important, however, to remind the patient that as yet you both do not know what is causing the symptoms and encourage positive thought.
  - 'I completely understand that you are upset about the possibility of cancer. But until we get the test results back, including the scans at the hospital, we can only speculate. I know it is easy to say, but it is very important to try and remain positive.'

O⊷ Key summary
- Manage an angry patient and understand his concerns about waiting for his appointment.
- Elicit the symptoms of obstructive jaundice.
- Be familiar with the causes of jaundice.
- Manage the uncertainty of a potentially life-changing diagnosis with the patient.

Jaundice

- Jaundice is the yellowish discolouration of the skin, sclera and mucous membranes due to hyperbilirubinaemia.
- Of bilirubin 80% is produced from the breakdown of haem from haemoglobin in red blood cells (RBCs), and 20% from the breakdown of haem in myoglobin and cytochromes.

Causes of jaundice

a Prehepatic causes

- Sickle-cell anaemia.
- Glucose-6-phosphate dehydrogenase (G6PD) deficiency.
- Spherocytosis.
- Malaria.

b Hepatic causes

- Acute hepatitis and liver cirrhosis of any cause result in reduced hepatic metabolism of bilirubin.
- Enzymopathies (Gilbert's and Crigler–Najjar syndrome) resulting in reduced biliary excretion.

c Posthepatic causes

- Biliary obstruction can be intrahepatic or extrahepatic and leads to the build up of bile products.

INTRAHEPATIC	EXTRAHEPATIC
PBC	Gallstones
PSC	Pancreatic carcinoma
Drugs	Parasites

Investigations in jaundice

TABLE 3.4 Biochemical features of the three categories of jaundice

	PREHEPATIC	HEPATIC	POSTHEPATIC
Bilirubin	↑	↑	↑
Conjugated bilirubin	N	N/↓	↑
Unconjugated bilirubin	↑	↑	N
Urobilinogen	↑	↑	↓
Colour of urine	N	Dark	Dark
Colour of stool	N	N	Pale
AST/ALT	N	↑	Normal
ALP	N	N	↑
Reticulocyte count	↑	N	N
Haptoglobulins	↓	N	N

* N means normal, ↑ means increased, ↓ means decreased

Investigations

a Blood tests

- FBC.
- LFTs.
- Haptoglobulins.
- Reticulocyte count.
- Coombs' test.
- Clotting studies.
- Autoimmune screen.
- Viral screen.

b Further tests

- USS abdomen.
- CT abdomen.
- Endoscopic retrograde cholangiopancreatography (ERCP).
- Liver biopsy.

Clinical features of chronic liver disease

TABLE 3.5 Clinical features of chronic liver disease

SYSTEM	SIGNS
Face	Jaundice
Hands	Clubbing
	Leukonychia
	Hyperpigmentation
	Excoriation
	Purpura
	Xanthomata
	Dupuytren's contracture
	Palmar erythema
	Hepatic flap
Abdomen	Hepatomegaly
	Splenomegaly
	Hepatosplenomegaly
	Ascites
	Caput medusa
Chest	Spider naevi
	Gynaecomastia
Other features	Tattoos
	Testicular atrophy
	Ankle oedema
	Needle marks suggesting IVDU

Causes of liver disease

- Alcohol.
- Viral hepatitis (hepatitis B or C).
- Biliary obstruction.
- Primary biliary cirrhosis.
- Autoimmune chronic active hepatitis.
- Budd–Chiari syndrome.
- Drugs (methyldopa, amiodarone, methotrexate).
- Metabolic disorders (haemochromatosis, Wilson's disease, α_1-antitrypsin deficiency).

Investigations

a Bloods

- LFTs and gamma-glutamyltransferase (GGT).
- Iron and ferritin.
- FBC.
- Autoantibody screen.
- Clotting.
- Alpha-fetoprotein (AFP).
- Hepatitis B and C screen.
- Caeruloplasmin.

b Analysis of ascitic fluid

- Determine whether an exudate or transudate.
- Microscopy and culture.

c Liver biopsy

d Imaging

- USS of liver and biliary tract.

Further reading

- British Liver Trust website. www.britishlivertrust.org.uk/home.aspx (accessed 24 November 2010).
- Simon C, Everitt H, van Dorp F. *Oxford Handbook of General Practice.* 3rd ed. Oxford: Oxford University Press; 2010.
- Longmore M, Wilkinson I, Davidson E, *et al. Oxford Handbook of Clinical Medicine.* 8th ed. Oxford: Oxford University Press; 2010.

Station 3.6

Candidate's notes

Name	Steven Pritchard
Age	21
Medical history	Nil
Medication	Mefloquine 250 mg once weekly (start two weeks before foreign travel and continue four weeks after return)
Allergies	Nil
Last consultation	Hepatitis A vaccination with nurse

Actor's notes

Background
- You are Steven Pritchard, a 21-year-old gentleman who has just finished university.

Opening statement
- 'Doctor, I feel like I've got the flu.'

History
- Over the last 48 hours, you have felt feverish and developed a mild, generalised headache.
- You have also had generalised muscle aches and pains.
- You feel more tired than usual and generally unwell.

Ideas, concerns and expectations
- You think you have the flu.
- You have an interview in three days with an engineering company and are concerned that if you do not get better soon, you will be unable to prepare for the interview, and will be unsuccessful.
- You want the doctor to prescribe you some antibiotics so the infection clears up.

Further history candidate may elicit
- You went to Africa at the end of your final-year university examinations for a seven-week holiday.
- You toured through South Africa, Zimbabwe, Tanzania and Kenya with three of your friends.
- Prior to the holiday, you saw the travel nurse in the surgery who advised some vaccinations, and tablets to take to prevent malaria.
- You had the vaccinations and started taking the anti-malarial tablets as advised, to prevent developing malaria. Unfortunately, when you were on holiday, you left the tablets in one of the hostels in Zimbabwe, and so did not take any further tablets for the rest of the holiday.
- You remained well for most of the trip, although did have a bout of diarrhoea a few weeks ago. There was no blood in the stool and no vomiting. This resolved in a few days.
- You did not use mosquito nets but did use mosquito repellent sprays. You were bitten several times over the course of your holiday, mainly on your arms and legs.
- You arrived back in the UK from Kenya three days ago. You started to feel unwell 48 hours ago, with a fever and headache, which has persisted. You have not measured your temperature.
- You have a mild generalised headache, which is getting worse. You do not have any associated nausea or vomiting, migrainous features, neck stiffness or photophobia.

- You do not have a cough, cold, earache, abdominal pain, diarrhoea, vomiting, urinary symptoms or jaundice. You have not taken any painkillers or antipyretics.
- You applied for over 50 jobs before you went travelling, and this is the only one you have been short-listed for. Your interview is with a multinational oil company.
- You achieved a first-class honours degree in engineering, but are aware of the difficulty in getting a job because of the recession. None of your friends have managed to secure a job.
- You have a large student debt and are desperate to secure a job. Your father lost his job recently and he expects you to support the family financially now you are no longer a student. You are keen to get the job so you can help support your parents and pay off your student loan.

Medical history
- Nil relevant.

Family history
- Nil relevant.

Drug history
- Mefloquine 250 mg tablets once weekly.
- You started taking the tablets two weeks before your holiday but stopped taking them a few weeks ago because you left them behind at a hostel.
- You have not taken any medication for the headache or fever.

Social history
- You smoke occasionally with your friends.
- You enjoy a 'few beers' with your friends but do not drink heavily.
- You do not use recreational drugs.
- You live with your parents and younger brother in a two-bedroom house.
- Your father was a postman but lost his job seven months ago due to staff cutbacks.
- Your mother is a part-time librarian and looking for more work to support the family financially.
- Your younger brother is in his last year at school and wants to apply to university.
- You are keen to offer your brother financial support.

Approach to scenario
- At the start of the consultation, you explain you think you have the flu. You request a course of antibiotics to get better.
- You only mention your recent travels abroad if the doctor comes across well **or** specifically asks you about foreign travel.
- If the doctor refuses to give you any antibiotics, you become agitated, and explain you need to get better soon because 'I have to get on with things'.
- If the doctor informs you that you may have malaria or another infectious disease, you become alarmed and ask how you picked it up, and how it can be treated.
- You want to know if you can pass it on to the family, and if they need treatment.
- In particular, you want to know how long it will take for you to get better, and if the infection has any complications.
- If the doctor suggests you need to go to hospital, you refuse and ask to be managed at home so you can prepare and attend your interview in two days.
- However, if the doctor is empathic and sensitive, and underlines the importance of attending hospital today, you will agree.

Information gathering
Presenting complaint
a Fever
- Enquire how long he has had the fever.
- Check when the fever started.
- Ask if he has measured his temperature, and if so how high it was.
- Does it respond to paracetamol or ibuprofen?
- Does the fever fluctuate at different times of the day?

b General symptoms
- Ask about other symptoms in detail:
  — headache, rash, neck stiffness, photophobia
  — earache and sore throat
  — cough or cold
  — jaundice
  — abdominal pain
  — diarrhoea and vomiting
  — urinary symptoms.

Travel history
- When did he depart and return to the UK?
- Where did he go on his trip (all countries)?
- Why did he go abroad?
  — tourism
  — business
  — visit family.
- What precautions did he take before he went?
  — immunisations
  — antimalarial use.
- What precautions did he take whilst there?
  — safe sex
  — safe eating
  — mosquito nets and repellent.
- What did he do there?
  — freshwater contact.
- Who else went with him?
- Who else got ill?

Medical history
- Any other medical condition.

Family history
- Ask about health conditions affecting the family.

Drug history
- Immunisations and use of antimalarials.

Social history
- Occupation.
- Alcohol and smoking.
- Use of recreational drugs.

Patient's agenda
- Explore his concerns about his symptoms.
- Explore his understanding of malaria.
- Explore his reluctance regarding hospital admission.

Examination
- Offer to check his temperature, examine his ears, throat, chest, heart, lungs, abdomen and dipstick his urine.
- 'If it's okay with you, I'll check your urine for infection and measure your temperature. I'll also check your ears, throat, heart, lungs and tummy to find out where the infection is coming from.'

Examination card

General examination	Temperature = 39.2 °C
	BP = 110/70 mmHg
	Pulse = 110/minute
	Urine dipstick = negative
	Multiple mosquito bites on legs
Systemic examination	No abnormalities detected

Clinical management
1 Discuss the likely diagnosis of malaria
- Explain to the patient that he does not have the flu. He is likely to have malaria in view of:
  — fever
  — multiple mosquito bites
  — history of travel to areas endemic for malaria
  — lack of antimalarials during his holiday
  — lack of other findings on examination today.

2 Explain what malaria is and its complications
- Explain that:
  — Malaria is an infection that is commonly found in Africa, Asia and South America.
  — It is caused by a parasite called *Plasmodium* that lives in mosquitoes and is transferred to humans through mosquito bites.
  — The parasite lives in RBCs.
  — Malaria from Africa can be potentially very serious.
  — Reassure the patient that malaria cannot be passed from human to human.
  — Symptoms usually occur one to four weeks after becoming infected.
  — Usually patients have fever, headaches, muscle aches and diarrhoea or vomiting.
  — However, more serious complications can occur, e.g. impaired consciousness, seizures, renal failure, liver failure, pulmonary oedema, haemolysis and shock.

3 Explain how malaria is diagnosed
- Explain that malaria can be confirmed by a blood test – often three blood samples may be needed.
- Using microscopy, the parasite can be directly visualised in the RBCs.

4 Explain how malaria can be treated
- Explain that:
  — Antimalarial medicines are used to treat malaria.
  — It should be treated quickly to prevent serious complications developing.

— The duration of treatment and the type of drugs used vary from person to person.
— In view of the high temperature and tachycardia, he needs to be admitted to hospital.

5 Discuss admission for inpatient management

- Explain that:
    — Examination suggests he could have a severe form of malaria (*Plasmodium falciparum*), which needs to be promptly diagnosed and treated.
    — Antibiotics will not work as they do not affect parasites.
    — Delay in treatment could result in one or more serious complications developing, and could be fatal.
    — He may need intravenous drug treatment and may need to be monitored.
    — Each patient responds differently, so it is unclear how long he will need to be admitted for.
    — The quicker he is admitted, the quicker he will be treated and so discharged.
    — It is likely that he will make a good recovery with treatment.
    — Treatment with oral antimalarials cannot be started without knowing the type of malaria he has, since different forms of malaria require different treatment regimens.

Interpersonal skills

- The key to this station is to negotiate inpatient admission for diagnosis and treatment. Failure to do so could result in the patient developing serious complications or death. Take a history, initially by asking open questions, then following up with more closed questions.
    — 'You mentioned you have been travelling. Tell me about your trip.'
    — 'How has this illness affected you?'
    — 'Have you experienced any headaches? What about any rashes?'
- With patients who have capacity, it is important to respect their autonomy and refusal of any treatment, including refusal to be admitted to hospital. However, in this case, inpatient admission can be agreed by discussing the benefits of admission versus the risks of not attending hospital, and eliciting his reasons for wanting to avoid hospital admission.
    — 'I am concerned you may have a serious type of malaria, which can only be managed in the hospital. By admitting you today, there are several advantages.'
    — 'We would be able to confirm if you have malaria, and the type you have. That way, you can be treated quickly and correctly. The quicker you are treated, the quicker you can go home.'
    — 'You would be closely monitored to prevent any serious complications from occurring. If they did occur, you would be treated quickly.'
    — 'If the tests show you do not have malaria, then other blood tests and investigations, such as a chest X-ray, would be performed to determine the sort of infection you have.'
    — 'If you do not go to hospital, you will get very sick pretty soon, and develop more serious problems such as breathing difficulties, kidney and liver failure.'
    — 'It is difficult to know for sure how many days you would have to stay in hospital because that depends on the type of malaria you have, how you respond to the treatment and whether you develop any complications.'
    — 'Is there something that's playing on your mind and stopping you from going to hospital?'
    — 'I appreciate you want to able to get to your interview, and how important it is to you. However, your health is also very important, and the quicker we treat you, the more likely you will be able to attend. What do you think?'
    — 'If you are not treated, you are likely to miss the interview because you will be too sick.'
- If it becomes clear that there is an important factor contributing to the patient's reluctance to hospital admission, gather further information.
    — 'So, tell me more about what the interview is for?'
    — 'I gather this is very important for your career?'
- Show an interest in the patient's predicament about wishing to attend an interview.

— 'Have you considered contacting the company interviewing you? They may be able to reschedule another date.'
— 'I would be happy to write to the company explaining your circumstances if you are not able to attend your interview and request an alternative date. How does that sound?'

⊶ Key summary
- Take a travel history and recognise the likely diagnosis of malaria.
- Explain the need for inpatient admission.
- Elicit the reasons for the patient refusing hospital admission.
- Negotiate inpatient admission, discussing the benefits and risks.

Malaria
- Endemic in Africa, Central and South America and Asia.
- Caused by infection with the parasite *Plasmodium* – four types: *falciparum, vivax, ovale, malariae*.
- Transmission occurs via bites from infected female *Anopheles* mosquitoes.
- The parasite infects RBCs and causes haemolysis. Each species infects RBCs with different capacity. *Plasmodium falciparum* can infect any red cell, so has severe effects, whereas *P. vivax* and *P. ovale* infect immature red cells, and *P. malariae* infects senescent red cells.
- Conditions such as sickle-cell disease, thalassaemia and G6PD deficiency provide some protection to the individual from the development of malaria.

Clinical features
a Mild malaria
- Fever.
- Myalgia.
- Sweats.
- Headache.
- Diarrhoea.

b Severe malaria
- Acidosis.
- Hypoglycaemia.
- Severe anaemia.
- Shock.
- Hepatic failure.
- Renal failure.
- Glomerulonephritis.
- Haemoglobinuria.
- Cerebral oedema and coma.
- Pulmonary oedema and respiratory distress.

Diagnosis
- Serology to detect malaria antigen.
- Repeated microscopy of thick and thin blood films – the disease is unlikely if there are three negative slides in 72 hours.

Treatment
a Drug treatment
- Treatment depends on the type of malaria. Drug resistance is an increasing problem.
- *P. vivax, ovale* and *malariae* can usually be treated on an outpatient basis. Chloroquine or primaquine are often used.
- All patients with *P. falciparum* must be initially admitted to hospital due to the possibility of rapid deterioration as the parasite replicates quickly.
- *P. falciparum* is resistant to chloroquine.
- Options include:
  — quinine and doxycycline
  — Co-artem® (artemether lumefantrine)
  — Malarone® (atovaquone and proguanil).

b Managing severe malaria
- Antipyretics.
- Intravenous fluids if dehydrated.
- Intravenous glucose if hypoglycaemic.
- Exchange transfusion if very high levels of parasites are found or complications develop.
- ITU admission is needed if complications such as acidosis, cerebral or pulmonary oedema occur.

Prophylaxis
a General measures
- Wearing long-sleeved shirts and trousers in the evening.
- Mosquito mats and nets impregnated with permethrin.
- Insecticides and diethyltoluamide (DEET) in lotions or sprays can be effective.

b Chemoprophylaxis
- This is not absolute. Infection can still occur with any of the recommended drugs.
- For areas with widespread chloroquine resistance, prophylaxis is with:
  — mefloquine
  — doxycycline or
  — Malarone (atovaquone and proguanil).
- For areas without chloroquine resistance, chloroquine and proguanil can be used.

Further reading
- World Health Organization (WHO). *Malaria*. WHO; 2010. Available at: www.who.int/topics/malaria/en (accessed 24 November 2010).
- The Travel Doctor. *Malaria Information Page*. The Travel Doctor; 2002–10. Available at: www.traveldoctor.co.uk/malaria.htm (accessed 24 November 2010).
- Eddleston M, Davidson R, Brent A, *et al. Oxford Handbook of Tropical Medicine*. 3rd ed. Oxford: Oxford University Press; 2008.

Station 3.7

Actor's notes

Background
- You are Amy Green, a 27-year-old artist.

Opening statement
- 'Doctor, my hands are hurting.'

History
- Initially, a few weeks ago, you noticed the pain after moving some furniture around at home.
- The pain got worse over the next few weeks and did not resolve.
- Over the last three weeks, both your hands have become more painful.

Ideas, concerns and expectations
- You are very concerned because the pain and stiffness in your hands has affected your ability to paint over the last three weeks.
- You have a contract with an art gallery for five paintings in one year. You are worried about meeting the deadline because you are behind schedule.
- You have heard about rheumatoid arthritis (RA) and are terrified this may be the underlying cause.
- You have come to the GP expecting to be referred urgently to see a specialist.

Further history candidate may elicit
- You are left handed.
- Over the last three weeks, there has been a gradual onset of pain and swelling affecting the joints on both hands. The pain is associated with stiffness, which is worse when you wake up in the morning and gradually improves over the course of the day.
- You feel that your fingers are a bit swollen since your fashion rings all feel tighter.
- You have started taking ibuprofen again to help control the pain in your hands, and noticed that smoking cannabis also eases the pain.
- Over the last few weeks, you have been very tired, but assumed this is because you are working long hours, painting until the early hours of the morning.
- You have no pain or swelling in any other joints, no weight loss, no fever and no other symptoms.
- Over the last few days you have struggled to open the lids on your paint bottles and now wear t-shirts so you do not have to fiddle with buttons.
- You burst into tears at home this morning when you could not open your bottle of shower gel.
- You love your artistic and creative side, passionately enjoying your work as a painter.

- You have just secured a contract with an art gallery, which has commissioned you for five paintings in the next year. This is a tight schedule and you 'do not have a minute to waste'.
- You can still hold a paintbrush, but cannot paint properly due to the pain in your hand. With every day lost, you know you will have to work harder to meet the art gallery's deadline.
- You remember learning about Renoir in your art history lessons. He developed RA and became 'a prisoner in his own wheelchair' because he could not walk even with crutches. You remember the art teacher explaining how his hands became completely deformed, 'like the claws of a bird', and were bandaged 'to prevent his fingernails from growing into the flesh'. You recall the dramatic finale to your art teacher's lecture – ultimately Renoir was unable to pick up a paintbrush. Could this be happening to you?

Medical history
- Nil.

Drug history
- Ibuprofen 400 mg tds.

Social history
- You are a 'social smoker', smoking three to four cigarettes on occasions when you are with your friends or surrounded by other artists.
- You smoke the occasional 'spliff' as you feel this helps 'to release creative juices' when you are painting, but do not use any other recreational drugs.
- You live with a flatmate in a small two-bedroom flat and work in a nearby art studio.
- Your family live locally.
- Your have one brother who works in the finance sector and your parents are both school teachers.

Family history
- There is no family history of autoimmune or joint problems.

Approach to scenario
- You are very concerned about your symptoms and are terrified that this is RA.
- You ask the doctor for an urgent referral to see a specialist early in the consultation, and ask for this repeatedly throughout the consultation until the doctor agrees.
- As the doctor asks you questions, you become more anxious and repeatedly ask what the diagnosis is, whether you have RA and what else the diagnosis could be.
- You ask the doctor what tests need to be done to find out what is causing the pain, and what treatment is available.
- You repeatedly ask the doctor 'I'm still going to be able to paint aren't I?' and say 'This isn't permanent is it?'
- You are not keen on taking other painkillers and would rather wait to see the specialist.
- If suggested, you agree to have some blood tests at the surgery.
- If the doctor comes across well, you will discuss all your ideas and concerns, emphasising the impact of the symptoms on your career.
- If the doctor does not seem empathic, you become very upset and say 'I'm going to be like Renoir!'
- If the doctor does not agree to you seeing a specialist as soon as possible then you become angry and demand a referral.

Information gathering
Presenting complaint
a Pain
- Ask her about the pain in her hands:
  - duration
  - stiffness of hands
  - swelling of joints
  - alleviating and exacerbating factors
  - better or worse in the morning.
- Check if other joints are affected:
  - knees
  - feet
  - elbows
  - wrists
  - neck
  - back
  - hips.

b Systemic features
- Fever.
- Weight loss.
- Malaise.
- Any nodules or skin rash.

Medical history
- Particularly autoimmune disease.

Drug history
- Use of painkillers and their effects.
- Current medications.

Family history
- Ask about autoimmune disease affecting the family.

Social history
- Enquire about alcohol, smoking and recreational drugs.
- Occupation.
- Home circumstances and activities of daily living:
  - house/flat/bungalow
  - lives alone or with someone.

Patient's agenda
- Explore impact of her symptoms at work and at home.
- Explore her understanding of RA.

Examination

- Offer to examine her hands.
- 'If it's okay with you, can I examine your hands? I promise to be gentle and you can stop me if I cause you any pain or discomfort.'

Examination card

General examination	Anxious
Hands	Slight swelling of PIPJs bilaterally
	Difficulty in holding a pen and writing
Elbows	No rheumatoid nodules

Clinical management

1 Explain the potential diagnosis

- Explain that the diagnosis may well be RA, but other conditions such as psoriatic arthritis or Reiter's disease may be causing the symptoms.
- Explain that if this is RA, early treatment is recommended.
- Explain that there have been many successful developments in the treatment of RA since Renoir's time, and although a cure is still not available, there are many drugs that greatly reduce or delay the progression of the disease.

2 Consider further tests

a Blood tests

- Explain that a blood test could help diagnose the condition.
- Explain you would request a full set of bloods including an autoimmune screen.
- Explain that rheumatoid factor is positive in only 70% of cases.

b Radiographs

- Explain that radiographs of the hands would be useful since they can detect RA and also show other causes of joint pain and swelling.

3 Discuss referral to a specialist

- Agree that you will refer her to a rheumatology specialist and will ask them to see her as soon as possible.

4 Discuss the management of rheumatoid arthritis

- Ensure she has adequate pain relief and offer other analgesics if NSAIDs are not effective alone.
- Explain that if this is RA, there are lots of medications available to treat this condition.
- Reassure her that RA can be controlled in many people.

5 Follow-up

- Offer follow-up appointments to discuss the results and/or after review by specialist.

Interpersonal skills

- This patient is distressed at the implications of developing a chronic condition with no set course.
- Use a wide range of open questions, whilst taking on board non-verbal and verbal cues.
  - 'How does the pain affect you at work and at home?'
  - 'You seem very concerned. Is there something in particular that is playing on your mind?'
  - 'Have you heard of rheumatoid arthritis before? What do you understand about it?'

- Managing uncertainty about the diagnosis and prognosis of a debilitating disease is difficult in any 10-minute consultation. It is important to be empathic to her situation.
  — 'The pain in your hands may be a temporary problem, or it could be due to rheumatoid arthritis – we can't be certain at the moment. There are several conditions that may present in this manner.'
  — 'Even if you do have rheumatoid arthritis, it is difficult to know how you will be affected. Some people only have minor flares throughout their life and so lead pretty normal lives. Others unfortunately have a more severe form of the disease, which can affect other joints in the body.'
  — 'The only way we can tell is by doing some more tests and waiting to see what happens.'
  — 'However, there are many recent drugs that have helped patients dramatically, and research is going on all the time.'
  — 'I can see how frightening this all is for you, particularly because you are an artist. Tell me some more about how your painting might be affected by all of this.'
  — 'Let's make sure we try and get all the tests done quickly so you are clearer about what is happening.'
- Discuss the limitations of a blood test in RA and suggest an X-ray of the hands.
  — 'There are some tests that would help us find out if you have rheumatoid arthritis. For example, I can arrange a blood test to check for rheumatoid arthritis and other conditions that can affect your joints. What do you think?'
  — 'Like any test, the test for rheumatoid arthritis is not 100% accurate. If I find 100 people with rheumatoid arthritis, only 70 of them will test positive for the condition. That means, it will not pick up 30 people in the group who do have rheumatoid arthritis. So for that reason, I would also recommend some X-rays of your hands. Does that seem to make sense?'
  — 'The X-ray will let us look at the bones in the hands and see if they are affected, and if so, where they are affected. X-rays can help us to determine whether you have rheumatoid arthritis or not.'

O⊶ **Key summary**
- Consider the cause of small-joint pain, including RA.
- Explore and understand the effect of painful hands on her work and home life.
- Address her concerns about RA.
- Manage uncertainty about the diagnosis and prognosis of a debilitating disease.
- Negotiate a shared management plan.
- Be empathic and supportive during the patient's journey.

Rheumatoid arthritis
- This is a chronic, inflammatory, autoimmune disease mediated by the formation of IgG antibodies produced by plasma cells in the joint synovium.
- This leads to the production of pro-inflammatory mediators, e.g. tumour necrosis factor (TNF)-α, which causes joint destruction.
- It affects 1% of the population with a female to male ratio of 3:1.
- The peak incidence is from 25 to 55 years.
- Early referral to a rheumatologist and early treatment improves prognosis.

Diagnostic criteria
The American College of Rheumatology requires four out of the following seven criteria to be present to diagnose RA:
1 Morning stiffness >1 hour for >6 weeks
2 Swelling of at least three types of joints for >6 weeks*
3 Swelling of hand joints for >6 weeks

4 Symmetrical joint involvement for >6 weeks
5 Nodules
6 Rheumatoid factor +ve
7 Radiological features such as joint erosions.

* Joints can be proximal interphalangeal joint (PIPJ), metacarpophalangeal joint (MCPJ), the wrist, elbow, knee, ankle or metatarsophalangeal joint (MTPJ).

Clinical features

TABLE 3.6 Clinical features in RA

Hands	• Palmar erythema • Triggering of the fingers • Z deformity of the thumb
Musculoskeletal	• Elbow, knee and foot involvement • Cervical spine involvement • Atlantoaxial joint subluxation can lead to spinal cord compression • Bursitis • Tenosynovitis
Respiratory	• Pleural effusions • Pulmonary fibrosis • Pulmonary nodules • Caplan's syndrome • Bronchiolitis obliterans
Neurology	• Peripheral neuropathy • Mononeuritis multiplex • Cervical myelopathy • Carpal tunnel syndrome
Eyes	• Episcleritis • Scleritis • Cataracts • Scleromalacia and scleromalacia perforans
Cardiovascular	• Pericarditis • Myocarditis
Dermatology	• Nail-fold infarcts • Pyoderma gangrenosum • Leg ulceration • Raynaud's phenomenon
Other	• Cushingoid features due to steroid therapy • Secondary amyloidosis • Other autoimmune disorders such as Sjögren's syndrome

Management of rheumatoid arthritis
a Conservative management
• Education.
• Exercise and physiotherapy.
• Splinting to protect joints.
• Occupational therapy.

b Drug management
- NSAIDs.
- Disease-modifying antirheumatic drugs (DMARDs).
- Steroids (oral or intra-articular injections).
- Inhibitors of TNF-α action.

c Surgery
- Joint replacement.
- Tendon transfer.

Side effects of steroids
- Bruising.
- Weight gain.
- Hirsutism.
- Acne.
- Moon face.
- Cataract.
- Hypertension.
- Glaucoma.
- Impaired glucose tolerance.
- Osteoporosis.
- Peptic ulcer disease.
- Infections, especially recurrent fungal infections.

Anti-TNF-α drugs

a Etanercept
- Indications include rheumatoid arthritis, ankylosing spondylitis and psoriatic arthritis.
- This is a fusion protein consisting of a recombinant TNF-α receptor and the Fc constant region of human IgG.
- It is administered through subcutaneous injection twice a week when other DMARDs have failed.
- It can be given alone or with methotrexate.
- It can cause reactivation of TB.

b Infliximab
- Indications include RA, ankylosing spondylitis, psoriasis and Crohn's disease.
- Infliximab is a chimeric mouse anti-TNF monoclonal antibody that binds to and inhibits human TNF-α.
- It is administered intravenously when other DMARDs (including methotrexate) have failed.
- It is given at zero, two and six weeks and then every eight weeks thereafter.
- It must be used in combination with methotrexate.
- It can cause reactivation of TB.

Further reading
- National Rheumatoid Arthritis Society website. www.nras.org.uk (accessed 24 November 2010).
- Arthritis Research UK website. www.arthritisresearchuk.org/ (accessed 24 November 2010).
- Adebajo A, editor. *ABC of Rheumatology.* 4th ed. Oxford: Wiley-Blackwell; 2009.
- Hakim A, Clunie G, Haq I, editors. *Oxford Handbook of Rheumatology.* 2nd ed. Oxford: Oxford University Press; 2006.

Station 3.8

Actor's notes

Background
- You are Joseph Sergeant, a 33-year-old chartered accountant.

Opening statement
- 'I don't want to waste your time, Doctor, but my brother said I must come and see you about my hand-washing problem.'

History
- For the last six months, you've felt like you have to keep washing your hands.
- The problem has worsened in the past two months and you now wash your hands five times an hour.
- Your hands have started becoming sore recently.

Ideas, concerns and expectations
- You recognise that the hand washing is a problem and you want help. You are embarrassed that others have noticed how often you wash your hands. Some work colleagues have started making jokes about it.
- Your main concern when you need to wash your hands is primarily with hygiene and a belief that the hands are contaminated with dirt or germs. You are particularly worried about swine flu.
- Several work colleagues were affected by the swine flu virus. This increased your worries about hand hygiene. You carry several tubes of alcohol gel and use it repeatedly.
- Recently your line manager commented that the standard of your work is slipping. This upset you as you are a high performer, consider yourself a perfectionist and want your senior colleagues to think of you in a positive manner.

Further history candidate may elicit
- The hand-washing problem started when you were 16 years old and took your GCSE exams. At that stage, you washed your hands two to three times an hour. This resolved after your exams, but during times of stress, such as exams, or starting a new job, the problem becomes worse.
- Until six months ago, the hand washing did not interfere with your life and you concealed the problem from others. When there were no major stressful factors, you spent less than a minute washing and drying your hands. Nowadays you spend up to 5 minutes washing your hands and find you spend most of that time lathering the hands with soap to ensure they stay clean.
- Sometimes, immediately after leaving the bathroom you feel an overwhelming need to revisit.

- Once the thought to wash your hands occurs, you find it hard to avoid obsessing about the cleanliness of your hands. You develop images in your head about the germs, and feel compelled to wash your hands. You become very preoccupied with these thoughts. Recently, if the thoughts are there for more than a few minutes, you start sweating and your heart starts to beat faster.
- Once you have washed your hands, the anxiety settles and your mind feels calmer until the cycle repeats itself.
- You work in a highly pressurised environment. You were promoted into a more senior position about six months ago. Soon after this, you started to wash your hands more frequently and for longer periods of time. The frequency of hand washing interferes with doing clients' accounts. You are no longer able to stay still at meetings or make contributions. You are embarrassed at having to leave meetings so often and have noticed many colleagues laughing at you.
- To try and make up for falling behind, you have started to work into the early hours at home. This has made you very tired and you have been arriving late for work.
- You live with your brother. He has noticed how often you are washing your hands, and how disruptive this is to your everyday life. He suggested you visit the doctor. You are a tidy and clean person. Your brother can be rather messy and you often have arguments with him about keeping things clean.
- When you come home from work during the week you often spend a large part of the evening in the bathroom. You have stopped socialising in public places since you are concerned that you will not be able to wash your hands cleanly in a public toilet.
- If pressed to elaborate further on your feelings about recurrent hand washing, you will say that it gives you a sense of feeling in control. You have no symptoms of depression or suicidal ideation.
- You find a couple of pints of beer help the hand-washing problem.

Medical and psychiatric history
- Nil.

Drug and family history
- Nil.

Social history
- You are a non-smoker, do not use recreational drugs and drink up to 12 units of alcohol/ week.
- You share a house with your older brother and have lived together for three years.
- You have been single all your life and not had a partner. You are attracted to women but are too shy to strike up a conversation.
- Your parents are both alive and well in their 60s. Your mother is a full-time housewife and your father is manager of a local supermarket store. Your relationship with your mother has been strained in the past. She was not happy for you to move away from home. She has tended to make the big decisions in your life and you find her controlling. She can become angry when you try to stand up to her, and so usually you back down. Your father is a quiet person and your relationship with him is amicable but very low key.

Approach to scenario
- You feel embarrassed to speak to the doctor and state 'I don't want to waste your time'.
- Your main concern is the impact this is having on your work performance. You are also preoccupied with swine flu and are particularly worried about catching it. You mention several times 'I don't want to catch swine flu'.
- You realise that the hand-washing problem needs to be overcome and you are willing to accept help for it but prefer to manage the symptoms 'in a natural way rather than rely on

artificial substances'. You are ready to engage with CBT (if offered) but unsure of medication at this stage.

- You are a private person, and if the doctor delves into your family dynamics, you become defensive. If the doctor suggests there is a connection between your life circumstances and the hand-washing problem, you say 'I don't see how this is relevant to my hand problem'.
- If the doctor responds sympathetically, seems genuinely interested in the difficulties you face and does not appear judgemental, you agree to explore the issues further.
- If the doctor communicates well what the problem is and helps to alleviate your feelings of embarrassment, then you will be prepared to accept the recommended help.
- However, if the doctor is unable to make you feel at ease, or fails to effectively explain what is wrong, then you will be guarded and continue to feel embarrassed.
- Depending on how well the consultation is going, you may agree to come back and see the doctor once you have had time to research your condition.

Information gathering
Presenting complaint
a Discuss the issues with hand washing
- Enquire about:
  — frequency
  — time spent washing
  — triggers and alleviating factors.

b Obsessional thoughts
- Ask about obsessional thoughts causing anxiety:
  — images or impulses
  — recurrent repetitive thoughts.
- Explore what happens if he resists these obsessions.

c Compulsive behaviours
- Identify compulsive behaviours that reduce anxiety:
  — repetitive actions
  — rituals or mental actions.

d Other psychiatric features
- Psychotic features:
  — paranoid thoughts
  — hallucinations (particularly auditory)
  — perceptual delusions.
- Anxiety and depression.

Medical history
- Enquire about any other medical conditions.

Psychiatric history
- Depression.
- Anxiety.
- Obsessive-compulsive disorder (OCD).
- Substance misuse.

Family history
- History of psychiatric illness or substance misuse.

Drug history
- Antidepressants or antipsychotics.
- Over-the-counter preparations, e.g. St John's wort.

Social history
- Smoking history.
- Occupation.
- Marital status.
- Recent life events.
- Social network.
- Family dynamics and childhood.

Patient agenda
- Explore why he thinks this problem has become worse.
- Explore the impact on his work and personal life.
- Explore his understanding of OCD and treatment options.

Examination
- Offer to examine the patient's hands and perform a general check up.
- 'Can I examine your hands and perform a general check up of your blood pressure and pulse?'

Examination card

General examination	BP = 120/78 mmHg
	Pulse = 69/minute and regular
Hand examination	The hands are very dry
	No erythema or signs of inflammation

Clinical management

1 Explain the diagnosis of obsessive-compulsive disorder
- Inform the patient he has OCD, which is an anxiety disorder characterised by intrusive thoughts (obsessions) that produce anxiety and repetitive behaviours (compulsions) aimed at reducing anxiety.
- Explain many patients present with symptoms of recurrent hand washing, switching lights on and off or opening/closing a door repeatedly.
- Reassure him many patients find these 'rituals' time consuming and often they affect other areas of life such as socialising and work.

2 Explore the likely contributing factors
- Guide the patient through current stresses at work or in his relationships, e.g. with his parents.
- Suggest factors such as his recent promotion at work, the family dynamics and concerns about swine flu may have each contributed to the OCD.
- Explain the repeated use of soap and alcohol gels can lead to other problems such as dermatitis, which would require treatment with emollients and steroid creams.
- Encourage him to use moisturisers regularly to alleviate the dry skin and aim to reduce hand washing and alcohol gel application. Suggest he discards all the alcohol gels he owns.

3 Provide information about swine flu
- Explain this is a self-limiting viral illness.
- Reassure him the complication rates are no greater than for the usual winter flu.

- Explain it is appropriate to take precautions such as hand washing when sneezing and disposing of dirty tissues, but repetitive hand washing will not make a difference to further spread of the virus.

4 Discuss options for treatment
- CBT is useful to help manage the unhelpful thinking patterns that perpetuate this condition. This can be offered through group or individual CBT with or without self-help materials.
- Local self-help and support groups, e.g. OCT-UK (www.ocduk.org), OCT Action (www.ocdaction.org.uk).
- SSRI drugs – explain how they work, their onset of action and that they are usually taken for at least a few months.
- Referral to a psychiatrist if the previous options are not successful.
- This patient prefers minimal intervention, so starting with CBT would be a reasonable first option.

5 Offer support with his job
- Suggest he speaks to his employer.
- If he would like time off work, offer to write a sick note to explain his diagnosis.

6 Offer general lifestyle advice
- Advise him about simple relaxation techniques such as meditation, exercise, hobbies and interests.
- Suggest the patient exercises to help deal with any stress.
- Encourage him to speak to any family members he would feel comfortable telling.
- Inform him that because alcohol can reduce the anxiety associated with OCD, there is a higher incidence of alcohol abuse in OCD sufferers. Reiterate the recommended weekly allowance and discourage him from increasing his alcohol intake to avoid alcohol dependence.

7 Offer follow-up
- Arrange to see the patient again to monitor symptoms and to monitor response to any treatments.
- Offer to see the patient with family members (e.g. his brother) and explain the problem to them.
- Provide the patient with information leaflets to take away.

Interpersonal skills
- Help the patient feel at ease from the start, especially since he feels as if he is wasting your time.
  - 'You aren't wasting my time at all. Please, take your time and tell me about the problem.'
- Explore relevant cues through open questions.
  - 'In what way does this problem make you feel helpless?'
  - 'You mentioned your colleagues have noticed the problems. How has that affected you?'
- To diagnose the condition, the history should elicit obsessions and compulsions, together with preserved insight. To achieve this, you may need to use a mixture of open and closed questions.
  - 'What's going through your mind when you feel you the need to wash your hands?'
  - 'Do you think that the number of times you wash your hands is a problem?'
  - 'Would you like help to manage this problem?'
- Be supportive of the patient attending for help.
  - 'I would like you to know that I think it is really good that you have come here for help.'
- Sensitively raise issues that might be related to his symptoms.
  - 'I'd like to know a bit more about you. How are things with the rest of your family?'

— 'You mentioned you only recently moved away from home. Has that helped you become more independent?'
- If the patient does not like personal questions, be respectful of this and offer an explanation.
  — 'I'm sorry for upsetting you with these questions . . . (pause) . . . We can stay away from any topics you do not wish to discuss.'
  — 'The reason for asking these questions is that problems like this can develop due to various factors, such as our relationships with others. Recognising them can help unravel things.'
- Explain the diagnosis of OCD in lay terms, using easy-to-follow language.
  — 'Obsessive-compulsive disorder or OCD is a condition where the patient experiences repetitive thoughts that lead them to carry out unwanted behaviours. These experiences are distressing and can start to interfere with daily life. Patients recognise these behaviours are not right.'
  — 'The OCD could be due to a combination of reasons. It can run in families; it might be a result of a chemical imbalance in the brain. Stress can make it worse.'
- Continue to follow a patient-centred approach to develop a shared management plan.
  — 'There is a special technique called cognitive behavioural therapy. Have you heard of it?'
  — 'We could try a few sessions. What are your thoughts about this so far?'
  — 'One of the problems in OCD is a chemical imbalance in the brain, rather like in depression. Certain drugs used for depression are also good for treating OCD. This would be another option we could try along with CBT if you would like?'
- Gently advise him to involve his family.
  — 'I realise you do not wish to tell family members about this condition. A lot of patients keep OCD secret for fear of embarrassment. Does this apply to you?'
  — 'Most patients find it helpful to involve close family. What do you think about this?'
- Emphasise to the patient that he is not alone in all this.
  — 'Now that you have identified the problem, you do not have to go through it alone. As I said, involving those close to you, like your brother, can help, but you can come and see me for support when you like. There are a number of other sufferers out there, and support groups and helpful resources such as books, internet sites and forums are also useful.'

O⚊ **Key summary**
- Confirm the diagnosis of OCD.
- Address his main concerns, particularly about work and swine flu.
- Sensitively explore family dynamics and encourage him to speak to close family members.
- Discuss management options with psychological treatments +/– SSRI drugs.
- Consider other associated problems, e.g. his dry hands.

Obsessive-compulsive disorder
Main features
- The main features of this condition are obsessions and compulsions. It can also be characterised by general indecisiveness.
- There is an association with anxiety, depression and other mental health conditions.

Epidemiology
- One to two per cent of the population suffer from OCD.
- Female to male ratio is 3:2.
- OCD usually presents in young adults, although patients may have had symptoms for a number of years before they present.
- Precipitating factors include stress and adverse life events. It is more common in those with high standards/expectations of themselves.

Clinical features

- Common obsessions can include:
  — fears of dirt, germs or contamination
  — fears of performing violent acts and of harming others.
- Patients will act on these obsessions to decrease the anxiety that they provoke. Common compulsive behaviours include:
  — excessive hand washing
  — excessive cleaning
  — checking things repeatedly, e.g. that the door is locked, that the gas heating is switched off, counting and keeping things tidy.

Management

Who is responsible for care	What is the focus?	What do they do?
Step 6 Inpatient care of intensive treatment programmes CAMHS Tier 4	OCD or BDD with risk to life, severe self-neglect or severe distress or disability	Reassess, discuss options, care coordination SSRI or clomipramine, CBT (including ERP), or combination of SSRI or clomipramine and CBT (including ERP), augmentation strategies, consider admission or special living arrangements
Step 5 Multidisplinary care with expertise in OCD/BDD CAMHS Tier 3 and 4	OCD or BDD with significant comorbidity or more severely impaired functioning and/or treament resistance, partial response or relapse	Reassess, discuss options **For adults:** SSRI or clomipramine, CBT (including ERP), or combination of SSRI or clomipramine and CBT (including ERP); consider care coordination, augmentation strategies, admission, social care **For children and young people:** CBT (including ERP), then consider combined treatments of CBT (including ERP) with SSRI, alternaitve SSRI or clomipramine. For young people consider referral to specialist services outside CAMHS if appropriate
Step 4 Multidisplinary care in primary or secondary care CAMHS Tier 2 and 3	OCD or BDD with comorbidity or poor response to initial treatment	Assess and review, discuss options **For adults:** CBT (including ERP), SSRI, alternative SSRI or clomipramine, combined treatments **For children and young people:** CBT (including ERP), then consider combined treatments of CBT (including ERP) with SSRI, alternaitve SSRI or clomipramine
Step 3 GPs, primary care team, primary care mental health workers, family support team CAMHS Tier 1 and 2	Management and initial treatment of OCD or BDD	Assess and review, discuss options **For adults:** Brief individual CBT (including ERP) with self-help materials (for OCD), individual group of CBT (including ERP), SSRI, or consider combined treatments; consider involving the family/carers in ERP **For children and young people:** Guided self-help (for OCD), CBT (including ERP), involve family/carers and consider involving school
Step 2 GPs, practice nurses, school health advisors, health visitors, general health settings (including hospitals) CAMHS Tier 1	Recognition and assessment	Detect, educate, discuss treatment options, signpost voluntary support organisations, provide support to individuals/families/carers/work/school, or refer to any of the appropirate levels
Step 1 Individuals, public organisations, NHS	Awareness and recognition	Provide, seek and share inforamtion about OCD or BDD and its impact on individuals and families/carers

FIGURE 3.1 The stepped-care model for the management of OCD

(Reproduced with permission of National Institute for Health and Clinical Excellence.)

National Institute for Health and Clinical Excellence. Obsessive Compulsive Disorder (OCD) and Body Dysmorphic Disorder (BDD): NICE guideline 31. London: NIHCE; 2005. www.nice.org.uk/CG031 (accessed 25 November 2010).

Further reading

- National Institute for Health and Clinical Excellence. *Obsessive Compulsive Disorder (OCD)and Body Dysmorphic Disorder (BDD): NICE guideline 31.* London: NIHCE; 2005. www.nice.org.uk/CG031 (accessed 25 November 2010).
- Semple D, Smyth R. *Oxford Handbook of Psychiatry.* 2nd ed. Oxford: Oxford University Press; 2009.
- Self-help groups: www.ocduk.org/ and www.ocdaction.org.uk (accessed 25 November 2010).

Station 3.9

Latest discharge report

Reason for admission	Infective exacerbation of pulmonary fibrosis
Treatment	Steroids
	Nebulisers
	Intravenous antibiotics

Comment
- She has had five similar admissions over the past 18 months with a further deterioration in her baseline function and exercise tolerance.
- Investigations revealed very poor lung function.
- The consultant explained to her that the prognosis is very poor, and a decision was made to treat palliatively.
- Mrs Patel decided to die at home and has said 'no' to having CPR or any intensive care admissions.

Actor's notes
Background
- You are Jyoti Patel, a 75-year-old lady and lifelong housewife.

Opening statement
- 'Doctor, I seem to be getting much worse. Can you help me?'

History
- You have felt increasingly breathless for the past few days and have been coughing.

Ideas, concerns and expectations
- You are longing to see your daughter, who lives in Australia and is hoping to fly to the UK soon.
- You were shocked to hear the consultant tell you that your breathlessness would worsen and you may die soon. You understand that your condition is likely to deteriorate further.
- You do not want to go back into the hospital and want to die calmly and peacefully.
- When you get breathless at night you feel very scared and as if you are about to die.
- You have asked for a home visit because you want something to help settle your breathlessness.

Further history candidate may elicit
- Your breathing has gradually worsened over the past several months. You cannot walk long distances and have a wheelchair. You are very breathless with all activities, including speaking and getting dressed.
- Now you are breathless at rest, despite using oxygen. In the last day or two, you have used the oxygen more than usual. Normally you use it 18–20 hours a day but now are only having a break from it for an hour a day. In addition, you have been using salbutamol nebulisers every 2 hours.
- You have a dry unproductive cough most of the time. This has not changed lately. Over the last few days, your ankles have become slightly swollen.
- You sleep using three pillows at night. Over the last few weeks you sometimes wake up 'gasping for air' and feel very scared.
- You have no palpitations or chest pain.
- During the latest hospital admission, the consultant explained there was not much more that could be done, and told you it was likely that your breathing would continue to become worse. The consultant offered to keep you in hospital if you wished, but you declined and said you would rather be at home. You dislike going into hospital because there are too many people, the food is not pleasant and you cannot rest properly.
- The palliative care team are now involved in your care. A nurse visited yesterday and said she would visit again in a few days' time.
- You have been quite down recently, your appetite is poor and you have been increasingly tearful in the past week.
- You were raised a Hindu, and until the decline in your health, used to attend the temple several days a week. You are a religious person and believe that everything happens for a reason.
- You have one daughter, who is your next of kin. She moved to Australia 10 years ago. Having heard the news, she is hoping to fly to the UK to see you in the next few days.
- Your husband died five years ago and you miss him dearly, especially at this vulnerable time.

Medical history
- Idiopathic pulmonary fibrosis – diagnosed three years ago.
- Type 2 diabetes – diagnosed 10 years ago.

Drug history
- Salbutamol nebules 5 mg prn.
- Atrovent nebules 5 mg qds.
- Salbutamol inhaler 100 mcg prn.
- Symbicort 200 mcg two puffs bd.
- Prednisolone 7.5 mg daily.
- Metformin 850 mg bd.
- Gliclazide 80 mg bd.

Social history
- You have never smoked and do not drink alcohol.

- You live alone in a ground floor flat.
- Your husband died five years ago following a heart attack.
- You have very helpful neighbours who visit regularly.
- You have carers who visit three times a day and manage the cleaning, shopping and cooking. They also help wash and clothe you.
- The palliative care nurse also visits you every few days to monitor your progress.

Family history
- Nil significant.

Approach to scenario
- As a result of your breathing difficulties you find it a big effort to speak and answer questions.
- You are fed up and frustrated about your symptoms and this comes across when you are speaking to the doctor.
- You will double check with the doctor if there is any cure 'for my lungs' and if the consultant was correct when he explained your condition will worsen.
- You want to see your daughter and worry you may not see her before you die.
- You wish to die peacefully, in minimal pain and discomfort.
- You do not want admission to intensive care or hospital, and certainly do not want anyone trying to re-start your heart if it stops beating.
- If the doctor raises the issue of admission to a hospice or back into hospital, you will say that you prefer to remain at home.
- You are not aware of the difference between a hospital and a hospice.
- If the doctor explains that hospices are generally calm, peaceful places with specialist staff to provide high-quality care for patients in your situation, you will consider this option.
- If the doctor offers to arrange your admission to a hospice, and comes across well, you agree.
- If the doctor does not raise the issue of hospice care, you explain you wish to die at home.
- In this case, you will continue to emphasise the issues about feeling uncomfortable with breathing difficulties.
- If the doctor is sensitive to this, listens to your concerns and offers to communicate with other relevant teams (e.g. palliative care, district nurses), you accept any help offered, including morphine-based medicines.
- If, however, the doctor communicates poorly, does not listen to your concerns, or ask about your symptoms, you are sceptical about receiving morphine-based drugs.
- If you feel the consultation is going badly, then you will say 'I feel I'm being left to die alone at home, Doctor.'

Information gathering
Presenting complaint
- Ask about chest pain and palpitations.
- Ask about her difficulty breathing:
  — changes in exercise tolerance
  — progress since discharge
  — alleviating and exacerbating factors.
- Ask about use of nebulisers and home oxygen.

Medical history
- Type 2 diabetes and idiopathic pulmonary fibrosis.

Drug history
- Clarify she is taking all her prescribed medicines.

Social history
- Smoking status (not safe with home oxygen).
- Support networks:
  — family
  — friends
  — carers
  — district nurses
  — palliative care nurses.
- Housing issues:
  — Ask if anyone else lives with her.
  — Ask about home and walking/mobility aids.
- Activities of daily living.
- Confirm next of kin.
- Enquire about any advanced directives.

Patient's agenda
- Explore her understanding of her current condition and prognosis.
- Discuss her reasons for declining hospital admission.
- Explore her understanding of hospice care.
- Explore her anxieties about breathlessness and 'gasping for air'.

Examination
- Offer to examine her cardiovascular and respiratory system, and check her vital signs.
- 'I would like to check you over and examine your heart and lungs – is that okay?'

Examination card	
General examination	Breathless at rest
	Peripherally cyanosed on 4 L of O_2 via nasal cannula
	Respiratory rate = 22
	Pulse = 110/minute and regular
	BP = 100/60 mmHg
	Oxygen saturation = 93% on oxygen
Systemic examination	Bilateral fine end-inspiratory crepitations from mid-zones down
	Decreased air entry
	Mild pitting oedema of the ankles

Clinical management
1 Discuss her condition and prognosis
- Ensure the patient has capacity to make decisions about her overall management.
- Discuss the advice from the consultant and her prognosis.
- Explain that the only treatment available is palliation and symptom control, and is not curative.
- Offer to liaise with her specialist if there are any questions you are not able to answer.

2 Discuss options about where she can be cared for
- Discuss the pros and cons of remaining at home versus hospital or hospice admission.
- Explore how she will cope living by herself.
- Emphasise the difference between a hospice and hospital, in particular that hospices offer personalised care with a high-quality team trained to look after patients in their last days.
- Suggest that her needs may be best managed by admission to a hospice.

- Advise her that you will make the necessary referrals and speak to the relevant teams straight after the consultation.
- Reassure her that whether she is at home or in a hospice, she would be reviewed on an ongoing basis by the palliative care team.
- However, if she decides to stay at home suggest you will:
  — speak to the palliative care nurse to discuss a management plan
  — liaise with the community respiratory nurse specialist to attend to issues such as home oxygen and nebulisers
  — offer to speak to her social worker to urgently review her care package
  — consider speaking to hospital-at-home services
  — arrange appropriate handover to out-of-hours services.

3 Offer symptomatic treatments

- Offer lorazepam for the anxiety she experiences at night.
- Consider increasing her steroids as a short-term measure – the evidence for this is limited but it may offer some short-term relief.
- Approach the subject of commencing opiates, e.g. Oramorph® to alleviate symptoms of distress.
- Mention to her that alleviating her symptoms with opiates is likely to also reduce her life span.
- Explain that if she remained distressed despite using opiates a syringe driver would be available.
- Explain side effects of these treatments.

4 Final preparations

- Discuss the option of having a pundit (priest) come to help guide her through this difficult time.
- Enquire if she has a will or if there are other issues that need finalising before she passes away.
- Check if she has considered how her remains should be dealt with, i.e. cremation or burial (Hindu custom is usually cremation).
- Offer to discuss the patient's condition with any friends or relatives.
- Offer to complete a form to allow her to benefit from attendance allowance (DS1500; *see* page 261).

5 Offer follow-up

- Reassure the patient that she will be followed up at home and monitored regularly.
- Offer to telephone or visit again to monitor her response to any treatments and update her about hospice admission.

Interpersonal skills

- The dynamic for the home visit is different from that at the surgery. You are in someone else's home. Be flexible in terms of how you conduct your consultation, for example, in the real-life setting you may need to stand or find a stool to sit down.
- Open with a simple statement to establish rapport.
  — 'Hello Mrs Patel, I don't believe we have met. My name is Dr Care. I was told your breathing has become worse.'
- Adopt an empathic and caring approach from the outset.
  — 'I'm sorry to hear things are worse. Tell me about your symptoms – I'm here to help.'
- During your enquiry about the patient's condition, be led by the patient and make sure you respond to cues in the process.
  — 'You mentioned the specialist said the prognosis is not good. What did you understand them to mean by that?'

- Carefully establish the patient's understanding of the terminal nature of her condition.
  — 'Just so we are clear, you do understand what is meant when the consultant said that the condition is terminal?'
- Assess the impact of the symptoms on her psychological health as well as any functional impact.
  — 'The breathlessness is there all the time now, you say. How is it affecting you in terms of looking after yourself?'
  — 'Do your symptoms ever frighten you?'
- Approach the subject of potential further management and resuscitation, with sensitivity.
  — 'If your oxygen levels were to fall further and you became sicker, would you under any circumstances wish to return to hospital?'
  — 'How about carrying out tests such as blood tests or X-rays? Is that something you wish to avoid too?'
  — 'Obviously we cannot say when this will happen, but if your heart stops beating would you want attempts made to re-start your heart?'
- Help guide the patient through the various management options, recognising that she may not be able to take everything in. Remain supportive of her wishes.
  — 'Clearly there is a lot for you to take in. Don't worry, I'll speak to the various team members to make sure you get what you need at home.'
  — 'I can see you are quite distressed by your symptoms. It might be a good idea for you to take something to help alleviate some of the distress . . . (silence) . . . We could try a small dose of something called morphine – are you familiar with this medicine?'
- Help draw the patient's attention to the advantages of hospice care so that she can make an informed decision about where she would like to die.
  — 'Hospice care is very different to what you've experienced so far. In a hospice there is a calm, peaceful atmosphere where the nurses and doctors have time to address all your needs and to relieve your symptoms.'
- If the patient opts to remain at home, share your concerns with the patient and help reassure her before leaving the house.
  — 'I am worried about you being alone at home. I think we need to increase the care you are receiving. Could I have your permission to contact the local hospital-at-home services to put in place extra provisions for you?'
  — 'I'll call you first thing tomorrow to touch base and see how your are. How does that sound?'

O━ **Key summary**
- Ensure the patient understands the terminal nature of her condition.
- Involve members of the primary healthcare team, including palliative care and care coordinator.
- Address the patient's concerns, including her symptoms and psychological well-being.
- Ensure the patient is informed about the pros and cons of hospice admission.
- Aim for good end-of-life care, ensuring the patient dies peacefully and with dignity.

Terminal care
- Terminal care applies to patients with liver, renal or heart failure, and other advanced medical conditions, including cancer.

Definitions
a World Health Organization (WHO) definition of palliative care
- 'Palliative care is an approach that improves the quality of life of patients and their families facing the problems associated with life-threatening illness, through the prevention and relief of suffering by means of early identification and impeccable assessment and

treatment of pain and other problems, physical, psychosocial and spiritual.' (World Health Organization, 2005).

b Department of Health definition of end-of-life care
- 'End-of-life care is care that helps all those with advanced, progressive, incurable illness to live as well as possible until they die. It enables the supportive and palliative care needs of both patient and family to be identified and met throughout the last phase of life and into bereavement. It includes management of pain and other symptoms and provision of psychological, social, spiritual and practical support.' (Department of Health, *End of Life Care Strategy England, 2008*).

c Liverpool Care Pathway (LCP) reference
- This was devised to help guide healthcare professionals in primary and secondary care to manage dying patients in their last days or weeks.
- The LCP sets in place a care pathway with five elements:
  1. an explicit statement of goals/key elements of care based on evidence and best practice
  2. facilitating communication among team members, patients and families
  3. coordinating the roles and sequencing the activities of the MDT, patients and carers
  4. documentation, monitoring and evaluation of variances and outcomes
  5. identification of the appropriate resources.

d DS1500
- This is a medical report form for patients who are considered to be terminally unwell, and in need of extra support.
- For the purposes of benefit entitlement, terminal illness is defined as life expectancy ≤6 months.
- Under special rules, the patient is given priority. Their application is fast tracked for Disability Living Allowance (DLA) and Attendance Allowance (AA).
- Normally, patients applying for DLA and AA have to prove the care they require, but with the DS1500 this is not the case.
- The DS1500 asks for details about the diagnosis and management plan, as well as the patient's clinical state.

Further reading
- Department of Health, *End-of-Life Care Strategy*. Available at: www.dh.gov.uk/en/Publicationsandstatistics/Publications/PublicationsPolicyAndGuidance/DH_086277 (accessed 23 November 2010).
- The Marie Curie Palliative Care Institute. *Liverpool Care Pathway for the Dying Patient (LCP)*. Liverpool: The Marie Curie Palliative Care Institute; n.d. Available at: www.mcpcil.org.uk/liverpool-care-pathway (accessed 13 December 2010).
- Murphy D, Ellershaw J, Jack B, *et al*. The Liverpool Care Pathway for the rapid discharge home of the dying patient. *Journal of Integrated Care Pathways*. 2004; **8**(3): 127–8.
- Patient UK. *Benefits for the Terminally Ill*. Patient UK; 2010. Available at: www.patient.co.uk/health/Benefits-for-the-Terminally-Ill.htm (accessed 13 December 2010).
- World Health Organization definition of palliative care. Available at www.who.int/cancer/palliative/definition/en/ (accessed 23 November 2010)

Station 3.10

Candidate's notes

Name	Tim Federer
Age	40
Medical history	Nil
Medication	Nil
Allergies	Nil
Last consultation	Telephone consultation two weeks ago, outlined as follows:
	Lumbar back pain for one week – no red flags
	Sounds like mechanical low back pain
	Will take over-the-counter ibuprofen
	Sick note issued for two weeks
	To attend surgery if no better in two weeks

Actor's notes

Background
- You are Tim Federer, a 40-year-old gentleman who works in a warehouse.

Opening statement
- 'Hello Doctor, this back pain doesn't seem to be going away. Not sure if anything needs doing.'

History
- You have had back pain for the past three weeks, which is not settling.
- You occasionally have to take ibuprofen to help control the pain.

Ideas, concerns and expectations
- You are worried that the pain has not yet resolved.
- You are unsure about what you should do or avoid. You have significantly restricted your activities to mainly lying down and staying still at home.
- You would like the GP to give you a sick note and offer treatment to help the pain resolve.

Further history candidate may elicit
- You work in a warehouse, lifting and transferring boxes. For a few weeks leading up to the onset of the pain, you were experiencing a dull ache in the lower back but ignored it.
- The back pain began suddenly when bending to do up your shoelaces. For the first few days you had to lie down most of the time.
- You self-certified off sick for the first week following the pain. You were then issued a sick note for a further two weeks by a GP whom you spoke to on the telephone.
- You have taken ibuprofen when the pain gets worse, and this helps.
- The pain has gradually improved and you only have a mild ache now.
- If asked to rate the severity of the pain, it is now 3/10 at worst whereas two weeks ago it was 7/10.
- The pain is located around the lower back and does not radiate anywhere.
- It is exacerbated by sudden movements, bending and lifting.
- You have no problem passing urine or controlling your bowel motions.
- There is no loss of feeling when you wipe around the anal region after going to the toilet.
- There is no numbness or tingling in the feet or legs.

- The pain does not disturb you at night and you sleep well. There has been no history of trauma.
- For the past month, you have not done very much with your time, except watch television.
- A friend has been helping with tasks such as the shopping.
- You have worked for the same company for 20 years in the same role, which you find monotonous. You applied for a senior role three years ago but were unsuccessful. The company recruited a man seven years younger than you. You were upset not to have been promoted, given your years of service and loyalty to the company. You find it difficult to take orders from someone younger than you. This has led to tension and animosity with your boss as well as arguments over how things should be done. Consequently, you feel quite reluctant to return to work at this stage.
- The problems at work and the back pain have got you down but you are not depressed or anxious.
- Your main financial commitments include paying child support for your two children and rent for the small flat you live in.
- You would like a sick note to cover more time off from work.

Medical history
- Lower back pain 10 years ago requiring two weeks off work.

Drug history
- Ibuprofen 400 mg taken as required for back pain.

Social history
- You are a non-smoker and drink alcohol socially.
- You live alone, having divorced your wife five years ago. She has subsequently remarried.
- You have two children who are eight and ten years old who live with their mother and visit you at the weekends.

Family history
- Nil significant.

Approach to scenario
- You feel anxious about persuading the doctor to issue you an extension of your sick note for work.
- If asked how much time off you would like, you seem unsure and ask for a 'few more weeks.'
- You are fed up with work. You feel let down and unappreciated, given your years of service. You do not like your boss and feel that he would not take into consideration your latest problems.
- If challenged about wishing to take more time off work, you become defensive and repeat your concerns about heavy lifting. You will also become worried and serious.
- You feel that if you go back to heavy lifting now, you could cause serious permanent damage.
- You are sure that your boss will make you carry weights as heavy as 20–30 kg.
- If the doctor takes the time to explore your worries about work in a friendly and calm manner, and explains what is wrong with your back, then you accept any help that is offered.
- If the doctor is flexible about your request for a sick note, then you are prepared to take up any suggestions about returning to work on restricted duties.
- However, if the doctor is insensitive to your worries about returning to work, antagonises you about your request for a sick note or makes you feel the back pain has not been taken seriously, then you will remain worried and serious and leave the consultation visibly unhappy.

Information gathering
Presenting complaint
a Pain
- Ask about general progress since the last consultation.
- Ask about the pain:
  — trauma
  — location
  — severity
  — radiation
  — intensity
  — alleviating factors, e.g. NSAIDs
  — exacerbating factors, e.g. lifting, bending.

b Features of inflammatory pain
- Early morning stiffness.
- Systemic features, e.g. fevers and malaise.

c Red flags
- Bladder or bowel dysfunction:
  — urinary retention
  — faecal incontinence.
- Perianal anaesthesia.
- Thoracic pain.
- Fever and unexplained weight loss.
- History of carcinoma.
- Progressive neurological deficit.

d Yellow flags
- Ask if the patient thinks back pain is severely disabling.
- Ask about reduced activity levels.
- Ask about depression, low morale and social withdrawal.
- Ask about social or financial problems.

Medical history
- Back or other musculoskeletal problems.

Drug history
- Ask about analgesia taken for back pain.
- Enquire about allergies and contraindications to NSAIDs.

Family history
- Back problems or autoimmune joint disease.

Social history
- Smoking and alcohol history.
- Occupation, e.g. manual work.
- Time off work, e.g. sick leave.
- Support networks, e.g. family and friends.

Patient's agenda
- Explore the impact of back pain on his work.
- Explore the impact of back pain on his personal and professional life.
- Explore his expectations of the consultation, e.g. referral, sick note, investigations.

Examination

- Offer to examine the patient's back, lower limbs and check his weight.
- 'I would like to examine your back and legs to help identify what is causing this pain.'

Examination card

General examination	Normal gait
	BMI = 24.5 kg/m²
Back	Tenderness at the right paralumbar region at the level of L2/3
	Straight-leg raising is painful on the right side but intact
	Full range of movements of the back
Lower limbs neurological	Normal

Clinical management

1 Offer an explanation about the back pain

- Advise the patient he has signs of mechanical back pain.
- Explain that this kind of pain may be due to a sprain, ligament or muscle problem, likely precipitated by the heavy lifting.
- Reassure the patient that this kind of pain is usually self-limiting and not serious. Patients would be expected to return to normal activities within six weeks.

2 Discuss the management of mechanical back pain

a Mobilisation

- Encourage him to keep mobilising gently and avoid strenuous activity. This will help with pain and recovery.
- Advise him to avoiding heavy lifting and bending for now.

b Offer drug therapy

- Suggest taking a course of regular analgesia such as stronger NSAIDs like diclofenac.

c Exercises and physiotherapy

- Offer to refer him for physiotherapy.
- Offer advice on simple back exercises that might help, and provide written information.

3 Discuss options about sick notes and returning to work

- Emphasise the benefits of resuming normal activities and returning to work as soon as possible.
- Explore alternative options about how he may manage at work, e.g. administrative or lighter duties.
- Encourage him to speak to his line manager and negotiate a phased or adjusted return to work.
- If his employer has an occupational health department, suggest he attends for further advice and assistance such as training in manual handling.
- Explain that his company would conduct an assessment and try to help him to work if at all possible.
- Discuss the option of sick notes, e.g.:
  — Provide him with a sick note for a limited time (e.g. two weeks); arrange follow-up to review his progress and suggest a date to return to work.
  — Provide him with a sick note specifying a phased return to work, e.g. with desk work only, for a defined time.

4 Offer follow-up

- Offer to see him again, e.g. when the sick note runs out, or following a fixed period like two to three weeks.
- Advise him to return earlier if he develops any red flags, e.g. difficulties passing urine or incontinence of stool.
- Offer information leaflets on mechanical back pain.

Interpersonal skills

- Show the patient you are listening by addressing the patient's opening statement directly.
  - 'I am sorry to hear the pain is not settling. Let's work out what might need doing. How about you start off by telling me some more about the pain.'
- Identify any hidden agendas there may be.
  - 'Is there something else you would like today?'
  - 'You mentioned time off work. Do you feel ready to return to work or were you looking to have some more time off?'
- If the patient remains vague about his reasons for wanting more time off from work, adopt a sensitive approach whilst at the same time exploring any verbal or non-verbal cues. Use open questions as much as possible.
  - 'Are there any problems you've had at work that have put you off going back?'
  - 'You seem upset at my suggestion to return to work. What's going through your mind?'
- When necessary, use closed questions, particularly in relation to ruling out red flags.
  - 'Would it be okay if I ask you some "yes or no" questions for a moment?'
  - 'Have you had any loss of feeling or tingling in your feet or legs at all?'
- If you feel the patient would benefit from returning to work soon, be prepared to negotiate, addressing any of his worries in the process.
  - 'You mentioned to me that you are worried about carrying out any activities that might aggravate the pain. I can understand that, and I agree with you that you shouldn't start carrying heavy items straight away ... (silence) ... How about we discuss the possibility of a gradual return to work, doing only non-manual work to start with?'
- Aim to address the patient's concerns, ensuring the explanations are simple to follow, and allow him the chance to feedback to you.
  - 'I know you are concerned about the pain still being there. Mechanical back pain of this nature is usually due to the muscles becoming very tight. It usually gets better within six weeks. Is there anything you would like to ask before I continue? ... (silence) ...'
  - 'Part of the way to relieve the tightness is to take the anti-inflammatory medication we spoke about, but also to allow yourself to move about as much as you can, pain permitting, of course.'
  - 'I know you mentioned you are avoiding almost all movements now. (silence) ... In fact, I would suggest that your back would benefit more from increasing your activity, according to pain. What do you think about that?'
- Offer shared management options.
  - 'You could continue with the ibuprofen as required, but it seems it isn't effective enough. Another option we could try is a regular course of an anti-inflammatory drug for a week or two ... (silence) ... How does that sound?'
- If the outcome seems complicated for the patient or yourself, summarise at the end.
  - 'So just to clarify then. I have adjusted the painkiller ... (silence) ... I'll refer you for physiotherapy ... (silence) ... and here's a sick note for two weeks. How is that? ... (silence) ... And then you'll to come and see me in two weeks and we'll discuss you returning to work on lighter duties?'

🔑 Key summary

- Diagnose mechanical back pain and rule out red flags.
- Identify yellow flags and address these factors.
- Reassure the patient about his back pain and manage it conservatively in the first instance.
- Negotiate how best to return to work and offer suggestions in the process, e.g. suggesting amended duties and an occupational health assessment by his employer.

Back pain

Yellow flags

- These refer to risk factors that may make someone more likely to have chronic pain and disability, usually in connection with back pain.

TABLE 3.7 Yellow-flag signs for back pain

YELLOW-FLAG SIGNS	
Poor social support or an overprotective family	Problems at work or low job satisfaction
Jobs involving manual work with heavy lifting	Work with unsociable hours
A belief that the pain or activity is bad for their back, resulting in reduced activity levels	Signs of social isolation, e.g. staying at home, not socialising
A history of back pain and sick leave	Depressive symptoms or negative thoughts
Patients with social or financial issues	

- In this case, the patient has several yellow-flags, which suggests he is at risk of remaining off work permanently or for a prolonged period of time. This should be recognised and appropriately addressed.
- Patients falling in this category have been shown to be at increased risk of:
  — mental health illness, e.g. depression
  — social isolation
  — low self-esteem
  — becoming de-skilled.
- Such patients have economic implications for society at large.

Red flags

- These are important signs to rule out when a patient presents with back pain.
- They often warrant an urgent or emergency referral.

TABLE 3.8 Red-flag signs for back pain

RED-FLAG SIGNS	
Age <20 years or >55 years	Inflammatory-sounding pain
Thoracic pain	Systemic signs, e.g. weight loss, night sweats
Neurological signs	Steroid use
HIV	History of neoplastic disease
Spinal deformity	

Sick certificates

- On 6 April 2010, the sick note was changed to a 'fitness to work' certificate.
- The certificate offers the doctor the option of either specifying the patient is 'not fit for work' or stating the patient 'may be fit for work'. This latter statement is a new addition to the certificate.
- Doctors no longer need to issue statements saying a patient is fit for work.
- If the note states the patient 'may be fit for work', there is scope for the doctor to specify the kinds of duties the patient could return to, including:
  — a phased return to work
  — flexible working
  — workplace adaptations
  — adjusted duties.
- The old Med 3 and Med 5 have been combined into this one certificate, providing greater flexibility and fewer forms for the doctor to fill in.

Further reading

- Hakim A, Clunie G, Haq I. *Oxford Handbook of Rheumatology.* 2nd ed. Oxford: Oxford University Press; 2006.
- National Institute for Health and Clinical Excellence. Low Back Pain: NICE guideline 88. London: NIHCE; 2009. www.nice.org.uk/guidance/CG88 (accessed 25 November 2010).
- ACC. *New Zealand Acute Low Back Pain Guide.* Wellington: ACC; 2004. Available at: www.nzgg.org.nz/guidelines/0072/acc1038_col.pdf (accessed 13 December 2010).
- Department for Work and Pensions. *Sick Note to Fit Note: helping people stay in work.* Available at: www.dwp.gov.uk/fitnote (accessed 25 November 2010).

Station 3.11

Actor's notes

Background

- You are Josephine Bailey, a 30-year-old lady working as a personal assistant (PA) in the city.

Opening statement

- 'I've been given the wrong medication for my hay fever! I cannot believe how this happened!'

History

- You saw another GP at the practice five days ago with symptoms of sneezing and itchy eyes.
- The doctor diagnosed you with hay fever and prescribed what you thought were antihistamines.
- As requested, you took the tablets daily but found no relief from your symptoms.
- Yesterday, your colleague pointed out that you had been prescribed benzodiazepines.

Ideas, concerns and expectations

- You have been significantly bothered with hay fever symptoms over the last month and are concerned that you will not be able to attend your brother's wedding in four weeks because it is in a country house with large gardens and many flowers, which trigger your symptoms.
- You are worried that the lorazepam will have a long-term effect on your brain.
- You are keen to receive the correct treatment but have lost confidence in the system after receiving the incorrect medication, which could have serious side effects.
- When you were a teenager, your parents took you to a private ENT specialist who administered a steroid injection. This seemed to give you relief from hay fever for several months. You had the treatment for two consecutive seasons, but did not continue as the symptoms settled down.
- Considering the extent of your symptoms, and the prescription error by the previous GP, you expect the GP today to administer the steroid injection for you.

Further history candidate may elicit

- You last suffered from hay fever quite badly in your teenage years. Following an injection at the age of 18, and again at 19, you continued to suffer only mild hay fever symptoms, which were controlled by over-the-counter antihistamines.
- However, this summer the symptoms have returned with a vengeance. The sneezing, runny nose and itchy eyes are interfering with everyday life, including your job and personal life.
- Over the past few weeks, you left several meetings at work early due to the continuous sneezing, which has caused embarrassment. In addition, you have had difficulty sleeping most nights due to the sneezing and nasal congestion. This has made you tired during the

day and it is significantly affecting your efficiency at work. You have stopped wearing contact lenses as your eyes are itchy and have resorted to wearing glasses, which you do not like cosmetically.

- You associate the hay fever symptoms with grass, but also with most plants and flowers, so have therefore avoided attending garden events, such as barbeques and social lunches, to avoid being around high-pollen areas.
- You tried several over-the-counter antihistamines, but these did not help.
- Eventually, you took the day off work to see the GP, who prescribed another antihistamine. You agreed to try this before requesting the steroid injection.
- You took the prescribed tablets daily for five days. They did seem to cause some drowsiness but you put this down to being sensitive to antihistamines. You did not experience any other side effects as far as you are aware (you have checked the drug leaflet for all the stated side effects).
- The hay fever symptoms continued to worsen.
- One of your colleagues saw the medication box yesterday and asked if you were suffering from anxiety. On further discussion, she explained that you were taking benzodiazepines that 'act on the brain' and are given for anxiety. You felt embarrassed that a colleague thought you were suffering from anxiety, and denied this. You read the information leaflet and realised you had been prescribed the wrong medication. You felt very upset and contacted the surgery to make an appointment for today.
- You have no other physical or psychological symptoms.

Medical history
- Childhood eczema and hay fever.
- No history of asthma.

Drug history
- Lorazepam 1 mg od.

Social history
- You are a lifelong non-smoker and drink alcohol occasionally.
- You work long hours for a city trader whose workload has increased recently. This has had a knock-on effect on your own workload and you sometimes have to visit the office at weekends.
- You are single and live alone. Your parents live locally and are in their late 50s.

Family history
- You have a younger brother who suffers from asthma, and a strong family history of hay fever.

Approach to scenario
- You begin the consultation angry and demand an explanation for what went wrong. You want to complain about the locum doctor and ask about how to go about this. You repeatedly say, 'I cannot believe this has been allowed to happen. Who was the doctor? I want his name.' You ask lots of questions about the mistake, and question the doctor at a fast pace.
- You were horrified to discover you had been prescribed the wrong medication and embarrassed that a colleague at work initially thought you were suffering from anxiety.
- You feel debilitated by your hay fever and let down by the practice.
- You expect the GP to help resolve the problem by giving you a steroid injection.
- If the doctor asks you about your symptoms, you answer one or two questions, but then raise your voice and say, 'Look, we are wasting our time going through what's wrong. I did that the other day and look where I'm at now – worse than last time!'
- If the doctor seems caring, apologises for what happened and comes across as being

competent, you calm down in the latter half of the consultation. If the discussion continues to go well, and you are assured the practice will take your complaint seriously, you accept the treatment options offered. You would be prepared to hold off having a steroid injection, provided your symptoms improve within two weeks.

- If, however, the consultation is not going well, the doctor does not apologise, is unable to communicate effectively or does not spend much time exploring the effect of hay fever on your personal and professional life, you remain angry throughout the consultation and will not be prepared to leave without an injection. If that does not happen, you say 'Fine, I'm getting nowhere, I'll go private. Is it too much to ask for a private referral letter then?' You then leave unhappy without saying goodbye.

Information gathering
Presenting complaint
a Clinical error
- Clarify the mistake and offer an apology.
- Determine how the mistake was discovered.
- Confirm how long and how many incorrect tablets she took.

b Adverse effects
- Drowsiness.
- Confusion.
- Light-headedness.

c Hay fever symptoms
- Ask about:
    — time course and duration of symptoms
    — over-the-counter medications used
    — severity of symptoms
    — sneezing
    — nasal symptoms
    — watery, sore, red eyes.

d Associated symptoms
- Hives.
- Wheeze.
- Breathlessness.
- Cough.

e Triggers
- Pollen (allergic).
- House dust (perennial).
- Occupational, e.g. working with flour.

Medical history
- Eczema, asthma, hay fever.
- Treatments used in the past.

Family history
- Eczema, asthma, hay fever.

Drug history and allergies
- Antihistamines, nasal sprays, eye drops, inhalers.

Patient agenda
- Identify how this clinical error has affected her.
- Explore what her expectations are, e.g. she may want to complain formally, leave the practice or be content with an apology from the doctor concerned.
- Explore how the symptoms are affecting her personally and professionally.
- Explore her understanding of hay fever and treatment options.

Examination
- Offer to examine her ears, nose and throat as part of her rhinitis symptoms.
- Offer to perform a respiratory examination and ask for a peak flow test.
- 'If it's okay with you, I would like to examine your ears, nose and throat, your eyes, and listen to your chest. After that, I'll explain how to use a special monitor to check the strength of your puff.'

Examination card

ENT examination	Inflamed turbinates and rhinorrhoea
	No other abnormalities
Eyes	Mild bilateral conjunctivitis
Chest examination	Unremarkable, good air entry and no added sounds
	Peak flow 450 L/min (normal value)

Clinical management
1 Address the patient's concerns and offer an explanation
- Apologise sincerely for the prescription error and reassure her that she is very unlikely to suffer any physical or psychological effects from having taken the lorazepam.
- Agree that from the history and examination, she appears to have hay fever – briefly explain your examination findings.
- Explain hay fever results from the release of histamine when the body's immune system recognises pollen, hence antihistamines are a useful treatment.
- Explain ways to prevent onset of symptoms. These include remaining indoors during peak times, ensuring windows remain shut, avoiding flowery and grassy areas and shielding eyes with glasses when outside.

2 Deal with her decision to make a complaint
- Support her if she wishes to complain, but also offer alternatives.
  — Explain you will contact the locum doctor concerned and speak to him to find out how the mistake occurred.
  — Offer a meeting with the doctor for an explanation – if necessary make yourself available at the meeting.
  — Encourage her to try and address this in-house before taking it further, e.g. PCT or General Medical Council (GMC).
  — Offer to run through the complaints procedures if she wishes (discussed on page 274).
- If she wishes to make a formal complaint, advise her to put something in writing and assure her that this will be investigated and that she will get a response.
- Explain to her that the practice will address this problem openly and honestly by carrying out a significant-event analysis – this will look at exactly what went wrong and how improvements can be made to prevent such problems in future.

3 Treat the hay fever symptoms
- Ensure the patient is given the appropriate treatment for her hay fever.
- Explore options of antihistamines, nasal sprays, eye drops or a combination of some of these.
- Reassure her that she can use all three treatments at the same time.
- Provide an explanation about how to administer these treatments.

4 Address her request for steroid injection
- Explain that there is a very good chance that her symptoms will be relieved by these treatments before her brother's wedding without the need for a steroid injection.
- Explain steroid injections are not advised nowadays because of uncertainty about how long effects last for (generally considered to be several weeks), and the potential systemic side effects.
- Advise her if the other treatments are unsuccessful at controlling her symptoms, she could be given a course of oral steroids over the period of her brother's wedding.
- Explain oral steroids are highly effective in controlling allergy symptoms and are reserved for situations such as this. However, they are not used as first-line treatment of hay fever because they can cause systemic effects.
- Suggest she tries the antihistamine/nasal spray/eye drop combination and if the symptoms are not controlled within two weeks, a course of oral prednisolone could be prescribed to cover her for her brother's wedding.

5 Arrange follow-up
- Have a plan of action set up, e.g. arranging a meeting with the locum doctor.
- Emphasise everything will be done to prevent the same mistake happening in future.
- Follow-up will enable the patient to review her hay fever symptoms and hopefully help her feel she is being well managed.
- Provide her with fact sheets and information leaflets.

Interpersonal skills
- Dealing with an angry patient requires a good demeanour, remaining calm under pressure and demonstrating to the patient that she is being listened to and taken seriously.
- If the patient becomes angry or raises her voice, respond by lowering the tone of your voice. Be as non-confrontational as possible, using verbal and non-verbal communication skills.
  — 'Talk me through how you are feeling.'
- It is important to use active listening skills, ensuring you pick up on cues and explore her concerns and expectations.
  — 'You mentioned you feel let down by us. I am truly sorry about that. Is there anything you feel that I can do to help put things right?'
- Avoid berating your colleague or making excuses for what has happened, whilst remaining professional. Offer an apology and constructive suggestions as to how to deal with her complaint.
  — 'I am really sorry this has happened. I would like to reassure you that this problem will be taken seriously within the practice and we will also contact the locum doctor.'
- Show the patient you are concerned about her hay fever through open questions.
  — 'Tell me about your hay fever symptoms. How have they been since the last visit?'
- Handle her request for a steroid injection with sensitivity, offer an explanation about why you are reluctant, but also be aware of her expectations.
  — 'I know the symptoms are really bad now and the worry is that they may go on longer. Also, I realise you have your brother's big day next month. We can get these symptoms under control very quickly with the right treatment, which I can prescribe for you now ... (silence) ... Steroid injections are very rarely used as a treatment for hay fever nowadays because of their side effects ...'

— 'How about we try the three treatments we spoke about and see you in two weeks or so? If the symptoms are still bad, then we can consider a short course of oral steroids, which would be a highly effective option. How does that sound?'
- Offer the patient options in your overall management, but also demonstrate that you care by offering follow-up.
  — 'We can use eye drops as well as tablets to treat this. There are also nasal sprays to treat the sneezing and runny nose aspect. Would you like me to run through these in a bit more detail?'
  — 'Let's meet again in two weeks. How does that sound?'
  — 'I'll get in touch with the locum doctor as soon as possible and ask him to respond to what happened.'

O⚬⅃ Key summary
- Reassure the patient that she will not suffer any long-term effects from the error.
- Address the hay fever symptoms.
- Negotiate about how to proceed in terms of a possible complaint.
- Assure the patient that the clinical error will be taken seriously.
- Aim to restore her trust in the doctor–patient relationship.

Common causes for complaints in primary care
- Prescribing errors.
- Refusal to perform a home visit.
- Delayed diagnosis, e.g. cancer.
- Refusal to refer.

Complaints procedures in primary care
- In the first instance, patients should speak to their GP or practice manager.
- If this is not satisfactory, the patient should complain verbally (with a staff member recording the complaint) or in writing. The practice should respond within three days. Thereafter, the surgery has six months to complete its investigation into the complaint.
- If the patient is still not happy then the complaint can be referred to the PCT, parliamentary or health service ombudsman.
- The patient can also take advice about complaints handling at any stage from the:
  — PCT complaints manager
  — local Patient Advice and Liaison Services (PALS)
  — local Citizens Advice Bureau
  — local Independent Complaints and Advocacy Service (ICAS).
- The Department of Health issued guidance in February 2009 for dealing with complaints in the document *Listening, Responding, Improving: a guide to better customer care*.
- From April 2009, a single approach to dealing with complaints was organised within the NHS and adult social care. This was intended to reduce the time taken to handle complaints and encourage greater flexibility for organisations in handling them. Advice sheets and leaflets are available for professionals to help in this process.

Injectable steroids in allergic rhinitis
- In the past, the steroid triamcinolone acetonide was used as an IM injection to treat resistant hay fever symptoms.
- A preparation called Kenalog®, containing triamcinolone, is licensed for the treatment of seasonal and perennial allergic rhinitis. The evidence for the overall benefits of Kenalog®

is mixed, and the current consensus is to try conservative measures first. In exceptional circumstances, oral steroids are highly effective as a short course (Scadding, *et al.* 2008).

- The main concerns about the steroid injections are the uncertainty about how long effects last for (generally considered to be several weeks) and the potential for systemic side effects.
- In 2008, the British Society for Allergy and Clinical Immunology (BSACI) published guidelines stating that systemic steroids are rarely indicated in the management of rhinitis, except for:
  — severe nasal obstruction
  — short-term rescue medication for uncontrolled symptoms on conventional pharmacotherapy
  — important social or work-related events, e.g. examinations, weddings.
- Oral steroids should be used only for short courses and should be administered together with topical nasal steroids. It was suggested that injectable steroids be avoided as much as possible.

Further reading

- Scadding GK, Durham SR, Mirakian R, *et al.* BSACI guidelines for the management of allergic and non-allergic rhinitis. *Clin Exp Allergy.* 2008; **38**(1): 19–42.
- British Society for Allergy and Clinical Immunology website. www.bsaci.org (accessed 25 November 2010).
- Department of Health. *Listening, Responding, Improving: a guide to better customer care.* London: Department of Health; 2009. Available at: www.dh.gov.uk/prod_consum_dh/groups/dh_digitalassets/documents/digitalasset/dh_095439.pdf (accessed 25 November 2010).

Station 3.12

Actor's notes

Background
- You are Priya Sharma, a 20-year-old lady, currently studying for a law degree.

Opening statement
- 'I've been getting these terrible headaches lately, Doctor.'

History
- The headaches began four months ago.
- You have tried taking various types of analgesia including paracetamol and ibuprofen.

Ideas, concerns and expectations
- You are fed up with the symptoms and now want to know what is wrong.
- You are worried there could be something serious going on. A family friend had a large brain haemorrhage when you were eight years old and you are worried this could easily happen to you.
- You have an assignment coming up at the end of the week. You have struggled to complete the work and do not think you will make the deadline.
- You want an MRI scan of the head. You have read on the internet that longstanding headaches should be investigated with a brain scan.

Further history candidate may elicit
- You have had headaches over the last four months.
- The headaches have become more frequent over the past month, occurring at least once or twice a week and last up to an hour.
- The headaches start from the neck and come on gradually.
- When you have a headache, you have to lie down. Sometimes you have to take the rest of the day off from lectures or studying.
- The pain radiates in a band-like distribution around the head to the forehead area.
- The pain can be quite sharp and at its most severe you would rate it at 6/10 severity.
- The headache comes on at any time of the day. It is not related to position or movements.
- You use painkillers occasionally but have not taken a course for more than a day.
- You sometimes experience nausea with the headaches but no vomiting.
- You do not experience any visual disturbances or any abnormal sensation or warning signs before the headaches.
- University is becoming particularly stressful with an increasing number of assignments, coursework and exams. You study for long hours, often until 3–4 a.m. and then attend 9 a.m. lectures. To keep awake, you have used Pro-Plus® increasingly more often over the past couple of months.

- You are currently re-sitting your first year because you failed it the first time. The university has said you have to pass all your exams this year and achieve at least a 2:2 standard, or else you will not be able to continue on the course.
- If asked about exams, you acknowledge you did not work hard last year and spent too much time socialising instead. Recently, most of your time has been spent studying.
- When your parents found out you had to re-sit the year, they were upset. You feel guilty that you have let them down.
- You come from a high-achieving family. Both your parents are barristers in the city. You are the youngest of three siblings. Your brother is training to be a barrister and your sister is currently in her final year at medical school. This places a lot of expectation upon you and you find it difficult to follow in their footsteps.
- You have not informed your parents about your headaches and most recent difficulties.
- You were never interested in law and only did it because your parents expected you to study either law or medicine and you thought this was the easier of the two.
- You had a passion for music whilst at school and played the violin in the school orchestra, but your parents discouraged you from pursuing a career in music.
- Your mood is reasonably stable. Apart from feeling tired during the day, you do not have any features of depression.

Medical history
- Nil significant.

Drug history
- Paracetamol and ibuprofen as required.

Social history
- You are a non smoker and only drink alcohol occasionally. You do not use recreational drugs.
- You are single.
- You live with friends in university accommodation.

Approach to scenario
- Your main focus of concern coming into the consultation is the headaches. You try to steer away from questions about your general circumstances and come back to your physical symptoms as you are very preoccupied by these.
- You are particularly worried about the chances of having a brain haemorrhage. If the doctor specifically addresses this you recount the family friend who suffered recurrent headaches and eventually went on to suffer a serious bleed. You recall she was admitted to hospital for many weeks and, although she survived, she is now confined to a wheelchair.
- You read on the internet that people with long-term headaches should be investigated with a brain scan. You are under the impression that this is the best test to have because it would look for a bleed or abnormal blood vessel. You ask the doctor for a scan several times during the consultation.
- If the doctor perseveres in exploring your social circumstances and makes you feel at ease, then you open up and discuss the difficulties you have had with your law degree.
- If the doctor also makes a point of taking an interest in your current difficulties with studies, you feel more trusting of any advice you are given.
- If the doctor declines your request for a scan, you become upset.
- However, if the doctor provides an explanation for the headache, provides advice on how to manage the headaches and reassures you there is no sinister underlying cause, you agree to follow the doctor's advice. You are not keen to use antidepressants but agree to consider these in the future if the other suggestions do not help.
- However, if doctor does not explore your studies or family situation, does not provide an explanation about the cause of the headaches, fails to reassure you about having an

abnormal blood vessel or does not develop good rapport with you, you continue to demand a brain scan. If this request is refused, you state 'Well this isn't good enough, I'd like a second opinion please.'

Information gathering
Presenting complaint
a Pain
- Nature of pain (dull, sharp, tight).
- Onset (acute or gradual).
- Site and radiation.
- Severity.
- Night pain.
- Symptoms of raised intracranial pressure (ICP).
  — morning headache
  — headache worse when leaning over.
- Alleviating factors, e.g. analgesia or relaxation.
- Exacerbating factors, e.g. stress, menstrual periods.

b Associated symptoms
- Fever and rash.
- Aura.
- Nausea and vomiting.
- Visual symptoms, e.g. zigzags, dots, loss of vision.
- Symptoms of anxiety or depression.

Medical history
- Migraines.
- Hypertension.

Drug history
- Analgesic use.
- Contraceptive pill.

Family history
- Migraine.
- Subarachnoid haemorrhage (SAH).

Social history
- Smoking and alcohol history.
- Recreational drug use or other stimulants, e.g. caffeine.
- Education, e.g. degree, exams, studying routine.
- Occupation, e.g. part-time work.
- Social support from friends and family.
- Friends and family details.
- Housing and financial issues, e.g. student loans.

Psychological
- Explore the impact of headaches on her studies and personal life.
- Explore any other stress she may be experiencing.
- Identify her thoughts about why she is getting the headaches.

Examination

- Offer to examine her cranial nerves, perform fundoscopy and check her BP.
- 'If it is okay, I would like to check your blood pressure and the nerves to your face and eyes.'

Examination Card

General examination	BP = 124/65 mmHg
	Temperature = 36.9 °C
	No signs of meningism
Cranial nerves	Normal

Clinical management

1 Discuss the likely diagnosis

- Explain the nature and timing of the headaches, combined with the classical symptoms she describes, suggest that she has 'tension headaches'.
- Reassure her the history suggests tension headaches, and not brain haemorrhage.
- Explain her neurological examination is normal and there are no signs of any other underlying brain pathology.

2 Explore likely triggers and offer solutions

- Help the patient reflect on the possible connection between psychosocial circumstances and her physical symptoms.
- Offer simple advice about her current work–life balance and sleep patterns.
  — Encourage her to find time to relax.
  — Suggest she takes up hobbies or regular exercise.
  — Underline the importance of having a full night's sleep.
- Explain that Pro-plus® contains high levels of caffeine, which could be contributing to her symptoms. Therefore, the tablets may help her to stay awake in the short term, but her body will remain sleep deprived. In the long run this will lead to impaired ability to work and perform, so she should ideally stop taking them.

3 Discuss the management of tension headache

- Offer analgesia, e.g. paracetamol, aspirin or ibuprofen. Consider a short course of treatment for one to two weeks. Advise the patient about analgesic-induced headaches.
- Negotiate to defer requesting an MRI scan, whilst reassuring her that there are no sinister features in the history or examination. Suggest that if the initial measures are unhelpful and she is not getting better, you would then reconsider the diagnosis and refer for a second opinion.
- Suggest counselling or cognitive therapies to help her manage stress, which she could access through university student support services or other local services.
- Advise her to involve close family in her current difficulties to improve support.
- Offer to write a medical note requesting an extension for her imminent deadline.
- Explain that preventive drug therapies such as TCA, e.g. amitriptyline, can be used to prevent the headache coming on. These drugs can take a few weeks to take effect, and thereafter they should be used for several months before being stopped.

4 Offer follow-up

- Offer a follow-up appointment at a short interval, e.g. after one to two weeks.
- Offer her the opportunity to bring her parents along.
- Provide her with information sheets about tension headaches to take away, e.g. from Patient UK (www.patient.co.uk).

Interpersonal skills

- Explore her concerns using open questions.
  - 'So you are worried about having a brain haemorrhage. I'll check you over for that. Have you had any personal experiences with this amongst friends or family?'
- Ensure you rule out any relevant red flags through a combination of open and closed questions, but also by picking up on relevant cues.
  - 'You mention the headaches are terrible . . . (silence) . . . Tell me some more about them?'
  - 'Tell me how a typical headache tends to come on.'
  - 'Do the headaches come on gradually or suddenly?'
- If the patient is reluctant to open up on certain areas you feel are relevant, then maintain friendly encouragement, and reveal your interest in her circumstances through positive verbal and non-verbal cues.
  - 'Tell me some more about the law degree. It sounds very tough.'
  - 'How does the lack of sleep impact on things day to day for you?'
- The patient may not have discussed some of her personal circumstances before. Allow her to reflect and work through these issues herself, by asking stimulating questions, and keeping them patient centred.
  - 'You speak very fondly about playing the violin. Looking back, do you think you would rather have pursued a music career? . . . (silence) . . .'
  - 'It may be that you are not enjoying your course because it's not the best for you. There are always options in the future whatever happens in your exam.'
- Show empathy in your approach.
  - 'It must be very tough having so many high-flyers around you.'
- Explain your diagnosis in simple, easy-to-follow terms, ensuring the patient understands you.
  - 'I think you have been suffering from tension headaches. They are quite common. Would you like me to explain some more?'
  - 'They can result from many factors. In your particular case I believe there are several factors that are not helping the headaches.'
- Ensure that the patient's agendas are met.
  - 'I know you mentioned to me that you were worried about having a brain haemorrhage. I am pleased to say that you do not have any signs of this.'
  - 'I can understand your reasons for requesting a brain scan. The good news is that when I examined you, there were no signs of any internal brain problems. I don't think a scan would reveal any new information. However, I take on board your concerns, so how about we treat this as tension headache and then review how you are in two weeks?'
- Keep the patient well informed of the management options, aiming to arrive at a shared agreement. Avoid coming across in a judgemental manner or as if you are preaching.
  - 'We talked about the possibility that your current difficulties with studies are likely to be having an effect on you. One way of addressing this might be by way of a letter for your faculty to help get an extension to your next assignment. Do you think that would help?'
  - 'It seems a real shame that you haven't pursued any interests or hobbies lately. Do you think taking time out every day might help you feel more relaxed?'
- Help the patient feel at ease before she leaves by offering her the chance to be followed up.
  - 'How about we try these various things and then you come back and see me in two weeks?'

⊶ Key summary
- Diagnose tension headache and rule out red flags.
- Address the likely triggers for her headaches, e.g. poor sleep, caffeine, stressful degree.
- Be sensitive to her request for a brain scan and reiterate the normal findings to reassure her.
- Treat her with a course of analgesia and arrange psychological treatment, e.g. CBT.
- Arrange early follow-up to check whether she would benefit from preventative treatments, e.g. TCAs.

Tension headaches

- These are often associated with stress, anxiety and depression.

Classification

- There are two main subtypes:
  - **Episodic**: these tend to occur less frequently than one day in two. Headaches can last anything from half an hour to a week.
  - **Chronic**: these tend to occur more frequently than one day in two, for more than six months.
- The patient in this case comes into the first category (episodic) because she has one to two headaches per week and has done so for less than six months.

History

- It is often experienced as a tightness or pressure, and described as a band-like pain coming from the neck and radiating to the frontal region.
- It is usually bilateral.
- Severity is mild to moderate.
- Patients may experience nausea, photophobia or phonophobia.
- It does not interfere with activity.
- There is no associated aura, visual disturbance or vomiting.
- There may be overlap with migraine.

Management

- Reassurance of no underlying pathology.
- Relaxation therapies: patients often have tense neck muscles and massage may alleviate this.
- Psychological support, e.g. cognitive therapies, counselling.
- General lifestyle measures: avoid alcohol, target stress, engage in regular exercise.
- Physiotherapy for any primary neck problems.
- Treat any other underlying factors, e.g. anxiety and depression.
- Use analgesics symptomatically, but with caution as there is a risk of analgesic-overuse headaches.
- Prophylactic treatments, e.g. amitriptyline can be used for frequent episodic or chronic tension headaches.

Further reading

- Manji H, Connolly S, Dorward N, *et al*. *Oxford Handbook of Neurology*. Oxford; Oxford University Press; 2006.
- British Association for the Study of Headache (BASH). *Guidelines for All Healthcare Professionals in the Diagnosis and Management of Migraine, Tension-type, Cluster, and Medication-overuse Headache*. 3rd ed. Hull: BASH; 2007. Available at: http://217.174.249.183/upload/NS_BASH/2010_BASH_Guidelines.pdf (accessed 13 December 2010).

TABLE 3.9 Comparison between the common and serious kinds of headache

	TENSION HEADACHE	CLUSTER HEADACHE	MIGRAINE	MENINGITIS	SAH	INTRACRANIAL TUMOUR
History						
Onset	Gradual	Acute	Gradual	Acute or subacute	Sudden	Varies
Natural history	Continuous. Occurs nearly every day. May worsen as the day passes. Episodic or chronic	Lasts from 20 minutes to 3 hours. Occurs frequently during the day, often in 3-month 'clusters' with long intervals of remission	Episodic – lasts 6–24 hours, no aura present. Classical – preceding aura lasting up to 30 minutes	Progresses over several hours. Can also present as a more chronic form of headache	May progress quickly within hours, often resulting in reduced consciousness, collapse and fitting	May be asymptomatic. Commonest presentations: • Raised ICP • Endocrine features** • Seizure • Neurological features
Site and typical description	Dull ache or pressure feeling. Neck pain/stiffness radiates in a band-like distribution to the front	Unilateral, retro-orbital, extends to upper cheek and temporal region	Unilateral, generalised, throbbing pain. Usually interferes with activities	May be generalised or localised to frontal area	Occipital pain, classically described as a 'thunderclap' or 'vice-like' headache	Rarely presents with headache (3–4% of cases)
Severity	Mild–moderate	Severe	Moderate–severe	Varies	Severe	Varies
Associated features	Stress, anxiety or depression. Occasionally nausea, photophobia, phonophobia	Unilateral conjunctival irritation and lacrimation. Nasal congestion. Rhinorrhoea	Nausea, vomiting. Photophobia. Phonophobia. Aura*	Nausea, vomiting. Photophobia. Rash	Vomiting. Reduced conscious levels. Fitting	According to the type of presentation stated above
Exacerbating factors and triggers	Stress. Cervical pathology	Alcohol (during a cluster)	Light, movement, stress, periods, food sensitivity, bright lights, altered sleep patterns, alcohol, caffeine, COC, high BP, viral illnesses	Viral illness, not always obvious	Predisposed by hypertension	–

	TENSION HEADACHE	CLUSTER HEADACHE	MIGRAINE	MENINGITIS	SAH	INTRACRANIAL TUMOUR
Relieving factors	Relaxation	Very few	Rest	–	–	–
Examination						
Vital signs	Often normal	Often normal	Sometimes raised BP	Fever, tachycardic/ hypotensive if advanced stage	Raised BP	Often normal
Neurological examination	Often normal	Often normal Rarely Horner's syndrome	Focal neurology occasionally present, e.g. Horner's, loss of vision, hemiplegia	Meningism Altered consciousness	Meningism Focal neurology, e.g. III nerve palsy, papilloedema Altered consciousness	Focal neurology in half of cases at presentation
Other salient features	Neck tenderness	–	–	–	–	–
Management	Address psychosocial/ lifestyle factors Treat neck pathology Analgesics Consider TCAs if frequent/chronic	**Acute attack:** High-flow O$_2$ 5-HT$_1$ agonist, e.g. sumatriptan **Frequent attacks:** Prophylaxis, e.g. ergotamine	**Acute attack:** High-dose NSAIDs 5-HT$_1$ agonist, e.g. sumatriptan **Chronic/frequent attacks:** Prophylaxis, e.g. TCA, β-blockers, pizotifen	Emergency admission	Emergency admission	Refer for emergency or urgent neurological input

Notes

* Aura may include visual symptoms (e.g. zigzags, floaters, hemianopia), speech problems (e.g. dysphasia) or peripheral neurological features (e.g. hemiparesis).

** e.g. from a pituitary tumour.

Be aware of analgesic overuse as a cause/trigger of headaches.

Other common and important causes to consider include sinusitis, benign intracranial hypertension, other forms of intracranial bleed (e.g. subdural haematomas), temporal arteritis, glaucoma and trigeminal neuralgia.

Station 3.13

Name	Abdi Ali
Age	38 years
Medical history	TB diagnosed three weeks ago
Medications	Isoniazid 300 mg daily
	Pyrazinamide 2g daily
	Rifampicin 600 mg daily
	Ethambutol 1 g daily
	Pyridoxine 10 mg daily
Allergies	Nil
Last consultation	Uncomplicated gastroenteritis six months ago
Other information	Diagnosed with TB at the local hospital
	Under care of the respiratory consultant
	Seen by TB clinic three weeks ago, see letter below

City Hospital
City Road
City

Dear GP

This 38-year-old Somalian gentleman is under the care of the TB clinic.
He initially presented to us with a six-month history of weight loss, night sweats, anorexia and productive cough.
He does not have any haemoptysis or other symptoms of note.
He has travelled to Somalia twice in the past year. There are no other TB contacts of note.
Results of initial sputum tests confirm TB.
He is being treated with rifampicin, isoniazid, ethambutol, pyrazinamide and pyridoxine.
Blood tests, including renal and liver function, are unremarkable.
Visual acuity was also checked and this was normal.
His wife and children have been screened and all cleared of having TB.
We will follow him up in clinic in four weeks time.

Kind regards
Dr T Bee

Actor's notes

Background

- You are Abdi Ali, a 38-year-old unemployed gentleman.

Opening statement

- 'I am worried about my kidneys, Doctor.'

History

- Three weeks ago you were told that you have TB and were given a course of treatment to take.
- You have noticed your urine has turned an orange colour in the past two weeks.

Ideas, concerns and expectations

- You are scared the discoloured urine is blood and are worried the TB has spread to your kidneys.
- You do not understand much about TB or the reason for needing treatment for so long.
- You are considering stopping the treatment because you are worried about taking so many tablets.
- You are worried about passing on TB to your wife and children.
- You feel embarrassed that you cannot read or write English.

Further history candidate may elicit

- You have had a cough with yellow sputum for six months. There is no haemoptysis.
- You generally feel quite lethargic and tired. You have noticed you sweat a lot at night.
- You have lost a stone in weight in three months and have lost your appetite.
- A few weeks ago, you decided to go to the local casualty department to be seen by a doctor, who said you may have TB and referred you to the TB clinic where you had some tests. The doctor explained you had TB and needed to start several tablets. The doctor was quite rushed at the time and spoke fast.
- You are not fully fluent in English, and find it difficult to understand what is being said if someone speaks fast. As a result, you still do not really understand much about TB.
- You have forgotten to take several doses of your medication because you cannot read what is written on the labels and cannot remember how often the doctor told you to take them.
- Your next appointment to see the TB specialist again is in two weeks time.
- The clinic also tested your wife and two children. They do not have TB.
- You have no history of kidney problems and do not have any other urinary symptoms.
- You came to the UK six years ago and have lived in the same council flat with your family.
- The flat is quite run down but it was the only one the council had for you.
- You are concerned because the flat is poorly ventilated and the walls are damp. You feel the condition of the flat has contributed to your illness.
- You live on the 15th floor. The lifts frequently break down and it takes days before they are fixed. Walking up the stairs has become particularly difficult because you feel very run down.
- You have approached the council many times about the poor housing conditions but they always recommend you remain where you are because the alternative flats are in the same state.
- You have come to see the GP today and brought the medications and instructions.

Medical history

- TB diagnosed three weeks ago.

Drug history
- Isoniazid 300 mg daily.
- Pyrazinamide 2g daily.
- Rifampicin 600 mg daily.
- Ethambutol 1 g daily.
- Pyridoxine 10 mg daily.

Family history
- Your wife is being treated for depression. Her mood is currently stable.

Social history
- You do not drink alcohol or smoke.
- You arrived in the UK six years ago with your wife and two children (6 and 8 years old).
- The economic climate in Somalia became unbearable and you were finding it increasingly difficult to provide for your family.
- You have been unemployed for a year – previously you worked in a warehouse.
- You and your wife are claiming benefits to help support your family.

Approach to scenario
- You feel overwhelmed by the diagnosis of TB and feel helpless because you do not understand what is going on.
- You are embarrassed about not being able to read or write English.
- You only mention that you cannot read or write if the doctor comes across well **and** asks why you are not taking your tablets regularly.
- You can converse in English but need others to speak at a slow–medium pace.
- If the doctor speaks fast or starts using complicated terms, you will look blank and will eventually say you do not understand, but feel bad about having to admit this.
- You welcome any support that is offered to you regarding your housing, even though you realise the GP has limited influence regarding this.
- If the GP speaks slowly and clearly, explains the importance of the medications, and addresses your concerns about TB affecting the kidneys, you agree to continue treatment and would be willing to follow other advice.
- If you feel the doctor is rushed, does not explore your current housing difficulties or does not reassure you about your kidneys, you remain polite and respectful, but will not be willing to engage with any further treatment. You leave the consultation saying 'I will wait to speak to the doctor in the clinic in two weeks.'

Information gathering
Presenting complaint
a Urinary symptoms
- Enquire about discolouration of the urine.
- Ask if his saliva, semen or tears have become discoloured.
- Ask about urinary symptoms:
  — dysuria
  — frequency
  — nocturia
  — haematuria (painful versus painless)
  — loin pain
  — poor stream
  — post-terminal dribbling
  — hesitancy.

b Tuberculosis

- Clarify how he presented with TB.
- Clarify what information the specialist gave him.
- Enquire about unwell contacts.
- Ask if close contacts have been screened for TB.

Medical history

- History of TB.
- Other underlying medical conditions.

Drug history

- Clarify his understanding of treatments:
  — awareness of side effects
  — concordance
  — understanding about instructions for use.
- Ask if he has the drugs with him.
- Check if he is on any other medications.

Family history

- Particularly of TB.

Social history

- Smoking and alcohol.
- Marital status and dependents.
- Enquire about housing conditions, asking about:
  — housing conditions
  — rough sleeping
  — crowded conditions
  — type of housing, e.g. flat, house.
- Occupation and financial circumstance.

Patient's agenda

- Explore his reasons for worrying about his kidneys.
- Explore his understanding of TB and current treatments.
- Offer suggestions of how you can provide help.

Examination

- Offer to check his BP, examine his kidneys and dipstick his urine.
- 'Can I check your blood pressure and feel your abdomen and your kidneys? If you would like to provide me a urine sample, I could also check it for any blood or infection.'

Examination card	
General examination	BP = 128/78 mmHg
Abdominal examination	Normal
Urine dipstick	Negative

Clinical management

1 Address the patient's concern about his kidneys
- Explain the rifampicin has turned his urine orange, and other bodily fluids such as his saliva, semen and tears may also be affected.
- Reassure him this is a common side effect and does not reflect kidney damage from TB.

2 Offer explanation about tuberculosis
- Explain TB is an infection that spreads from person to person by droplets in the air.
- Explain TB can spread to other organs in the body.
- Underline the importance of treatment in preventing the spread of TB to other parts of the body and to other people.
- Explain poor concordance can lead to drug resistance and difficulty eradicating the infection.
- Reassure him tests on his wife and children showed they did not have TB.

3 Discuss tuberculosis treatment further
- Discuss the important side effects of the medications, including visual problems, peripheral neuropathy, vitamin B6 deficiency, kidney and liver dysfunction.
- Reassure him the TB clinic has checked his vision, kidney and liver function to make sure it is safe for him to be on these medications, and explain that he is taking pyridoxine to prevent vitamin B6 deficiency.
- Safety net by educating him to present to medical services immediately if he develops any fever, malaise, jaundice, vomiting or visual changes.
- Help the patient to understand the dosage of the medications.
- Provide useful suggestions to aid compliance.
  — Dosette box.
  — Directly observed therapy (DOT) – a fully supervised method of drug administration by the TB clinic. The clinic will often give the medicines three times a week.

4 Address any relevant psychosocial issues
- Explore housing conditions, and suggest you can write to the council stating his medical problems and supporting a move to better, more hygienic conditions.
- Offer to use interpreters or Language Line Services for future appointments.

5 Arrange a follow-up and management plan
- Offer to review the patient, to ensure he has followed the advice and to see how he is.
- Suggest writing to the TB specialist, alerting them to the psychosocial issues, including being unable to read and write English and any potential compliance issues.
- Offer to provide written information in his native language and details of any support groups or local Somali centres that may also be able to help, e.g. TB Alert (www.tbalert.org).

Interpersonal skills

- Explore the patient's initial statement with an open question.
  - 'What worries you about your kidneys?'
- Take on board his concerns and show you are taking them seriously.
  - 'I would just like to ask you, have you experienced any problems passing urine?'
- Identify any other worries the patient might have that may affect his treatment. Pay attention to cues using active listening skills and open questions.
  - 'You mentioned that the doctor in the hospital was a bit rushed. Was there anything that you feel was not addressed?'
  - 'What is it about the medication labels you aren't sure about?' ... (pause, gesture over to the medicines) ...
  - 'Living on the 15th floor must be very difficult for you and your family?'
- If it becomes apparent that the patient does not understand your comments or questions, be prepared to slow your rate of speech and use simple words. Pay particular attention to verbal and non-verbal cues for feedback.
  - 'I'm sorry, was I speaking a bit too fast? ... (silence) ... Please do interrupt me straight away or ask any questions if I don't make sense or speak too fast. So, as I was saying ...'
- Show an interest in the patient. This will help you to see the patient's problems in a more holistic context and to maintain rapport.
  - 'You mentioned that you came over to the UK six years ago. Tell me about life in Somalia before you came here.'
- Reassure the patient if he feels embarrassed about anything.
  - 'Don't worry about not being able to read and write English. Your spoken English is really good and you're not alone. We can still help you understand what TB is and support you with treatment.'
- Rather than lecture on the importance of concordance, try and engage him with the issues.
  - 'One of the issues with not taking treatment regularly is that this can cause something called resistance. ... (silence) ... Is this something that was explained to you?'
- Ensure the patient's concerns from the history are tackled in the management.
  - 'You are right to say that the housing is not helping your condition. If I write a letter to the council arguing for better housing, do you think that would be helpful?'
  - 'If I arrange to contact the specialist to discuss improving the way we provide your medication, do you think that will help you to take the treatment?'

O⎯ Key summary
- Address the patient's concerns about his kidneys.
- Ensure he understands what TB is and the importance of treatment.
- Understand drugs used to treat TB, and their important side effects.
- Explore ways to promote concordance with treatment, e.g. DOT.
- Recognise that communication needs vary in different populations.
- Address the relevant psychosocial factors affecting the patient, such as the housing difficulties.

Tuberculosis (NICE guidelines, 2006)
Screening
- Offer screening to patients considered to be at risk. This includes those:
  - in prisons
  - sleeping rough/living in hostels
  - coming into the country from high-risk areas.

Bacillus Calmette–Guérin (BCG) vaccination
- Considered in the following groups:
  — babies born in areas where there is a high incidence of TB
  — babies whose parents or grandparents were born in high-risk areas
  — those entering the country from high-risk areas
  — those exposed to pulmonary TB
  — prison employees
  — NHS clinicians
  — older children considered to be at higher risk
  — people visiting high-risk areas for more than a month, e.g. Asia and Africa.

Treatment
- Treatment of active TB can vary depending on several factors including resistance patterns.
- The standard treatment for active TB usually consists of:
  — **For the first two months**: isoniazid, rifampicin, pyrazinamide and ethambutol.
  — **Following four months**: isoniazid and rifampicin alone.
  — (Pyridoxine cover for isoniazid to help prevent neuropathy.)

TABLE 3.10 Adverse effects of the main antituberculous medications

DRUG	SIDE EFFECTS
Rifampicin	Orange-coloured body secretions including saliva and urine GI effects Impairment of liver function Renal failure Skin problems, e.g. Stevens–Johnson syndrome.
Pyrazinamide	Liver impairment GI effects Photosensitivity
Ethambutol	Mainly visual problems*, e.g.: • Visual field loss • Colour blindness • Impaired visual acuity
Isoniazid	GI effects Optic neuritis Peripheral neuropathy (resulting from vitamin B6 deficiency) Liver impairment
Pyridoxine	Prophylaxis against vitamin B6 deficiency (due to isoniazid)

* Ensure the patient's visual acuity is checked before treatment is initiated

Further reading
- National Institute for Health and Clinical Excellence. Tuberculosis: NICE guideline 33. London: NIHCE; 2006. www.nice.org.uk/CG033 (accessed 25 November 2010).
- Eddleston M, Davidson R, Brent A, *et al. Oxford Handbook of Tropical Medicine.* 3rd ed. Oxford: Oxford University Press; 2008.
- Patient leaflets in different languages, including Somali, can be found at the TB Alert website. www.tbalert.org (accessed 25 November 2010).

Index